Studies in Big Data

Volume 78

Series Editor

Janusz Kacprzyk, Polish Academy of Sciences, Warsaw, Poland

The series "Studies in Big Data" (SBD) publishes new developments and advances in the various areas of Big Data- quickly and with a high quality. The intent is to cover the theory, research, development, and applications of Big Data, as embedded in the fields of engineering, computer science, physics, economics and life sciences. The books of the series refer to the analysis and understanding of large, complex, and/or distributed data sets generated from recent digital sources coming from sensors or other physical instruments as well as simulations, crowd sourcing, social networks or other internet transactions, such as emails or video click streams and other. The series contains monographs, lecture notes and edited volumes in Big Data spanning the areas of computational intelligence including neural networks, evolutionary computation, soft computing, fuzzy systems, as well as artificial intelligence, data mining, modern statistics and Operations research, as well as self-organizing systems. Of particular value to both the contributors and the readership are the short publication timeframe and the world-wide distribution, which enable both wide and rapid dissemination of research output.

** Indexing: The books of this series are submitted to ISI Web of Science, DBLP, Ulrichs, MathSciNet, Current Mathematical Publications, Mathematical Reviews, Zentralblatt Math: MetaPress and Springerlink.

More information about this series at http://www.springer.com/series/11970

Aboul-Ella Hassanien · Nilanjan Dey ·
Sally Elghamrawy

Editors

Big Data Analytics and Artificial Intelligence Against COVID-19: Innovation Vision and Approach

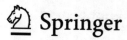 Springer

Editors
Aboul-Ella Hassanien
Department of Information Technology
Faculty of Computers and Artificial
Intelligence
Cairo University
Giza, Egypt

Nilanjan Dey
Department of Computer Science
and Engineering
JIS University
Kolkata, India

Sally Elghamrawy
Department of Computer Engineering
MISR Higher Institute for Engineering
and Technology
Mansoura, Egypt

ISSN 2197-6503   ISSN 2197-6511   (electronic)
Studies in Big Data
ISBN 978-3-030-55260-2   ISBN 978-3-030-55258-9   (eBook)
https://doi.org/10.1007/978-3-030-55258-9

This Springer imprint is published by the registered company Springer Nature Switzerland AG
The registered company address is: Gewerbestrasse 11, 6330 Cham, Switzerland

Preface

In the fight against COVID-19 pandemic, big data analytics and artificial intelligence (AI) techniques play a significant role in several aspects. The integration between both technologies will help healthcare workers for early and accurately diagnosing COVID-19 cases. Both technologies allow the application of machine learning, deep learning, computer vision, and robotics to develop computer-based models for predicting, forecasting, diagnosing, and devolving drugs of the SARS-CoV-2 virus. In addition, the strategic planning for crisis management is supported by the aggregation of big data to be used in the epidemiologic directions. Moreover, AI and big data-driven tools present visualization for COVID-19 outbreak information that helps in detecting risk allocation and regional transmissions. This book presents different approaches for fighting against COVID-19 reflected in different categories, namely forecasting and visualization, diagnosis and predictions, artificial intelligence (AI), deep learning, and big data analytics. The content of this book is divided into four parts:

- *Forecasting and Visualization*
- *Diagnosis and Predictions of COVID-19*
- *Artificial Intelligence (AI) Against COVID-19*
- *Deep Learning Against COVID-19.*

Each submission is reviewed by the editorial board. Evaluation criteria include correctness, originality, technical strength, and significance, quality of presentation, and interest and relevance to the book scope. Chapters of this book provide a collection of high-quality research works that address broad challenges in both theoretical and application aspects of COVID-19 big data analytical and AI including machine learning and deep learning technologies.

Giza, Egypt
Kolkata, India
Mansoura, Egypt

Aboul-Ella Hassanien
Nilanjan Dey
Sally Elghamrawy

Contents

About the Editors

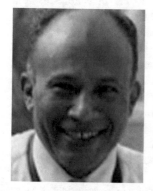

Aboul-Ella Hassanien is the founder and head of the Egyptian Scientific Research Group (SRGE) and a professor of Information Technology at the Faculty of Computer and Artificial Intelligence, Cairo University. He has more than 1000 scientific research papers published in prestigious international journals and over 50 books covering such diverse topics as data mining, medical images, intelligent systems, social networks, and smart environment. He won several awards including the Best Researcher of the Youth Award of Astronomy and Geophysics of the National Research Institute, Academy of Scientific Research (Egypt, 1990). He was also granted a scientific excellence award in humanities from the University of Kuwait for the 2004 Award and received the superiority of scientific in technology—University Award (Cairo University, 2013). Also, he was honored in Egypt as the Best Researcher in Cairo University in 2013. He also received the Islamic Educational, Scientific and Cultural Organization (ISESCO) prize on Technology (2014) and received the State Award of Excellence in engineering sciences 2015. He holds the Medal of Sciences and Arts from the first class from president of Egypt in 2017.

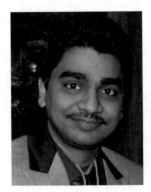

Nilanjan Dey is an associate professor, Department of Computer Science and Engineering, JIS University, Kolkata, India. He is a visiting fellow of the University of Reading, UK. He was an honorary visiting scientist at Global Biomedical Technologies Inc., CA, USA (2012–2015). He was awarded his Ph.D. from Jadavpur University in 2015. He has authored/edited more than 70 books with Elsevier, Wiley, CRC Press, and Springer and published more than 300 papers. He is the editor-in-chief of the International Journal of Ambient Computing and Intelligence, IGI Global, and the associated editor of IEEE Access and International Journal of Information Technology, Springer. He is the series co-editor of Springer Tracts in Nature-Inspired Computing, Springer, series co-editor of Advances in Ubiquitous Sensing Applications for Health care, Elsevier, and series editor of Computational Intelligence in Engineering Problem Solving and Intelligent Signal Processing and Data Analysis, CRC. His main research interests include medical imaging, machine learning, computer-aided diagnosis, data mining, etc. He is the Indian ambassador of the International Federation for Information Processing—Young ICT Group and the senior member of IEEE.

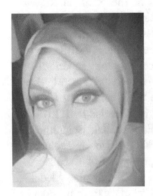

Sally Elghamrawy is the head of Communications and Computer Engineering Department at MISR higher Institute for Engineering and Technology and a part-time associate professor at Electrical and Computers Engineering Department, Faculty of Engineering, British University in Egypt BUE and at Computers Engineering Department, Faculty of Engineering, Mansoura University in Egypt. She received a Ph.D. degree in 2012 in Distributed Decision Support Systems Based on Multi Intelligent Agents from Computer Engineering Department, Faculty of engineering, Mansoura University, and received a M.Sc. degree in Automatic Control Systems Engineering in 2006 from the same department, and received B.Sc. in Computers Engineering and Systems in 2003. She has been delivering lectures, supervising graduation projects, master's thesis, and doctoral dissertations. She was a practical trainer in the grants from the Ministry of Communications and Information Technology with collaboration with IBM. She is certified in Cloud Application Developer 2018 Mastery Award for Educators, Mobile Application Developer Mastery Award for Educators 2017, and A+ International Inc. CompTIA. She is a member in Scientific Research Group in Egypt. Her research focuses on big data analysis, artificial intelligence, information retrievals, and software engineering. She is the author of number peer-reviewed publications, receiving best paper awards. She is also an IEEE member. She is an editor and reviewer in number of international journals and a judge on IEEE Young professionals' competitions.

Forecasting and Visualization

Coronavirus Spreading Forecasts Based on Susceptible-Infectious-Recovered and Linear Regression Model

Neha Tyagi, Naresh Dhull, Meenakshi Sharma, Vishal Jain, and Shashank Awasthi

Abstract An epidemiced environment is an occurrence of disease that spreads rapidly and disturbs many persons at the same time. Well, transmission of viruses is a big problem of today's era. Environmental conditions and habits of people are somehow responsible for the vulnerable conditions of the environment. In consequence, to find out the exact condition the study needs to know about the symptom of the person (like age, gender, current body temperature, dry cough duration, headache, and travel history). As per the study given by India today magazine, a very first case of coronavirus was found in Kerala's Thrissur district in India on January 30 2020. Thus, after 4–5 days, another two cases were found in Kerala too. Therefore, the state government took action and put these 3 patients in Isolation. Accordingly, with these 3 patients, the government quarantined their contacted persons (around 3400) too, who were suspected of symptoms of the coronavirus. Thereby, after the isolation and quarantine period, 3 patients among all were discharged upon recovery. Therefore, in this way, this study has to focus and trying to visualize the impact of isolation and quarantine on the health of the patients.

Keywords COVID-19 · Epidemic theory · SIR · Linear regression and coronavirus

N. Tyagi (✉) · S. Awasthi
G.L. Bajaj Institute of Technology and Management, Greater Noida, India
e-mail: nehacs1988@gmail.com

S. Awasthi
e-mail: shashankglbitm@gmail.com

N. Dhull · M. Sharma
Galgotias University, Greater Noida, India

V. Jain
BharatiVidhyapeeth's Institute of Computer Applications and Management, New Delhi, India

© The Editor(s) (if applicable) and The Author(s), under exclusive license to Springer Nature Switzerland AG 2020
A.-E. Hassanien et al. (eds.), *Big Data Analytics and Artificial Intelligence Against COVID-19: Innovation Vision and Approach*, Studies in Big Data 78, https://doi.org/10.1007/978-3-030-55258-9_1

3

1 Introduction

The 2020 year, which unstable the lives on the earth, will be considered in the history of pandemics. It was first reported by the Wuhan Health commission, in China on 31st December 2019. From the 31st December 2019, it blowouts all over the world and damage the lives of male, female, kids, etc. The pandemic COVID-19 may be a major world health threat. The novel coronavirus have been rumored because of the most damaging metabolism virus since the 1918 contagion pandemic. Consistent with WHO novel coronavirus state of affairs report as on March 2020, a complete of around 600, more than 150 confirmed cases and more than 300 deaths are rumored across the planet [1]. Therefore, World unfolds has been fast, with More than 150 countries currently having rumored a minimum of one case. Coronavirus sickness (COVID-19) is an associate in nursing communicable disease caused by severe acute metabolism syndrome coronavirus-2. Coronavirus belongs to a family of viruses that is to blame for unhealthiness starting from respiratory disease to deadly diseases as MERS and SARS that were 1st discovered in China (2002) and Saudi Arabia (2012).

In view of this, the novel Coronavirus or higher referred to as COVID-19 was rumored in a metropolis, China for the 1st time on thirty-first Gregorian calendar month 2019. Consistent with Jiang et al. the death rate for this virus has been calculable to be 9/5 except for the people 80, this has gone up to 0.086 whereas for those >80 it's been noted to be 15% [2]. This has junction rectifier to aged persons higher than the age of 40 plus with underlying diseases like polygenic disorder, Parkinson's sickness, and disorder to be thought-about at the best risk. Symptoms of this sickness will take 5–20 days to look and might vary from fever, cough, and shortness of breath to respiratory illness, nephropathy, and even death [1]. The spread is one individual to another via metabolism droplets among shut contact with the typical variety of individuals infected by a patient being 4–5% however the virus isn't thought-about mobile [3]. Choice makers are benefited from a higher geared towards MC outputs complemented through min-max policies that foretell about the acute degrees of destiny possibilities with admiring to the epidemic [4].

Although, there exist an outsized variety of pieces of evidence wherever machine learning algorithms has proved to offer economical predictions in care [5–7]. Nsoesie et al. have provided a scientific review of approaches accustomed forecast the dynamics of contagion pandemic [8]. Similarly, they need reviewing analysis papers supported settled principle models, regression models, prediction rules, Bayesian network, SEIR model, ARIMA statement model, etc. Recent studies on COVID-19 embrace solely searching analysis of the offered restricted knowledge [9–11].

Here, the Prediction Module is projected for predicting the power of the patient to reply to treatment supported various factors e.g. age, infection stage, metabolic process failure, multi-organ failure, and therefore the treatment regimens. The Module implements the Whale improvement rule for choosing the foremost relevant patient options [12].

Thus, operative and effective vaccinum against novel coronavirus has not been unreal and thus a key half in managing this pandemic is to decrease the epidemic peak, conjointly referred to as flattening the epidemic curve. Here, the role of knowledge of scientists and data processing researchers is to integrate the connected data and technology to higher perceive the virus and its characteristics, which may facilitate in taking right selections and concrete arranges of actions. As a result in an even bigger image of taking aggressive measures in developing infrastructure, facilities, vaccines, and restraining similar to epidemic in the future. The objectives of this study area unit are following as designing a SIR (Susceptible, Infectious, Recovered) models to judge the unfold of sickness; Concluding the speed of unfolding of the sickness in the Republic of India &Forecasting of COVID-19 irruption exploitation SIR and Regression models.

Accordingly, the upcoming future is much unknown about this virus. The scientists, researchers, many peoples only can do predictions based on data given by the World health organization to the world.

The Introduction and Theory part given in Sect. 1, In order to this, the model used in this study illustrate in Sect. 2. In such a way, Analysis, performance evaluation and experimental results explicate in Sect. 3. Section 4 enlightens the Methodology discussion followed by the conclusion in Sect. 5.

2 Pandemic Theory

Koykul et al. examine about focal points and inconveniences of utilizing savvy lattice in circulated restoration vitality age [13]. Pipattanasomporn et al. talk about giving knowledge to a savvy network through a multi-operator framework [14]. The ideas remain identified with one another and bolster a ton of work just as parts. Generally the collaboration among supplier and performer is rapidly however here and there the change in encompassing may influence the communication of the supplier and the performer. Similarly, the plague hypothesis is likewise supportive to depict the idea of the spread of worm from source to a goal by characterizing the infection just as contortion or clamor in data. Likewise the survey study can say that the plague hypothesis depicts the proliferation of infection or mutilation or commotion in the data. Generally, the data consistently transmit or get regularly, so if the worm is engendered in a similar normal way, at that point the infection additionally proliferates similarly because the immediate contact characterizes the spread of infection using a typical frequency.

On condition that, there should be an occurrence of investigation of science, during the compelling contamination at the masses scale, two philosophies or ideas are portraying the engendering of disease which is characterized as the stochastic procedures and the deterministic techniques. Generally, a mass of n individuals is divided into a couple of compartments, and the spread of the illness is thought about (Fig. 1).

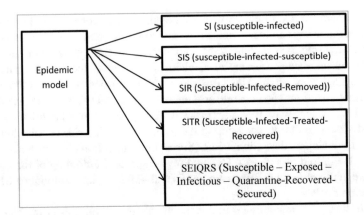

Fig. 1 Different types of epidemic models

3 SIR Model

The Kermack-McKendrick Model is very well known as the SIR model. Here for simulation, the study has used 3 variables, S–I–R to symbolize the total number of individuals in an epidemic environment at a given frame. Where susceptible individuals will depict by S, Infected individuals will depict by I and Recovered individuals or can say that the removed individuals from an epidemic environment that recovered by isolation or quarantine process by R.

Hence, these 3 kinds of persons may vary after some time frame. So, 't' will represent that time frame. The final number of functions of a specific time frame will be S (t); I (t) & R (t). In the same way, the SIR model is dynamic because of the number of people changing their state after the specified interval of time 't'.

On that account, to find out the value of conversion rate of I and S, then have to use the formula $\beta I/N$. β depicts the ordinary number of individuals contact per person per time that has to be multiplied by the disease spreading probability. Thus, the fraction of contact with individuals is depicted by I/N [15].

Where γ is the conversion rate of S and I i.e. rate of recovery. D is the duration of infection, at that juncture γ will depict by $1/D$ [15].

At this moment, a very important measurement of any disease prototypical is the R-Naught. It is the reproduction number of secondary contagions generated from one contagion individual in a total populace. As per the SIR model, $R0 = \beta N/\gamma$. The total population size will represent by $N = S+I + R$. In order to find out the value of β, then $\beta = R0\gamma/N$. R0 is property of breakout and does not change once calculated, as it's calculated assuming inclined inhabitants. The efficient copy quantity, "R" represents the typical collection of secondary infections in an inhabitant that can come with immune individuals. That is the metric this is wanted to be minimized via vaccination campaigns [15].

Thus, this is a very basic model but has effective assumptions. Very firstly, as a populace is shut and fixed, as such—nobody it included into the helpless gathering (means no births), all people that progress of from being contaminated to recuperated is for all time impervious to disease and there are no passings.

Similarly, as the populace considered as homogenous and just vary by their ailment state. At last third one, disease and that person's "infectiveness" or capacity to defect powerless people, happens at the same time [16, 17]. This section describes the simulating part of SIR model.

3.1   Simulation of SIR (the Susceptible-Infected-Removed) Model Using R Packages

As anticipated, the simulation study has used the deSolve R package for this simulation prediction. The study has used different variables here γ & β & t for several days. Here this research work had plotted the graph at 14 days for higher goals [15, 18].

Here, consider the R0 that is reproduction number. Because simulation found the data which is going to change day by day from COVID-19. As it a pandemic data onto the country, so, R0 represents the no. of cases produced by an infected person during the transmissible period. Thus, R0 is equal to cpd. So, with the help of R0, the value of β and exact information about the isolation period of the COVID-19 data can be calculated. For example, initially consider as the transmissible duration is equivalent to the period of contamination. It is notable that if one person is infected by a coronavirus, so that person will not infect the other persons immediately. It will take between 3 and 5 days as an incubation period and able to flacking the symptoms of coronavirus. For this reason, have to find out the value of β, i.e. $\beta = R0/\gamma$, where, R0 = 2.26 [15, 18].

Here, initially set the data onto 3 infected individuals. Then we will run R function of 14 days. The Study says that if R0 > one, the infection rate is greater than the recovery rate, and thus the infection will grow throughout the population. If R0 < one, the infection fast will die out since people are health-giving faster than they are transmitting it [15, 18].

Accordingly, Fig. 2 represents the stepwise step model for Susceptible-Infected-Removed, where, S (Susceptible), I (Infected), and R(No. of recovery people). Here this study is checking the top ten results come after applying the model on the discussed case. Findings have plotted the visualization by using the 't' parameter for 14 days [15, 18].

As a result, in Fig. 3, β gives the typical choice of contacts in line with the particular person in line with time multiplied by way of the likelihood of the disease spreading in a touch between I and S and γ is the conversion rate between I and S. Consequently, on the assumption of S = 0.9899906 I = 9.000750e−03 & R = 1.008659e−03, when β = 1.4247 and γ = 0.14286 [15, 18].

In order to this, Figs. 4 and 5, demonstrate the SIR model predictions in correspond

Model for Susceptible-Infected-Removed
SIR(14,0,0.32,1/7)
SIR<-function
(time,state,parameters)(with(as.list(c(state, parameters))
dS<- -(β*S*I)
dI<- ((β*S*I) - (γ*I))
dR<- γ*I
return list[dS,dR, dI]
β=1.427, γ=0.14286

Fig. 2 Model for susceptible-infected-removed using R packages

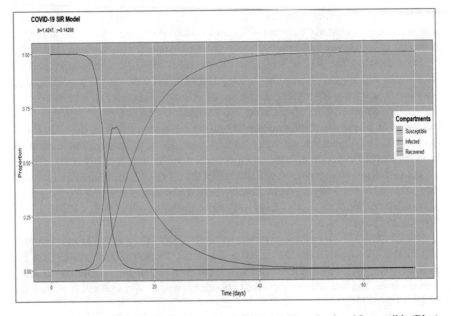

Fig. 3 Depicting the susceptible-infected-removed (SIR) model by using β and Susceptible (Blue), Infected (Red) and Removed (Green)

to the isolation period of the patients. This study also focuses on the isolation period which creates a great impact for the recovery of COVID-19 patients.

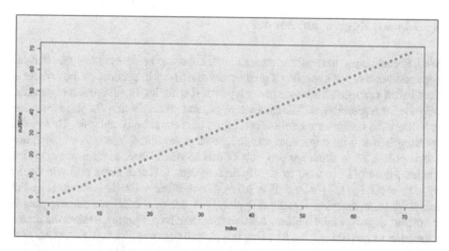

Fig. 4 SIR model in respect of time of isolation of populace

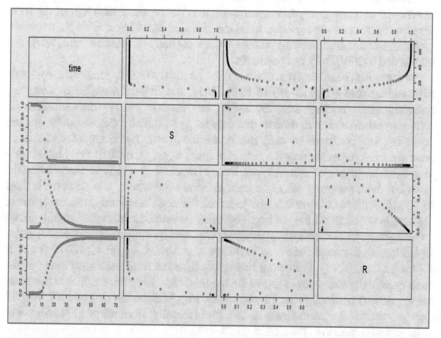

Fig. 5 SIR model representation in correspond to whole populace. The time span of simulation is 14 days

4 Linear Regression Model

Well, linear Regression approaches are numerical components of techniques that can approximation or are expecting a goal or variable that is dependent on the criteria of established variables. There are many types of Regression like Bayesian regression, polynomial regression, and linear regression, and so on. In this chapter regression type had used i.e. linear model for prediction of coronavirus pandemic. This model working is based on dependent and independent variables. The cost of slope and intercept is used to show the products of this model. Hence, in a linear regression model, $\beta 0$ and $\beta 1$ are used to signify an intercept & slope. Error rate will depict by ϵ. $Y = \beta 0 + \beta 1 x + \epsilon$ and $Y = \theta 0 + \theta 1 x + \theta 2 x 2 + \theta 3 x 3 + \theta n x n$, [19]. For this purpose, in the given equations depicts the value of coefficients that assigned to predictors & polynomial diploma has to be depicted by n. Figure 8 depicts the Linear regression model fitting line. By using this plotted figure author says that as the time goes the number of confirmed cases of COVID-19 also goes high.

Accordingly, for proposing the model, here author considers the pandemic COVID-19 as a case study/baseline from India. Hence, more than half of the India has already stopped commuting. India has replaced handshakes with Namaste and now, the new standard: social distance. Around the early of March month, WHO has been stated a COVID-19 is a pandemic.

By using Fig. 6 author gives outline of the processes used to predict the epidemic environment data (COVID-19) in India. Here, the Impact Analysis to study the epidemiological environment, the author has used nCov2019 data outbreak. It includes real-time data and historical data as well. Initially these simulations are deploying the packages to start the prediction work. By virtue of basic functions are used for extracting the data example as: get_nCov2019 () which is used to get the latest online information; load_nCov2019 () which is used to get the historical data; summary which is used to access the whole data and plot is used to visualize the whole data in the pictorial form. Subsequently, the deployment process, now install all the packages by using commands: Remotes::install_github ("GuangchuangYu/nCov2019"); require (nCov2019); require (dplyr). Initial Impression: Here author have fixed two Variables A and B. A ← getnCov2019 () and B ← load_nCov2019 (). Following this it will give the total confirmed cases of the country. Initially this study explores the required data then after prediction functions has applied on particular data [3]. Similarly, Fig. 7, elaborate that how COVID-19 data gets trained for predictions. Author gives learning from initial to N number of steps to find the optimal prediction results (Fig. 8).

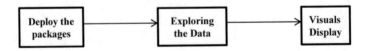

Fig. 6 Process followed for epidemic environment study

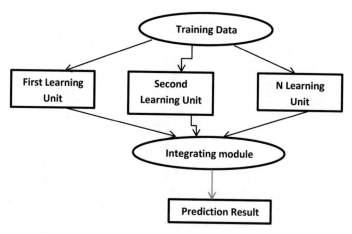

Fig. 7 Process to explore the COVID-19 training data

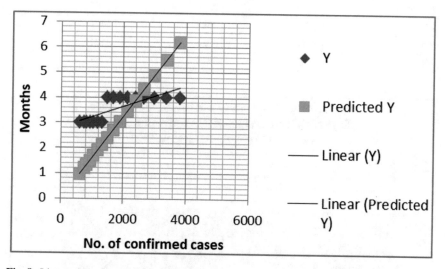

Fig. 8 Linear regression model fitting line

5 Comparison of SIR and Linear Regression Model

In Mentioned Table 1 is the Date-wise SIR, Linear Regression, and actual data comparison for 14 days; this chapter has used 14 days of training data onto prediction analysis. By using R packages for the SIR model depiction where with the help of this study found that $\beta = 1.4247$ and $\gamma = 0.14286$. Thereafter, Standard error in the linear regression model was 2.253 [17, 19]. The graphical assessment of Date-wise comparison of Susceptible-Infectious- Recovered, Linear Regression and actual data is given in Fig. 9. Subsequently, author finds out the linear regression model gives the

Table 1 Date-wise SIR, linear regression and actual data comparison for 14 days

Date	SIR	Linear	Actual
25/03/20	648	604	562
26/03/20	720	740	649
27/03/20	874	820	724
28/03/20	974	923	873
29/03/20	1081	1040	979
30/03/20	1199	1172	1071
31/03/20	1333	1321	1251
1/4/2020	1485	1488	1397
2/4/2020	1654	1676	1965
3/4/2020	1837	1887	2301
4/4/2020	2038	2127	2902
5/4/2020	2264	2396	3374
6/4/2020	2520	2669	4067
7/4/2020	2807	3007	4421
8/4/2020	3122	3386	5194
9/4/2020	3465	3814	5734

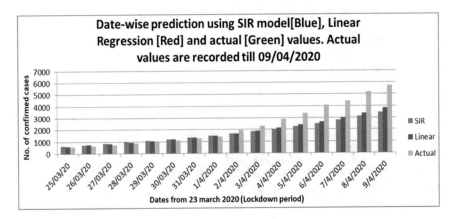

Fig. 9 Comparative graph of susceptible-infectious- recovered and linear regression model of COVID-19 Data

very close results to the actual one scenario. Similarly, Fig. 10, shows the COVID-19, actual data depiction in India before the period of lockdown and after the period of lockdown. So, it shows the change in the number of confirmed cases too.

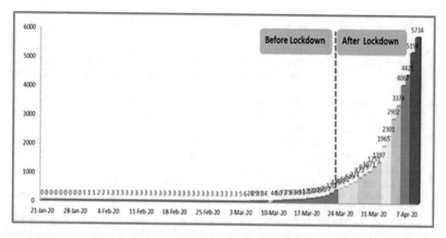

Fig. 10 Change in number of confirmed cases before and after lockdown period due to COVID-19 in India

6 Conclusion

This chapter focused on the COVID-19 initial case that occurs in India. Initially this chapter considered 3 cases of Kerala's district on January 30 2020. Thereupon, the government took steps to isolate or quarantine those 3 as well as the people those who had contact with those 3 individuals. Later, that 3 people have been recovered by the process of isolation or quarantine. As a consequence, by using the SIR model in the particular case mentioned by author, exploration work found that the recovery rate has grown by using the isolation process for infected people. Initially set the value of R is 0.000000e+00 after the SIR model application will find R = 1.008659e−03. Therefore, it shows the Isolation and quarantine help to improve the health condition of COVID-19 infected people. Similarly, the problem has solved by using a linear regression model. Simulation results shows that the standard deviation between SIR and actual is ±15% and the standard deviation between linear regression and actual is ±7%. Thus, it has been concluded that linear regression model predicts the very near results of the actual data.

References

1. World Health Organization.: Coronavirus disease 2019 (COVID-19): situation report, **67** (2020)
2. Jiang, F., Deng, L., Zhang, L., Cai, Y., Cheung, C.W., Xia, Z.: Review of the clinical characteristics of coronavirus disease 2019 (COVID-19). J. General Int. Med. 1–5 (2020)
3. Wu, Z., McGoogan, J.M.: Characteristics of and important lessons from the coronavirus disease 2019 (COVID-19) outbreak in China: summary of a report of 72 314 cases from the Chinese Center for Disease Control and Prevention. JAMA (2020)

4. Composite Monte Carlo decision making under high uncertainty of novel coronavirus epidemic using hybridized deep learning and fuzzy rule induction. Appl. Soft Comput. 106282 (2020)

5. Ye, Q.H., Qin, L.X., Forgues, M., He, P., Kim, J.W., Peng, A.C., Simon, R., Li, Y., Robles, A.I., Chen, Y., Ma, Z.C.: Predicting hepatitis B virus–positive metastatic hepatocellular carcinomas using gene expression profiling and supervised machine learning. Nat. Med. **9**(4), 416–423 (2003)

6. Mai, M.V., Krauthammer, M.: Controlling testing volume for respiratory viruses using machine learning and text mining. In: AMIA Annual Symposium Proceedings, vol. 2016, p. 1910. American Medical Informatics Association

7. Purcaro, G., Rees, C.A., Wieland-Alter, W.F., Schneider, M.J., Wang, X., Stefanuto, P.H., Wright, P.F., Enelow, R.I., Hill, J.E.: Volatile fingerprinting of human respiratory viruses from cell culture. J. Breath Res. **12**(2), 026015 (2018)

8. Nsoesie, E.O., Brownstein, J.S., Ramakrishnan, N., Marathe, M.V.: A systematic review of studies on forecasting the dynamics of influenza outbreaks. Influenza Other Respir. Viruses **8**(3), 309–316 (2014)

9. Pirouz, B., ShaffieeHaghshenas, S., ShaffieeHaghshenas, S., Piro, P.: Investigating a serious challenge in the sustainable development process: analysis of confirmed cases of COVID-19 (New Type of Coronavirus) through a binary classification using artificial intelligence and regression analysis. Sustainability **12**(6), 2427 (2020)

10. More, G.D., Dunowska, M., Acke, E., Cave, N.J.: A serological survey of canine respiratory coronavirus in New Zealand. New Zealand Vet. J. **68**(1), 54–59 (2020)

11. Wu, C., Chen, X., Cai, Y., Zhou, X., Xu, S., Huang, H., Zhang, L., Zhou, X., Du, C., Zhang, Y., Song, J.: Risk factors associated with acute respiratory distress syndrome and death in patients with coronavirus disease 2019 pneumonia in Wuhan. China, JAMA Intern. Med. (2020)

12. Diagnosis and Prediction model for COVID19 patients response to treatment based on convolutional neural networks and whale optimization algorithm using CT image. medRxiv 2020.04.16.20063990; https://doi.org/10.1101/2020.04.16.20063990

13. Akyildiz, I.F., Su, W., Sankarasubramaniam, Y., Cayirci, E.: Wireless sensor networks: a survey. Comput. Netw. **38**(4), 393–422 (2002)

14. Vahdat, A., Becker, D.: Epidemic routing for partially connected ad hoc networks. Duke University Technical Report CS-200006 (2000)

15. https://cran.rproject.org/web/packages/shinySIR/vignettes/Vignette.html

16. CSSEGISandData. CSSEGISandData/COVID-19 (2020) https://github.com/CSSEGISandData/COVID-19

17. Pandey, G., Chaudharya, P., Guptab, R., Pal, S.: SEIR and regression model based COVID-19 outbreak predictions in India (2020)

18. https://rpubs.com/choisy/sir

19. Gupta, R., Pal, S.K.: Trend analysis and forecasting of COVID-19 outbreak in India. Published online 30/03/2020 in preprint archive MedRxiv https://www.medrxiv.org/content/10.1101/2020.03.26.20044511v1 (2020)

Virus Graph and COVID-19 Pandemic: A Graph Theory Approach

H. R. Bhapkar, Parikshit N. Mahalle, and Prashant S. Dhotre

Abstract In the field of science and technology, the graph theory has offered several approaches to articulate any situation or concept. The use of graph theory enables the users to understand and visualize the situations like COVID-19. Looking at this pandemic disease, its impact and the preventing measures, the graph theory would be the most appropriate way to exercise the graph models with theoretical as well as practical aspects to control this epidemic. In the context of COVID-19, this chapter defines the variable set, variable graphs, and their types considering the variations in the vertex sets and edge sets. The virus graph and their type are discussed in this chapter that states that the Virus graph type I and III are not so perilous for all living beings, but virus graph type III and IV are extremely hazardous for the harmony of the world. Initially, the COVID-19 was in Virus graph-I type, but presently it is in Virus graph-II type. Given different aspects for expansion of pandemic, this chapter presents growth types of virus graphs and their variation as 1-1, 1-P, and 1-all growth types. This chapter provide the number of infected people after 'n' number of days concerning different values of P and growth rates with I0 = 100. At the end of this chapter, the country-wise starting dates of stages of the virus graph-I and II are specified. The concept of cut sets is applicable for the prevention of COVID-19 and the whole world is using the same analogy.

H. R. Bhapkar (✉)
Department of Mathematics, MIT ADT University's, MIT School of Engineering, Pune, Maharashtra, India
e-mail: hrbhapkar@gmail.com

P. N. Mahalle
Department of Computer Engineering, STES'S, Smt. Kashibai Navale College of Engineering, Pune, Maharashtra, India
e-mail: aalborg.pnm@gmail.com

P. S. Dhotre
Department of Information Technology, JSPM's Rajarshi Shahu College of Engineering, Pune, Maharashtra, India
e-mail: prashantsdhotre@gmail.com

© The Editor(s) (if applicable) and The Author(s), under exclusive license
to Springer Nature Switzerland AG 2020
A.-E. Hassanien et al. (eds.), *Big Data Analytics and Artificial Intelligence Against COVID-19: Innovation Vision and Approach*, Studies in Big Data 78,
https://doi.org/10.1007/978-3-030-55258-9_2

Keywords Virus graphs · COVID-19 · Pandemic · Epidemic

1 Introduction

COVID-19 is the transferrable disease caused by the recent coronavirus recently started in Wuhan, China. This virus and subsequently the disease were shadowy to the world before its outbreak. Considering the recent COVID-19 virus and its spread across the globe, it is important to understand and visualize the virus spread and impact. The disease caused by this virus has become pandemic and many countries are affected badly. Using the graph theory approach, this chapter helps users to understand and visualize this disease, impact and spread. The different graph method presented in this chapter shows a virus, its growth type is presented using graph theory. The number of persons who are affected and prevention is also presented in this chapter. This chapter concludes that there is an infinite scope of mathematics for the research as well as resolving social problems like COVID-19 and technical problems.

The reader will refer [1–4] for the absolute dealing with the subject matter. All Graphs considered in this chapter are simple as well as connected. The neighbor of the vertex v in graph H is the set of all the vertices adjacent to the vertex v in H. A graph with n vertices and without any edges is called the Null graph and it is denoted by Nn [1, 5–9].

A simple connected graph, in which the degree of each vertex is 2, is called a cycle graph. Cn is the cycle graph on n vertices [4]. A graph, in which one vertex is adjacent to n pendant vertices, is called the star graph. It is symbolized by K1, n. Here, I V(K1, n) I = n + 1 along with I E (K1, n) I = n [10].

The chapter is organized as follows. Basic terms of graph are presented in Sect. 1. Motivation and related work is presented in Sect. 2 and 3 respectively. Graphical theoretical model that emphasizes on Virus Graph I, II, III and IV is presented in Sect. 4. Sections 5 and 6 discusses on growth rate and its types. Country wise stages of Virus graph I and II is presented in Sect. 7. Growth rate of COVID-19 is predicted and presented in Sect. 8. This chapter is summarized with future outlook in Sect. 9 [10].

2 Motivation

Almost 2.5 million cases of COVID-19 (corona virus) and more than 160,000 deaths have now been reported worldwide [4]. The largest part of the epidemic in the world comes into sight to be steady or declining [3]. A good number countries are immobile in the early stages of their epidemics and few of them were affected early in the pandemic are now starting to see an improvement in cases. Hence, it is the most important and essential to prevent the spread of such types of epidemic [10]. As we know, mathematical modelling award different astonishing inspiration and tools to study different communal as well as technical problems and interpret solutions. This will lead to find the practical solutions of a variety of problems and helps to continue the harmony of the mankind.

3 Related Work

Let us consider following terminologies.

- **Partite Graphs**

A graph H is n- partite graph if $V(H) = V_1 \cup V_2 \cup ..., \cup V_n$, where all V_i are disjoint and every edge of H joins a vertex of V_i and V_j for $i \neq j$. If $n = 2, 3, 4$ then graphs are called Bipartite, Tripartite and four partite respectively [1].

- **Cut Sets**

A set of edges of a connected graph H, whose removal disconnects H, is called the disconnecting set of H. The smallest disconnecting set is called the cut set of H [2, 4].

- **Corona Product of Graphs**

The corona product of H and K is denoted by H ○ K and obtained from a copy of H and | V (H) | copies of K, joining each vertex of H to all vertices of the graph K. This graph product was initiated by mathematicians Frucht and Harary in 1970 [11, 12].

Giulia Giordano et al. [2] proposed an innovative epidemic model which distinguishes between infected people depending on whether they have been confirmed by considering their symptoms. Non diagnosed peoples can spread virus rapidly than diagnosed people. Therefore the divergence between diagnosed and non-diagnosed plays an important role for the deterrence of a pandemic. A fuzzy theory and deep learning networks help to enhance for acquiring superior stochastic insights concerning the epidemic growth is experimented [3]. A deep learning based Composite Monte-Carlo (CMC) showed better results than simple Monte Carlo (MC) which will be obliged for decision makers for greater ranges of the future promises of epidemic and pandemic [13]. In [14], it is studied that due less and incorrect information about COVID-19, there is no any exact model which can predict spread of the pandemic. Every model has different levels of predictive efficiency.

By analyzing data in few countries, it is noted that an infection reached to peak around 10 days after the controlling measures are initiated. The growth rate of infected people was slowly decreasing during this period. But, especially the growth rate in Italy remains exponential. Hence, quarantine is insufficient and need strict measures [15]. In [16], the authors have made a mathematical model for the epidemic by applying linear differential equations. By identifying patterns and analyzing desired data, it is concluded that the growth rate is dynamic or exponential depending upon precautions taken by people. Shinde Gitanjali et al. [17], presented and meticulously discussed different predictive analytic models as well as algorithms for the number infected cases in the near future. Moreover, the Prophet predictive analytics algorithm is implemented on the Kaggle dataset and its predictions are studied in their research work. The following new terms are defined for constructing the pedestal of mathematical modelling of any types of pandemic or COVID-19.

Critical decision making is difficult due to uncertainty caused by novel coronavirus epidemic. Fong et al. [10] presented deep learning and fuzzy based prediction method for the future possibilities of coronavirus and its impact. The present events and its future behavior is presented using Composite Monte Carlo simulation method. The difficult task is accurate forecasting of destiny of an epidemic is presented by Fong et al. [18] using augmentation of existing data, panel design for selection of best forecasting model and its fine tuning of parameters of each model. Deep learning method was presented by Hu et al. [19] for forecasting of COVID-19.

Based on the lung CT scan images, Rajinikanth [20] presented a system for detection of COVID-19. This proposed method is based on Otsu and a meta-heuristic Harmony search algorithm. Using graph theory, data classification was proposed by Kamal [21] which is based on De-Bruijn graph with MapReduce framework.

After evaluation of related work, there is a need for the mathematical modelling and visualization of COVID-19 using graph theory is essential to spread awareness among many stakeholders.

3.1   Variable Set

A set S is said to be Variable set if elements of the set S changes with respect to time or some rule. That is, the set S is not constant set. Its cardinality changes with respect to time. S_v is the notation of variable set. In the variable sets, time units depend upon its nature. According to the scenery of the cardinality of the set S, there are three types of sets.

- Increasing Variable Set: A variable set S_v is said to be increasing variable set if $|S_v(x)| < |S_v(y)|$, whenever $x < y$, where x and y are different times.
- Decreasing Variable Set: A variable set S_v is said to be decreasing variable set if $|S_v(x)| > |S_v(y)|$, whenever $x < y$.
- Non Decreasing Variable Set: A variable set S_v is said to be non-decreasing variable set if $|S_v(x)| \leq |S_v(y)|$, whenever $x \leq y$.
- Non Increasing Variable Set: A variable set S_v is said to be non-increasing variable set if $|S_v(x)| \geq |S_v(y)|$, whenever $x \leq y$.
- Stable Variable Set: A variable set S_v is said to be stable variable set if $|S_v(t)| =$ constant, for any time t. However, the set is a variable set. Elements of the set S vary according to time, but the $|S_v(t)|$ is steady, for any time t.

3.2 Variable Graph

A graph H is said to be a vertex variable graph if V (H) or E (H) is variable sets. Variable graphs are also known as V-graphs. Big network graphs are variable graph. There are two types of variable graphs.

3.3 Edge V-Graph

A variable graph H is said to be edge V-graph if E (H) is a variable set and V (H) is the stable variable set.

3.4 Vertex V-Graph

A variable graph H is said to be vertex V-graph if V (H) is a variable set and E (H) is the constant variable set.

3.5 N-Partite V-Graphs

A variable graph H is said to be n-partite V-Graph if

1. $V (H) = V_1$ U V_2 U V_3,...., V_n where V_1, V_2, V_3,..., V_n disjoint variable sets having different characteristics.
2. There exists a bond on the link or edge between vertices of Vi & Vj, for i, j and $i \neq j$.

3.6 Bipartite V-Graph

A variable graph H is said to be Bipartite V-Graph if

1. $V (H) = V_1$ U V_2, where V_1 and V_2 are disjoint variable sets with different characteristics.
2. There exists a bond on the link or edge between vertices of V_1 and vertices of V_2
3. There is no any bond among the vertices of V_1 only or V_2 only.

These types of graphs are denoted by BV_2. In BV_2, a vertex x of V_1 is said to be **Active Vertex** or element if there exists a bond between x and at least one vertex of V_2 or x is trying to build a bond or edges to the vertices of V_2. Moreover, x is ready for the sharing some characteristics. Other vertices of V_1 are known as the Passive

Fig. 1 Virus Graph I

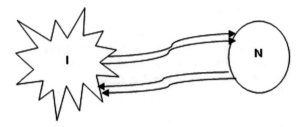

Vertices. A vertex y of V_2 is said to be Active Vertex or element if there exists a bond between y and at least one vertex of V_1 or y is aiming to build a bond or edges to the vertices of V_1. Other vertices of V_2 are known as the **Passive Vertices**.

4   Graph Theoretical Model

4.1   Virus Graph I

A Bipartite V-graph H is said to be Virus Graph I (VRG-I) if

1. $V(H) = I \cup N$, where, I be the variable set of vertices have some special properties or infected by virus and N be the variable set of vertices not having a virus.
2. If $x \in I$, creates a bond or an edge with the vertex $y \in N$ or vice versa, then y is shifted to I and $N = N - \{y\}$.
3. If $x \in I$, is recovered by treatment or lost properties of virus then, x is shifted to N and $N = N \cup \{x\}$. The diagrammatic representation of VRG-I is shown in Fig. 1.

4.2   Virus Graph II

A Tripartite V-graph H is said to be Virus Graph II (VRG-II) if

1. $V(H) = I \cup N \cup F$, where, I be the variable set of vertices having the virus, N be the variable set of vertices not having virus and F be the set of vertices which can never be shifted to I or N.
2. If $x \in I$, creates a bond or an edge with the vertex $y \in N$ or vice versa, then y is shifted to I and $N = N - \{y\}$.
3. If $x \in I$, is recovered by treatment or vanished properties of virus then, x is shifted to N and $N = N \cup \{x\}$.
4. Vertices of I are shifted to F if the vertices are infected forever. Therefore, S is the non-decreasing variable set. This is represented in Fig. 2.

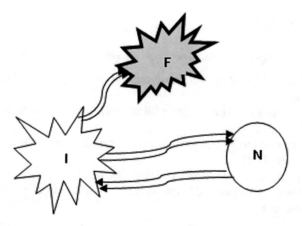

Fig. 2 Virus Graph II

4.3 Virus Graph III

A Tripartite V-graph H is said to be Virus Graph III (VRG-III) if

1. V(H) = I U N U S, where, S be the set of vertices which is never infected by the virus.
2. If x ∈ I. creates a bond or an edge with the vertex y ∈ N or vice versa, then y is shifted to\in I and N = N − {y}.
3. If x ∈ I. is recovered by treatment or lost properties of virus then, x is shifted to N and N = N U {x}.
4. Vertices of N, with some additional features, can be shifted to variable set S. Furthermore, the vertices of S are protected by a shield of antivirus or some special vaccines. The vertices of V can't be directly transformed into S, but transformed to N and N to S. Consequently, S is the non-decreasing variable set. This occurrence is shown in Fig. 3.

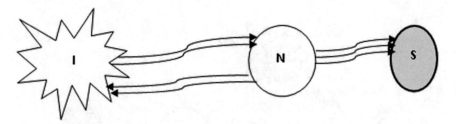

Fig. 3 Virus Graph III

4.4   Virus Graph IV

A four partite V-graph H is said to be Virus Graph IV (VRG-IV) if

1. V(H) = I U N U S U F, where, F be the set of vertices which can never be shifted to I or N or S.
2. If x ∈ I, creates a bond or an edge with the vertex y ∈ N or vice versa, then y is shifted to I and N = N − {y}.
3. If x ∈ I. is recovered by treatment or lost properties of virus then, x is shifted to N and N = N U {x}.
4. Vertices of N, with some additional features, can be shifted to variable set S. Furthermore, the vertices of S are protected by a shield of antivirus or some special vaccines.

Vertices of F can be never shifted to any other set. The elements of F are having philosophy "infected once is infected forever". It is shown in Fig. 4.

Virus Graph: A variable graph is said to be a Virus graph if it belongs to class of either Virus graph-I or Virus graph-II or Virus graph-III or Virus graph-IV.

5   Growth Rate

The growth rate of any V-graph is the rate of increase of active elements minus the rate of increase of passive elements.

6   Types of Growth

There are three types of growth of any virus, according to graph theory. Each type of growth is discussed as below.

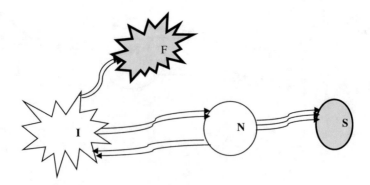

Fig. 4 Virus Graph IV

6.1 One–One Growth

A growth is said to be one–one or 1–1 growth if one active element of the variable set infects only one active element of another set at that instant. This growth is articulated as the corona product of cycle graph with K_1. Here Cm is the cycle graph having r active elements, which are elements of the variable set I. Additionally, K_1 is an individual active element of the variable set N. It is shown in Fig. 5.

- **Growth rate is constant**

Without loss of generality, assume that there are 30% active elements in each set. Also assume that the number of infected people is extremely less than the total population. In this growth type, every day 30% new patients are increased in the set I. Let I_0 be the number of people infected by the virus at initial stage. Let In be the number of people will be infected after n days. As a result,

$$I_1 = I_0 + (0.30) I_0 = 1.3 * I_0, \tag{1}$$

$$I_2 = I_1 + (0.30) I_1 = 1.30 * I_1 = 1.3(1.3 * I_0) = (1.3)^2 I_0 \tag{2}$$

In general, $I_n = (1.3)^n * I_0$.

Let R be the rate of the virus per unit tine and I_0 be an initial number of infected people. Therefore,

$$I_1 = I_0 + R I_0 = (1 + R) I_0, \tag{3}$$

After second time interval,

Fig. 5 One-One Growth

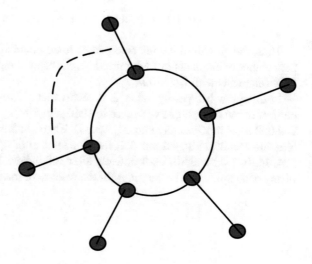

Table 1 Growth rate and time interval

After time ti	t1	t2	t3	t4	...	tn-1	tn
Growth rate Ri	R1	R2	R3	R4	...	Rn-1	Rn

$$I_2 = I_1 + R\,I_1 = (1 + R)\,I_1 = (1 + R)^2 I_0. \tag{4}$$

After n time intervals, the number of infected people will be

$$I_n = (1 + R)^n I_0 \tag{5}$$

- **Growth rate is not constant**

Now, assume that the growth rate is different in each time interval as given Table 1
After the second time interval,

$$I_2 = I_1 + R_2 I_1 = (1 + R_2)\,I_1 = (1 + R_2)\,(1 + R_1)\,I_0, \tag{6}$$

$$I_3 = (1 + R_3)\,(1 + R_2)\,(1 + R_1)\,I_0, \tag{7}$$

After n time intervals, the number of infected people is

$$I_n = (1 + R_n) \ldots (1 + R_2)\,(1 + R_1)\,I_0. \tag{8}$$

Moreover, at time t_i, growth rate is R_i and R_i is repeated m_i times in the given interval. Hence,

$$I_n = (1 + R_1)^{m_1}(1 + R_2)^{m_2} \ldots (1 + R_j)^{m_j}$$
$$\text{where } 1 \le j \le n \text{ and } m_1 + m_2 + \cdots + m_j = n. \tag{9}$$

Thus, the growth of the infected people is exponential. Consider the Table 2 for the number of elements in I after nth days corresponding to various percentages of active elements with $I_0 = 100$.

In this growth type, by Table 2, it seems that if growth rate is 30%, then the number of infected people will reach to 1060 after 9th day, 19,005 after the 20th day, 262,000 after the 30th day and 24,793,351,109,660 after 100th day. But if growth rates are 1%, 2%, 3%, 4% and 5%, then the number of infected people will be 245, 594, 1430, 3412 and 8073 respectively after 100th days. Therefore, the growth rate of any pandemic must be very less for the welfare of mankind.

Table 2 Number of elements in I after nth days with respect to active elements

No. of days	I_n (Growth 30%)	I_n (Growth 1%)	I_n (Growth 2%)	I_n (Growth 3%)	I_n (Growth 4%)	I_n (Growth 5%)	I_n (Growth 7%)	I_n (Growth 10%)	I_n (Growth 15%)	I_n (Growth 20%)
1	130	101	102	103	104	105	107	110	115	120
2	169	102	104	106	108	110	114	121	132	144
3	220	103	106	109	112	116	123	133	152	173
4	286	104	108	113	117	122	131	146	175	207
5	371	105	110	116	122	128	140	161	201	249
6	483	106	113	119	127	134	150	177	231	299
7	627	107	115	123	132	141	161	195	266	358
8	816	108	117	127	137	148	172	214	306	430
9	1060	109	120	130	142	155	184	236	352	516
10	1379	110	122	134	148	163	197	259	405	619
15	5119	116	135	156	180	208	276	418	814	1541
20	19,005	122	149	181	219	265	387	673	1637	3834
25	70,564	128	164	209	267	339	543	1083	3292	9540
30	262,000	135	181	243	324	432	761	1745	6621	23,738
35	972,786	142	200	281	395	552	1068	2810	13,318	59,067
40	3,611,886	149	221	326	480	704	1497	4526	26,786	146,977
50	49,792,922	164	269	438	711	1147	2946	11,739	108,366	910,044
60	686,437,717	182	328	589	1052	1868	5795	30,448	438,400	5,634,751
70	9,463,126,845	201	400	792	1557	3043	11,399	78,975	1,773,572	34,888,896
80	130,457,239,505	222	488	1064	2305	4956	22,423	204,840	7,175,088	216,022,846

(continued)

Table 2 (continued)

No. of days	I_n (Growth 30%)	I_n (Growth 1%)	I_n (Growth 2%)	I_n (Growth 3%)	I_n (Growth 4%)	I_n (Growth 5%)	I_n (Growth 7%)	I_n (Growth 10%)	I_n (Growth 15%)	I_n (Growth 20%)
90	1,798,463,828,896	245	594	1430	3412	8073	44,110	531,302	29,027,233	1,337,556,525
100	24,793,351,109,660	270	724	1922	5050	13,150	86,772	1,378,061	117,431,345	8,281,797,452
120	4,711,967,396,969,860	330	1077	3471	11,066	34,891	335,779	9,270,907	1,921,944,500	317,504,237,378

6.2 One-P Growth

If one active element of the variable set (I) infects at most -p active elements of another set (N) together at that instant, is called One-P growth or 1-P growth. In this case, Cm is the cycle graph having r active elements of variable set I and there is a group of P individual active elements of variable set N. Therefore, it is the corona product of the Cm with null graph having n vertices, which is shown in Fig. 6.

Without loss of generality, assume that there are R active elements in each set. R % new patients are increased every day in the set I. Let I0 be the number of people infected by the virus at initial stage. Let In be the number of people will be infected after n days.

As a result,

$$I_1 = I_0 + (R * P) I_0 = (1 + R * P) * I_0, \tag{10}$$

$$I_2 = I_1 + (R * P) I_1 = (1 + R * P)^2 * I_0 = (1.3)^2 I_0 \tag{11}$$

In general,

$$I_n = (1 + R * P)^n * I_0. \tag{12}$$

The number of infected people will be doubled in at most P number of days which will assist for confirming the greatest value of P.

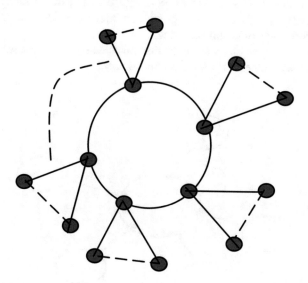

Fig. 6 One—P Growth

If R = 0.01 and n = 2, then the greatest value of P is the value where I_0 will become doubled. Therefore, The greatest value of P is $(e^{0.34657} - 1) * 100 \approx 42$. Hence, growth is 1–P type if the value of P ≤ 42. For the greater values of P, the growth type is 1-all growth.

6.3   One—All Growth

If one active element of the variable set infects all or more than 42 active elements of another set together at that instant, is called 1—all growth. Such types of growth occur through water or air only. This is extremely perilous for living beings. Cm is the cycle graph having r active elements of variable set I and the group of the active elements of the variable set N. This is the corona product of Cm with all individual elements of null graph having more than 42 vertices. Its graph is given in Fig. 7.

7   COVID-19

COVID-19 is a virus graph. At the initial stage, it was in the type virus graph-I. Let V (C) and E (C) are the variable vertex set (the set of people) and variable edge set of the COVID-19 graph C. Therefore, V(C) = I U N, where I be the variable set of people infected by the virus COVID-19 and N be the variable set of people not infected by the COVID-19. Some corona viruses can be transmitted from person to person, generally after close contact with an infected patient, for example, in a household workplace, or health care center.

The continuity of the graph C can be disconnected by the disconnecting set. So, keep all vertices of either set in the disconnecting set.

That is

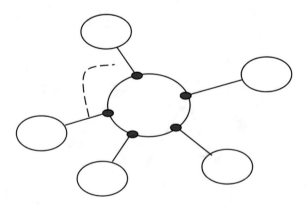

Fig. 7 One—All Growth

D = {set of all edges adjacent to active vertices of I} or

D = { set of all edges adjacent to active vertices of N}   (13)

Moreover, the cut set of C is {I} if | I | ≤ |N |, otherwise, the cut set is {N}. At present, every country of the world is doing the same for controlling the effect of COVID-19. We isolate people of set I as well as N or quarantine the people of set I or N, as per the necessities.

Presently, COVID-19 is in the virus graph-II type. Moreover,

$$V(C) = I \cup N \cup F \qquad (14)$$

where F be the set of people, who are infected permanently. The people of the set F will not be recovered by any medicine and will die in the near future. The whole world is suffering from the effect of this virus and everyone is fervently waiting for the vaccine of this virus.

Table 3 gives the country wise starting dates of stages of the virus graph-I and II.

It is observed that if we take desired precautions, then we can control the spread of the epidemic or pandemic. There are few countries still in virus graph-I and most of the countries rapidly reached to virus graph-II.

After discovering the vaccine on COVID-19, it will be shifted to virus graph-IV type. Therefore,

$$V(C) = I \cup N \cup F \cup S, \qquad (15)$$

where S be the set of vertices which can never be infected by virus. That is all people in the set S are vaccinated by desired medicines.

In this situation, we need to increase the number of elements of the set S up to the whole population of the universal set. Hence, everyone will be free from the effect of the virus.

Moreover, hope that there should not be such types of pandemic, but if so, that must be Virus graph-III. This will help to preserve excellent harmony of living beings.

8   Growth Rate of COVID -19

The growth type of the COVID-19 is 1-P growth. One person can infect at most P ≤ 42 persons at a time. For the superior values of P, this growth is also called Small Community Spread.

Table 4 gives the number of infected people after n days with respect to different values of P and growth rates with $I_0 = 100$.

If the growth rate is 1 % and P = 5, then the number of infected people will be doubled after 15 days, whereas, R = 5 and P = 5, then the number of infected people will be 244 after the 4th day, 1164 after 11th day, 10,842 after the 20th day and

Table 3 Country wise stages of the virus graph-I and II

Sr. No.	Name of country	Virus Graph-I from	Virus Graph-II from
1	Afghanistan	25-Feb-20	24-Mar-20
2	Africa	15-Feb-20	9-Mar-20
3	Australia	25-Jan-20	1-Mar-20
4	Bermuda	20-Mar-20	9-Apr-20
5	Bhutan	6-Mar-20	–
6	Bolivia	12-Mar-20	1-Apr-20
7	Brazil	26-Feb-20	18-Mar-20
8	Bulgaria	8-Mar-20	12-Mar-20
9	Cambodia	28-Jan-20	–
10	Canada	26-Jan-20	10-Mar-20
11	China	31-Dec-19	11-Jan-20
12	Colombia	7-Mar-20	22-Mar-20
13	Denmark	27-Feb-20	16-Mar-20
14	Egypt	15-Feb-20	9-Mar-20
15	Europe	25-Jan-20	15-Feb-20
16	Finland	30-Jan-20	22-Mar-20
17	France	25-Jan-20	15-Feb-20
18	Germany	28-Jan-20	12-Mar-20
19	Ghana	13-Mar-20	22-Mar-20
20	Greece	27-Feb-20	12-Mar-20
21	Greenland	20-Mar-20	–
22	Hungary	5-Mar-20	16-Mar-20
23	India	30-Jan-20	13-Mar-20
24	Indonesia	2-Mar-20	12-Mar-20
25	Iran	20-Feb-20	23-Feb-20
26	Iraq	25-Feb-20	14-Mar-20
27	Ireland	1-Mar-20	12-Mar-20
28	Israel	22-Feb-20	21-Mar-20
29	Italy	31-Jan-20	27-Feb-20
30	Japan	15-Jan-20	13-Feb-20
31	Kenya	14-Mar-20	27-Mar-20
32	Kuwait	24-Feb-20	5-Apr-20
33	Malaysia	25-Jan-20	25-Mar-20
34	Nepal	25-Jan-20	–
35	Netherlands	28-Feb-20	7-Mar-20
36	New Zealand	28-Feb-20	29-Mar-20

(continued)

Table 3 (continued)

Sr. No.	Name of country	Virus Graph-I from	Virus Graph-II from
37	North America	21-Jan-20	1-Mar-20
38	Oman	25-Feb-20	1-Apr-20
39	Pakistan	27-Feb-20	21-Mar-20
40	Peru	7-Mar-20	21-Mar-20
41	Poland	4-Mar-20	13-Mar-20
42	Russia	1-Feb-20	29-Mar-20
43	Rwanda	15-Mar-20	–
44	Singapore	24-Jan-20	29-Mar-20
45	South Africa	6-Mar-20	31-Mar-20
46	South America	26-Feb-20	8-Mar-20
47	South Korea	20-Jan-20	21-Feb-20
48	South Sudan	6-Apr-20	–
49	Spain	1-Feb-20	5-Mar-20
50	Sri Lanka	28-Jan-20	29-Mar-20
51	Sudan	14-Mar-20	15-Mar-20
52	Swaziland	15-Mar-20	18-Apr-20
53	Sweden	1-Feb-20	12-Mar-20
54	Switzerland	26-Feb-20	6-Mar-20
55	Taiwan	21-Jan-20	17-Feb-20
56	Thailand	13-Jan-20	1-Mar-20
57	Turkey	12-Mar-20	19-Mar-20
58	Uganda	22-Mar-20	–
59	United Arab Emirates	27-Jan-20	1-Apr-20
60	United Kingdom	31-Jan-20	6-Mar-20
61	United States	21-Jan-20	1-Mar-20
62	Vietnam	24-Jan-20	–
63	Yemen	10-Apr-20	–
64	Zimbabwe	21-Mar-20	24-Mar-20

1,00,974 after 31st day. Thus the growth rate as well as the P value play a vital role in prevention of any types of epidemics.

Table 4 Number of infected people with respect to R and P

Patient no.	I_n Growth rate 1%		I_n Growth rate 2%		I_n Growth rate 3%		I_n Growth rate 4%		I_n Growth rate 5%	
	P = 3	P = 5	P = 3	P = 5	P = 3	P = 5	P = 3	P = 5	P = 3	P = 5
1	103	105	106	110	109	115	112	120	115	125
2	106	110	112	121	119	132	125	144	132	156
3	109	116	119	133	130	152	140	173	152	195
4	113	122	126	146	141	175	157	207	175	244
5	116	128	134	161	154	201	176	249	201	305
6	119	134	142	177	168	231	197	299	231	381
7	123	141	150	195	183	266	221	358	266	477
8	127	148	159	214	199	306	248	430	306	596
9	130	155	169	236	217	352	277	516	352	745
10	134	163	179	259	237	405	311	619	405	931
11	138	171	190	285	258	465	348	743	465	1164
12	143	180	201	314	281	535	390	892	535	1455
13	147	189	213	345	307	615	436	1070	615	1819
14	151	198	226	380	334	708	489	1284	708	2274
15	156	208	240	418	364	814	547	1541	814	2842
16	160	218	254	459	397	936	613	1849	936	3553
17	165	229	269	505	433	1076	687	2219	1076	4441
18	170	241	285	556	472	1238	769	2662	1238	5551
19	175	253	303	612	514	1423	861	3195	1423	6939
20	181	265	321	673	560	1637	965	3834	1637	8674
21	186	279	340	740	611	1882	1080	4601	1882	10,842
22	192	293	360	814	666	2164	1210	5521	2164	13,553
23	197	307	382	895	726	2489	1355	6625	2489	16,941
24	203	323	405	985	791	2863	1518	7950	2863	21,176
25	209	339	429	1083	862	3292	1700	9540	3292	26,470
26	216	356	455	1192	940	3786	1904	11,448	3786	33,087
27	222	373	482	1311	1025	4354	2132	13,737	4354	41,359
28	229	392	511	1442	1117	5007	2388	16,484	5007	51,699
29	236	412	542	1586	1217	5758	2675	19,781	5758	64,623
30	243	432	574	1745	1327	6621	2996	23,738	6621	80,779
31	250	454	609	1919	1446	7614	3356	28,485	7614	100,974

8.1 Complexity

The Virus graph representation includes either adjacency matrix or adjacency list. The adjacency matrix is 2D matrix that has row and column combination. The combination may include growth rate and number of infected people. The complexity of representing this information will have $O(n^2)$. On the other side, if it is implemented using adjacency list, the complexity will be $O(v + e)$, where v is vertices and e is edges connecting those vertices.

8.2 Limitations

In this chapter, the data under consideration is enormous and varying, consequently the size of virus graph is extremely large. The cut sets of the graphs recommended for the prevention of the COVID-19 is large but if handled logically, will award superior results. The growth rate is high, so practically difficult to measure, but mathematically it is simple to analyze.

9 Conclusions and Future Outlook

To describe the different situations in the different contexts across different geolocations, the graph -theory has been useful. By applying different aspects of Mathematics, the world's universal problems have had been consistently resolved. This chapter presented the graph theory and its variations to understand the outbreak of COVID-19. The concepts of graph theory have provided the mathematical modeling of the COVID-19. The detailed discussion on Virus graph and its Types has revealed that the type I and II are not dangerous as compared with type III and IV. The growth rates are modeled using graphs that show the spread of contagious and active elements are exponential. In the view of COVID-19, the country wise starting dates of stages of the virus graph-I and II is presented and the spread of this pandemic can be reduced by taking necessary precautions.

If the growth rate is 1 % and P = 5, then the number of infected people will be doubled after 15 days. The growth rate will increase as 1164 after 11th day, 10,842 after the 20th day and 1,00,974 after 31st day. Thus the growth rate as well as the P value play a vital role in the prevention of some types of epidemics. This chapter presents methods to control the spread of some types of a pandemic. The analysis and study presented in this chapter indicate a special need to identify the minutiae of pandemic and apply astonishing theories for maintaining the smooth harmony of mankind. There is an infinite scope of mathematics for the research as well as resolving the social and technical problems of the world.

References

1. West, D.B.: An Introduction to Graph Theory. Prentice-Hall, Pearson Edison India (1995)
2. Giulia Giordano, G., Blanchini, F., Bruno, R., Colaneri, P., Di Filippo, A., Di Matteo, A., Colaneri, M.: A SIDARTHE model of COVID-19 epidemic in Italy. arXiv preprint arXiv: 2003.09861 (2020)
3. Akhtar, I.H.: Understanding the CoVID-19 pandemic curve through statistical approach. Cold Spring Harbor Laboratory (2020)
4. WHO: Novel Corona virus (2019-nCoV) Situation Report - 39. 2020 [cited 2020 April 20]; Available from: https://www.who.int/docs/defaultsource/coronaviruse/situationreports/20200228-sitrep-39-covid-19.pdf?sfvrsn=5bbf3e7d_2
5. Chung, F.R.K., Lu, L.: Complex graphs and networks, CBMS regional conference series in mathematics. Am. Mathe. Soc. **10** (2006)
6. Bhapkar, H.R., Salunke, J.N.: The geometric dual of HB graph, outerplanar graph and related aspects. Bull. Math. Sci. Appl. **3**(3), 114–119 (2014). ISSN 2278-9634
7. Bondy, J.A., Murty, U.S.R.: Graph Theory with Applications. Elsevier, MaccMillan, New York - London (1976)
8. Kamal, M.S., Parvin, S., Ashour, A.S., Shi, F., Dey, N.: De-Bruijn graph with MapReduce framework towards metagenomic data classification. Int J Inf Technol **9**(1), 59–75 (2017)
9. Deo, N.: Graph Theory with Applications to Engineering and Computer Science, Prentice-Hall of India (2003)
10. Mahalle, P.N., Sable, N.P., Mahalle, N.P., Shinde, G.R.: Predictive analytics of COVID-19 using information. Commun. Technol. Preprints 2020040257 (2020). https://doi.org/10.20944/preprints202004.0257.v1
11. Zmazek, B., 'Zerovnik, J.: Behzad—vizing conjecture and cartesian product graphs. Elect. Notes in Discrete Math. **17**:297–300 (2004)
12. Frucht, R., Harary, F.: On the corona of two graphs. Aequationes Math. **4**, 322–325 (1970)
13. DeCapprio, D., Gartner, J., et al.: Building a COVID-19 vulnerability index, medRxiv preprint https://doi.org/10.1101/2020.03.16.20036723
14. Fong, S.J. Li, G. Dey, N., et al.: Composite monte carlo decision making under high uncertainty of novel coronavirus epidemic using hybridized deep learning and fuzzy rule induction. Appl. Soft Comput.
15. Volpert, V., Banerjee, M., Petrovskii, S.: On a quarantine model of coronavirus infection and data analysis. Math Model Nat. Phenom. (2020)
16. Weber, A., Ianelli, F., Goncalves, S.: Trend analysis of the COVID-19 pandemic in China and the rest of the world (2020). arXiv preprint arXiv:2003.09032
17. Shinde, G.R., Kalamkar, A.B., Mahalle, P.N. Dey, N., Chaki, J., Hassanien, A.: Forecasting Models for Coronavirus (COVID-19): A Survey of the State-of-the-Art. TechRxiv. (2020). Preprint. https://doi.org/10.36227/techrxiv.12101547.v1
18. Fong, S.J., Li, G., Dey, N., Crespo, R.G., Herrera-Viedma, E.: Composite Monte Carlo decision making under high uncertainty of novel coronavirus epidemic using hybridized deep learning and fuzzy rule induction. Appl. Soft Comput. 106282 (2020)
19. Fong, S.J., Li, G., Dey, N., Crespo, R.G., Herrera-Viedma, E.: Finding an accurate early forecasting model from small dataset: a case of 2019-ncov novel coronavirus outbreak (2020). arXiv preprint arXiv:2003.10776
20. Hu, S., Liu, M., Fong, S., Song, W., Dey, N., Wong, R.: Forecasting China future MNP by deep learning. In: Behavior engineering and applications, pp. 169–210. Springer, Cham (2018)
21. Rajinikanth, V., Dey, N., Raj, A.N.J., Hassanien, A.E., Santosh, K.C., Raja, N.:. Harmony-Search and Otsu based System for Coronavirus Disease (COVID-19) Detection using Lung CT Scan Images (2020). arXiv preprint arXiv:2004.03431

Nonparametric Analysis of Tracking Data in the Context of COVID-19 Pandemic

D. A. Klyushin

Abstract Methods of statistical pattern recognition are powerful tools for analysis of statistical data on COVID-19 pandemic. In this chapter, we offer a new effective online algorithm for detection of change-points in tracking data (movement data, health rate data etc.). We developed a non-parametric test for evaluation of the statistical hypothesis that data in two adjacent time intervals have the same distribution. In the context of the mobile phone tracking this means that the coordinates of the tracked object does not deviated from the base point significantly. For estimation of the health rate it means the absence of significant deviations from the norm. The significance level for the test is less than 0.05. The test permits ties in samples. Also, we show that results of comparison of the test with well-known Kolmogorov–Smirnov test. These results show that the proposed test is more robust, sensitive and accurate than the alternative ones. In addition, the new method does not require high computational capacity.

Keywords COVID-19 · Time series · Change-Point problem · Mobile control · Health rate control · Nonparametric test · Homogeneity measure

1 Introduction

In the midst of the COVID-19 pandemic, an avalanche of information is crashing down on scientists and decision makers. Among this huge volume of data ones of the most important are geolocation data of millions of mobile phone users in different regions and health data obtained from wearable devices. This data allows tracking migration of isolated patients and prevent their uncontrolled walks. Also, it allows detection of significance changes in the health rate of a user (temperature, pulse etc.). As far these data have a random nature, quite high rate of arrival and volatility, it is

D. A. Klyushin (✉)
Faculty of Computer Science and Cybernetics, Taras Shevchenko National University of Kyiv, Akademika Glushkova Avenue 4D, Kiev 03680, Ukraine
e-mail: dokmed5@gmail.com

A.-E. Hassanien et al. (eds.), *Big Data Analytics and Artificial Intelligence Against COVID-19: Innovation Vision and Approach*, Studies in Big Data 78, https://doi.org/10.1007/978-3-030-55258-9_3

impossible to correctly process and analyze then manually, and therefore make the right decisions based on it without automatic analysis. In this regard, the development of artificial intelligence methods for the analysis of sequential data about isolated patient movements and analysis of health data of wearable devices users becomes an urgent task. In particular, now there were developed highly effective methods for decision making during the COVID-19 pandemic [1], diagnosis and prediction models for COVID-19 patients response to treatment [2], forecasting of coronavirus outbreak [3, 4], and methods of analysis of computer tomography images of COVID-19 patients [5]. But, the search of current publications in the repositories of preprints arXiv and medRxiv shows that yet there are no papers on analysis of data obtained via wearing gadgets.

Storing a huge amount of information is one of the main problems of big data. Offline algorithms using complete time series become impossible in such cases. Therefore, we must use online algorithms of time series analysis for detection of change points. In the context of tracking mobile phones and wearable devices the change of time series means the deviation of data from a reference point.

It is convenient to use sliding window to analyze such data. However, this approach has two draw backs. First, the sliding window size should be small enough to prevent the problems with storing data. Second, due to the small size of the sliding window algorithms of analysis must be quite sensitive and recognize changes using small samples. In this work, we develop such an algorithm and show its advantages over an alternative (the Kolmogorov–Smirnov statistics).

In the chapter it is proposed to use the novel nonparametric test for checking the statistical hypothesis that two given samples belong to the same distribution, i.e. they are homogeneous. This test is based on the measure of samples homogeneity, which is used to reject the hypothesis that the samples are identically distributed at a given significance level. The change-point detection is equivalent to change in distribution of data in adjacent intervals. Therefore, we reformulate this problem as the problem of two-sample homogeneity and solve it using the sliding window approach.

The motivation of this chapter is to describe a new approach to change-point detection in time series and demonstrate its application in the context of COVID-19 pandemic (analysis of geolocation tracking data, detection of changes in health data of patient etc.). Now, one of the most popular online statistical methods for solving such problems is the Kolmogorov–Smirnov test [6–10]. This non-parametric test is simple and effective when samples are not overlapping or they have small overlapping. But, it is very sensitive to outliers and may produce high level of false-positive responses when the samples are highly overlapping. The novelty of the proposed approach is that it is based on the Klyushin–Petunin non-parametric test for samples' homogeneity that allows very effective comparing not only non-overlapping samples but the samples with highly overlapping. It is the first application of the Klyushin–Petunin test for detection of change-point of time series and as it will be shown it provides more effective estimation of homogeneity of overlapping samples comparing with the Kolmogorov–Smirnov test. The contribution of this chapter is that it describes a fast, accurate and robust online algorithm to detect change-points in time series that may be an effective tool for measuring the violation of quarantine regime, keeping the social distance between people, and remote controlling the health data of patients suffering from COVID-19.

The chapter is organized in the following way. Section 2 describes the homogeneity measure for samples without ties. Section 3 describes the homogeneity measure for samples with ties. Section 4 contains the results of the experiments with samples from different distributions (normal, lognormal, uniform and gamma distributions) with different degree of overlapping (from completely overlapped samples to disjoined samples) with ties and without ties. Section 5 summarizes the chapter.

2 Homogeneity Measure for Samples Without Ties

Consider samples $u = (u_1, u_2, \ldots, u_n) \in G_1$ and $v = (v_1, v_2, \ldots, v_n) \in G_2$ from populations G_1 and G_2 with distribution functions F_1 and F_2 that are absolutely continuous. The null hypothesis states that $F_1 = F_2$ and the alternative hypothesis states that $F_1 \neq F_2$. There are several categories of criteria for testing such hypotheses: permutation criteria, rank criteria, randomization criteria, and distance criteria. In addition, these tests are divided into universal tests that are valid against any pair of alternatives (for example, Kolmogorov–Smirnov criterion [11, 12], and criteria that are correct against pairs of different alternatives of a particular class (Dickson [13], Wald and Wolfowitz [14], Mathisen [15], Wilcoxon [16], Mann–Whitney [17], Wilks [18] etc.). Also, they could be divided into two large groups: nonparametric and conditionally nonparametric ones. Nonparametric criteria are criteria for testing the hypothesis of the homogeneity of general populations regardless of their distribution assumptions [11–18]. Conditionally non-parametric criteria (Pitman [19], Lehmann [20], Rosenblatt [21], Dwass [22], Fisz [23], Barnard [24], Birnbaum [25], Jockel [26], Allen [27], Efron and Tibshirani [28], Dufour and Farhat [29]) use some assumptions on distributions.

According to Hill's assumption $A_{(n)}$ [30], if random values $u_1, u_2, \ldots, u_n \in G$ are exchangeable and belong to absolutely continuous distribution then

$$P\left(u \in \left(u_{(i)}, u_{(j)}\right)\right) = \frac{j - i}{n + 1}, \tag{1}$$

where $j > i, u \in G$ is a sample value, and $\left(u_{(i)}, u_{(j)}\right)$ is an interval formed by the i-th and j-th order statistics. This assumption was proved in papers of Yu.I. Petunin et al. for independent identically distributed random values [31] and for exchangeable identically distributed random values [32]. Also, it was developed a nonparametric test for detecting the homogeneity of samples without ties [33]. Later, this test was extended on the samples with ties [34].

These tests estimate homogeneity of samples $u_1, u_2, \ldots, u_n$ and $v_1, v_2, \ldots, v_n$ under the strong random experiment and does not depends on their distribution. Suppose that $F_1 = F_2$ and construct the variational series $u_{(1)}, u_{(2)}, \ldots, u_{(n)}$. Denote as $A_{ij}^{(k)}$ an event $\left\{v_k \in \left(u_{(i)}, u_{(j)}\right)\right\}$. According to the Hill's assumption, for $j > i$

$$P\left(v_k \in \left(u_{(i)}, u_{(j)}\right)\right) = p_{ij} = \frac{j - i}{n + 1}.$$

Let us construct the Wilson confidence interval (or any other confidence interval for binomial proportion in Bernoulli trials) for an unknown probability of the event $A_{ij}^{(k)}$:

$$p_{ij}^{(1)} = \frac{h_{ij}^{(n,k)}n + g^2/2 - g\sqrt{h_{ij}^{(n,k)}(1 - h_{ij}^{(n,k)})n + g^2/4}}{n + g^2},$$

$$p_{ij}^{(2)} = \frac{h_{ij}^{(n,k)}n + g^2/2 + g\sqrt{h_{ij}^{(n,k)}(1 - h_{ij}^{(n,k)})n + g^2/4}}{n + g^2}, \tag{2}$$

where $h_{ij}^{(n,k)}$ is the relative frequency of the occurrence of the event $A_{ij}^{(k)}$ in n trials. Then, construct the confidence interval $I_{ij}^{(n)} = \left(p_{ij}^{(1)}, p_{ij}^{(2)}\right)$ with a significance level defined by the parameter g. Note, that if g is equal to 3 than the significance level of $I_{ij}^{(n)}$ is less than 0.05 [33]. Also, the value of p-statistics very weakly depends on the choice of the confidence intervals for a binomial proportion [35]. Let B be an event $\left\{p_{ij} = \frac{j-i}{n+1} \in I_{ij}^{(n)}\right\}$. Put $N = (n-1)n/2$ and find $L = \#B$. Then, $h = L/N$ is a homogeneity measure of samples x and y which we shall call p-statistics.

Let us put $h_{ij}^{(n)} = h$, $n = N$ and $g = 3$, and construct the Wilson (for definiteness) confidence interval $I_n = (p_1, p_2)$ for $p(B)$. The confidence intervals $I_{ij}^{(n)} = \left(p_{ij}^{(1)}, p_{ij}^2\right)$ and $I = (p_1, p_2)$ are called *intervals based on the 3 s-rule*. The scheme of trials, where the events $A_{ij}^{(k)}$ can arise when the hypothesis that distributions are identical holds is true, called a *generalized Bernoulli scheme* [36–38]. If the hypothesis does not hold, this scheme is called a *modified Bernoulli scheme*. In general case, when the null hypothesis can be either true or false, the trial scheme is called *MP-scheme* (Matveychuk–Petunin scheme). If $F_1 = F_2$, $\lim_{n\to\infty} \frac{j-i}{n+1} \in (0, 1)$, and $\lim_{n\to\infty} \frac{i}{n+1} \in (0, 1)$, then the asymptotic significance level β of a sequence of confidence intervals $I_{ij}^{(n)}$ based on the 3 s-rule, is less than 0.05 [33]. Let $B_1, B_2, \ldots$ be a sequence of events that may arise in a random experiment E, $\lim_{n\to\infty} p(B_k) = p^*$, $h_{n_1}(B_1), h_{n_2}(B_2), \ldots$ be a sequence of relative frequencies of the events $B_1, B_2, \ldots$, respectively, and $\frac{k}{n_k} \to 0$ as $k \to \infty$. We shall call an experiment E a *strong random experiment* if $h_{n_k}(B_k) \to p^*$ as $k \to \infty$. In a strong random experiment the asymptotical significance level of the Wilson confidence interval I_n as $g = 3$ is less than 0.05. The test for the null hypothesis $F_1 = F_2$ with a significance level, which is less that 0.05, is following: if I_n contains 0.95, the null hypothesis is accepted, else the null hypothesis is rejected.

3 Homogeneity Measure for Samples with Ties

Unfortunately, the main assumption used in the test based on p-statistics is that the distributions F_1 and F_2 are absolutely continuous, i.e. the sample must not contain any repetitions. Therefore, it is necessary to extend the above ideas to samples with repetitions, i.e. *ties*.

Consider the sample $u = (u_1, u_2, \ldots, u_n)$ from distribution F obtained in a strong random experiment. A *tie* is a sample value u_k that has duplicates. *Multiplicity* $t(u_k)$ is the number of duplicates u_k in u. If a joint distribution function is absolutely continuous and there are no duplicates in a sample, then the probability of the tie in the sample is equal to zero. In practice, we obtain sample values as the result of measuring a quantitative features. The measurements have a restricted accuracy, so a sample may contain ties. We propose a modification of p-statistics that could be used to estimate homogeneity of samples containing ties.

Consider a sample $u = (u_1, u_2, \ldots, u_n)$ drawn from a population G with a distribution function that is absolutely continuous. If the sample values u_k are measured absolutely precisely we shall call the sample $u = (u_1, u_2, \ldots, u_n)$ *hypothetical*. If the sample values $\tilde{u}_k \in \tilde{u}$ are approximations of the elements of the hypothetical sample u, we shall call the sample $\tilde{u} = (\tilde{u}_1, \tilde{u}_2, \ldots, \tilde{u}_n)$ *empirical*. Population $\tilde{G}$ we shall call an *empirical population corresponding to G*. As a rule, real empirical samples contain ties.

Denote as P_α the flooring of a value:

$$|P(u) - u| \leq 10^{-\alpha} = \Delta$$

Let $u_{(1)} < u_{(2)} < \cdots < u_{(n)}$ and $\tilde{u}_{(1)} < \tilde{u}_{(2)} < \cdots < \tilde{u}_{(n)}$ be variational series corresponding to the hypothetical and empirical samples.

For a sample value u^* that is drawn from G independently from u the following equation holds [30]:

$$p\big(u^* \in [u_{(k)}, u_{(k+1)})\big) = \frac{1}{n+1}, \tag{3}$$

where $k = 0, 1, \ldots, n$, $u_{(0)} = -\infty$, and $u_{(n+1)} = \infty$.

This formula may be extended to empirical samples [34].

Theorem *If the distribution F is differentiable and Lipschitz continuous, i.e.*

$$|F(x) - F(y)| \leq K|x - y|$$

the sample value u^* is independent on u, and the order statistics $\tilde{u}_k = P_\alpha(u_{(i)})$, $k \leq i$ of the empirical sample $\tilde{u} = P_\alpha(u) = (\tilde{u}_1, \tilde{u}_2, \ldots, \tilde{u}_n)$ is a tie with multiplicity $t(\tilde{u}_k)$, then

$$\gamma\left(\tilde{u}_{(k)}\right) + \frac{1}{n+1} - K\Delta \le p\left(\tilde{u}^* \in \left[\tilde{u}_{(k)}, \tilde{u}_{(k+1)}\right)\right) \le \gamma\left(\tilde{u}_{(k)}\right) + \frac{1}{n+1} + K\Delta,$$

where $\tilde{u}^* = P_\alpha(u^*)$, $\tilde{u}_{(k)} = P_\alpha\left(u_{(i)}\right)$, $\gamma\left(\tilde{u}_{(k)}\right) = \frac{t(\tilde{u}_{(k)})-1}{n+1}$, $\lambda = t(\tilde{u}_k) - 1$, $1 \le k \le$
n, and $\Delta = 10^{-\alpha}$.

Corollary *With precision to the rounding error*

$$p\left(\tilde{u}^* \in \left[\tilde{u}_{(k)}, \tilde{u}_{(k+1)}\right)\right) \approx \gamma\left(\tilde{u}_{(k)}\right) + \frac{1}{n+1}. \tag{4}$$

Thus, if $p\left(\tilde{u}^* \in \left[\tilde{u}_{(i)}, \tilde{u}_{(j)}\right)\right)$, $i < j$, and $1 \le i, j \le n$, then

$$p_{ij} = p\left(A_{ij}\right) = p\left(\tilde{u}^* \in \left[\tilde{u}_{(i)}, \tilde{u}_{(j)}\right)\right) \approx \gamma_i + \gamma_{i+1} + \cdots + \gamma_{j-1} + \frac{j-i}{n+1}, \tag{5}$$

where $\gamma_l = \gamma\left(\tilde{u}_{(l)}\right)$, $A_{ij} = \left\{\tilde{u}^* \in \left[\tilde{u}_{(i)}, \tilde{u}_{(j)}\right]\right\}$.

Remark *If* $\tilde{u}_{(l)}$, $i \le l \le j - 1$ *is not a tie, then* $\gamma_l = 0$ *and* (5) *transforms to* (1).

Denote by H the null hypothesis on identity of absolutely continuous distribution functions F_1 и F_2 of populations G_1 and G_2 respectively. Consider $\tilde{u} = (\tilde{u}_1, \ldots, \tilde{u}_n) \in G_1$ and $\tilde{u}' = \left(\tilde{u}'_1, \ldots, \tilde{u}'_n\right) \in \tilde{G}_2$, and let $\tilde{u}_{(1)} \le \cdots \le \tilde{u}_{(n)}$, $\tilde{u}'_{(1)} \le \cdots \le \tilde{u}'_{(n)}$ be their variance series, where $\tilde{G}_1$ and $\tilde{G}_2$ are the empirical populations corresponding to G_1 and G_2. Suppose that $F_1 = F_2$ and denote by $A_{ij}^{(k)}$ $k = 1, 2, \ldots, n$ the random event $\left\{\tilde{u}'_k \in \left(\tilde{u}_{(i)}, \tilde{u}'_{(j)}\right)\right\}$. If $F_1 = F_2$ then the probability of $A_{ij}^{(k)}$ is equal to (5). Construct $I_{ij}^{(n)} = \left(p_{ij}^{(1)}, p_{ij}^{(2)}\right)$ as a Wilson confidence interval (1) for the unknown probability of the event $A_{ij}^{(k)}$. Denote by $N = (n-1)n/2$ the number of all possible confidence intervals $I_{ij}^{(n)} = \left(p_{ij}^{(1)}, p_{ij}^{(2)}\right)$, by B an event $\left\{p_{ij} = \frac{j-i}{n+1} \in I_{ij}^{(n)}\right\}$ and by $L = \#B$. Put $h^{(n)} = \frac{L}{N}$. Since $h^{(n)}$ is a relative frequency of B, then, for $h_{ij}^{(n)} = h^{(n)}$, $n = N$ and $g = 3$, using (1) we obtain the confidence interval $I^{(n)} = \left(p^{(1)}, p^{(2)}\right)$ for the probability $p(B) = 1 - \beta$. The statistics $h^{(n)}$ is called *empirical p-statistics*. It estimates the homogeneity of samples $\tilde{u}$ and $\tilde{u}'$.

4 Experiments and Results

Let us divide the time series in portions of size n and consider two windows of lengths n:

$$\underbrace{x_1, x_2, \ldots x_n}_{window1}, \underbrace{x_{n+1}, \ldots, x_{2n}}_{window2}$$

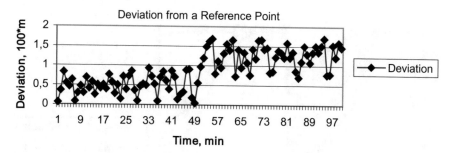

Fig. 1 Random deviation of data from a reference point (1–50 min—in a range of 100 m, 51–100—there is suspicion o violation of self-isolation)

In this experiment we use samples generated with the given distribution. If the samples $x_1, x_2, \ldots, x_n$ and $x_{n+1}, x_2, \ldots, x_{2n}$ are heterogeneous, i.e. they have different distributions, then the point x_{n+1} is a change point, that is a tracked date deviate from the reference point significantly (Fig. 1). The windows must have equal sizes but may have different starting points. As an initial point we selected two windows with the same left end, let one window be fixed and the second window be moving with the step l (for example, $l = 1$) overlapping with the first window. As a variant, we can consider adjacent non-overlapping windows also.

Hereinafter $N(m, v)$ is a normal distribution, where m is the expected value and v is the variance, $LN(m, v)$ is a lognormal distribution, where m is the expected value and v is the variance, $U(a, b)$ is the uniform distribution on an interval (a, b), and $G(a, b)$ is a two-parameter gamma distribution. For comparison we selected p-statistics and wide-used Kolmogorov–Smirnov statistics. The width of sliding window is equal to 40 (due to the requirement that the significance level of Klyushin-Petunin test must be less than 0.05). The sliding step is equal to 1. The averaging was made on 10 experiments. The results demonstrate the high effectiveness of the proposed method (see Figs. 2, 3, 4 and 5).

Here, we selected the distribution parameters such that to demonstrate the deviation of the expected values of the samples from the reference point, but the same experiments may be conducted with the same means and various standard deviation. As was shown in [33] the p-statistics has great advantage in these cases.

As we see, the curves of p-statistics and the Kolmogorov–Smirnov statistics decrease from the left upper corner (corresponding to the same samples which imply the high homogeneity measure) toward right lower corner (corresponding to the very different samples which implies the low homogeneity measure). The sensitiveness is estimated by the slope of these curves (the more steep curve means the more sensitive homogeneity measure). The monotonicity is estimated visually.

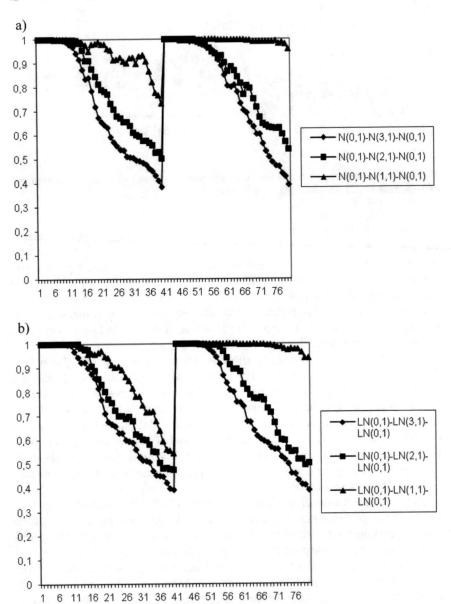

Fig. 2 P-statistics for **a** normal and **b** lognormal distribution functions

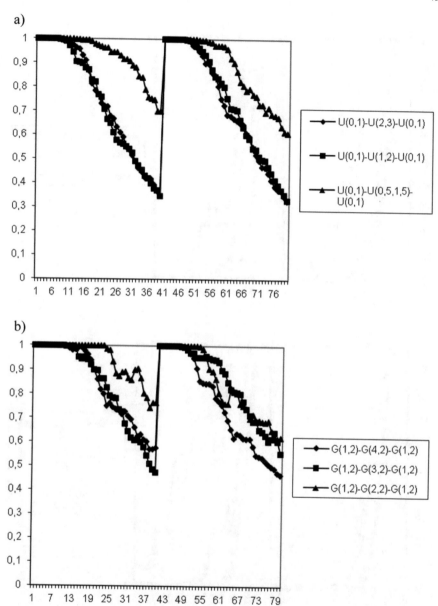

Fig. 3 P-statistics for **a** uniform and **b** gamma distribution functions

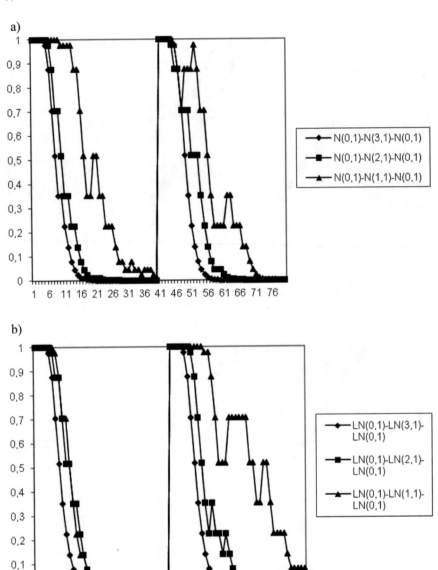

Fig. 4 *P*-value of the Kolmogorov–Smirnov test for **a** normal and **b** lognormal distribution functions

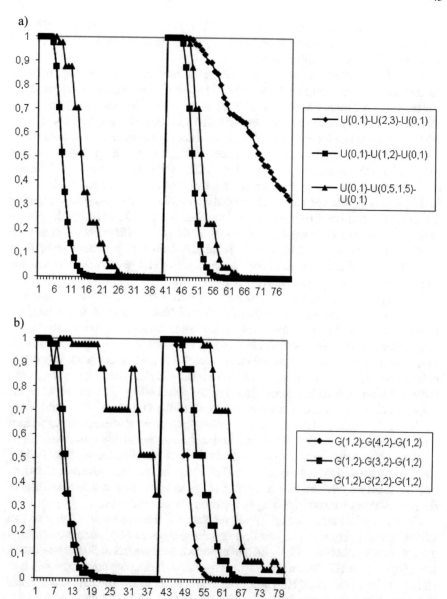

Fig. 5 *P*-value of the Kolmogorov–Smirnov test for **a** uniform and **b** gamma distribution functions

The results show that the *p*-statistics is monotonic, sensitive, and robust homogeneity measure. Since the step of sliding window is equal to 1, at every time step the first sample becomes more "contaminated" by the sample values of the second sample. Thus, we handle the variants with different degrees of overlapping between samples: from total coinciding to disjoining. As we see, in many variants of distributions the Kolmogorov–Smirnov statistics as opposed to the p-statistics demonstrate non-monotonic and nor-robust behavior.

There is one more method to estimate the sensitiveness of the test statistics. Remember, that the null hypothesis about identity of distribution functions in the Kolmogorov–Smirnov test is rejected if the Kolmogorov–Smirnov statistics is less than 0.05. Vice versa, in the Klyushin–Petunin test the null hypothesis is rejected when the confidence interval for the p-statistics does not contain 0.95. As we see on Fig. 2 and Fig. 4 (shifted normal and log-normal distributions), the p-statistics rejects the null hypothesis starting from the half point, while the Kolmogorov–Smirnov statistics rejects the null hypothesis starting from the one quarter point. Therefore, in the cases of shifted normal and lognormal distributions the Kolmogorov–Smirnov test is more sensitive. From the other side, Figs. 3 and 5 demonstrate the advantage of the p-statistics in the case when distributions are different but significantly overlapping. As previously, the p-statistics rejects the null hypothesis starting from the half point but in the cases of overlapped uniform and gamma distributions the Kolmogorov–Smirnov test cannot distinguish them.

We may conclude that the Kolmogorov–Smirnov statistics is more preferable when the distributions are shifted (i.e. they have different expected values) and the p-statistics in useful in the same cases but overcome the Kolmogorov–Smirnov test in the cases when the distributions have significant overlapping (for example, normal distributions with the same expected values and different variances or uniform distributions on overlapping intervals). It may be explained by the different nature of these statistical tests. The Kolmogorov–Smirnov test detects the difference between the empirical distributions functions and is more sensitive to shifts of distributions and outliers. Instead, the p-statistics uses the information on permutations and can detect both shifting and changes of the shapes of distributions remaining robust to outliers.

Next, let us consider two quasi-real experiments imitation the deviation of the tracked object from the reference point. Obviously, the real experiment requires real data but there are private and inaccessible, so we just demonstrate the capabilities of the proposed test for solving such problems on the artificial data.

Case 1 is illustrated by Fig. 1. We simulate the time series consisting of two slightly overlapping samples: the first sample consists of 50 random values from the uniform distribution $U(0,1)$ and the second sample consists of 50 random values from $U(0,1)$ plus 0.7. We compare two consecutive sliding windows. The width of sliding window is equal to 10. The sliding step is equal to 10. The largest difference is expected between 5th and 6th segments (5th row of Table 1). Indeed, in this case we obtain the minimal value of p-statistics (0.8444) and according to the Klyushin–Petunin test [33] the null hypothesis on homogeneity of the sample is rejected because the confidence interval for the p-statistics does not contain 0.95). The Kolmogorov–Smirnov test demonstrates the over-conservativeness. According to its p-value the null hypothesis is rejected in the first, second, fourth, sixth and eights cases besides that by assumption first five segment and the second five segments were drawn from

Table 1 Empirical p-statistics (h) and its left (hl) and rights (hu) confidence bounds, p-statistics without ties (ro) and its left (ro_l) and right (ro_u) confidence bounds, the Kolmogorov–Smirnov statistics (ro_ks) and its p-value in Case 1

h	h_l	h_u	ro_p	ro_l	ro_u	ro_ks	p-value
0.9778	0.7983	0.998	0.9778	0.7983	0.998	0	0
0.9111	0.7077	0.9775	0.9111	0.7077	0.9775	0.1	2e-005
0.8889	0.6803	0.9678	0.8889	0.6803	0.9678	0.5	0.112
0.9333	0.7363	0.986	0.9333	0.7363	0.986	0.3	0.00556
0.8444	0.6283	0.9457	0.8444	0.6283	0.9457	0	0
1	0.8333	1	1	0.8333	1	0.4	0.03008
0.9778	0.7983	0.998	0.9778	0.7983	0.998	0.5	0.112
0.9556	0.7663	0.993	0.9556	0.7663	0.993	0.7	0.664
1	0.8333	1	1	0.8333	1	0.4	0.03008

the same distributions respectively. It may be explained by that the Kolmogorov–Smirnov test based in the difference between the empirical distributions functions and is very sensitive to outliers.

In order to demonstrate the difference between empirical p-statistics and original p-statistics let us consider the case for samples rounded up to two decimal digits.

As we see, the original p-statistics overestimate the homogeneity of the rounded samples (see Table 2). The Kolmogorov–Smirnov statistics demonstrate the same properties as in Case 1. But these results may be explained by the small size of samples. Thus, we must consider the case with more large samples.

In Case 2 we simulate the time series consisting of ten alternating samples: the odd samples consist of 50 random values from the uniform distribution $U(0,1)$ and the even samples consist of 50 random values from $U(0,1)$ plus 0.7. Now the width of sliding window is equal to 50 and the sliding step is equal to 50.

Table 2 Empirical p-statistics (h) and its left (hl) and rights (hu) confidence bounds, p-statistics without ties (ro) and its left (ro_l) and right (ro_u) confidence bounds, the Kolmogorov–Smirnov statistics (ro_ks) and its p-value for rounded Case 1

h	h_l	h_u	ro_p	ro_l	ro_u	ro_ks	p-value
1	0.8333	1	0.9778	0.7983	0.998	0.2	0.00064
1	0.8333	1	1	0.8333	1	0.2	0.00064
0.9778	0.7983	0.998	0.9556	0.7663	0.993	0.6	0.3088
1	0.8333	1	1	0.8333	1	0.1	2e−005
0.9111	0.7077	0.9775	0.9111	0.7077	0.9775	0.3	0.00556
1	0.8333	1	1	0.8333	1	0.3	0.00556
0.7778	0.5556	0.9074	1	0.8333	1	0.6	0.3088
1	0.8333	1	1	0.8333	1	0.7	0.664
1	0.8333	1	1	0.8333	1	0.3	0.00556

Table 3 Empirical p-statistics (h) and its left (hl) and rights (hu) confidence bounds, p-statistics without ties (ro) and its left (ro_l) and right (ro_u) confidence bounds, the Kolmogorov–Smirnov statistics (ro_ks) and its p-value for Case 2

h	h_l	h_u	ro_p	ro_l	ro_u	ro_ks	p-value
0.4082	0.3669	0.4508	0.4082	0.3669	0.4508	0.1	0
0.4612	0.4189	0.5041	0.4612	0.4189	0.5041	0.32	0
0.4204	0.3788	0.4631	0.4204	0.3788	0.4631	0.24	0
0.3902	0.3493	0.4327	0.3902	0.3493	0.4327	0.24	0
0.4114	0.37	0.4541	0.4114	0.37	0.4541	0.1	0
0.422	0.3804	0.4648	0.422	0.3804	0.4648	0	0
0.4751	0.4326	0.5179	0.4751	0.4326	0.5179	0.1	0
0.3494	0.3098	0.3912	0.3494	0.3098	0.3912	0	0
0.3665	0.3263	0.4087	0.3665	0.3263	0.4087	0.2	0

As we see in Table 3, all statistics demonstrate the stable results. All pairs of segments are recognized as heterogeneous. Therefore, as a practical recommendation we may state that the sample size must exceed 40.

5   Conclusions and Future Work

The new online algorithm implementing the Klyushin–Petunin test on streaming geolocation data is effective, sensitive, and robust. It does not depend on assumptions about distributions of samples and equally sensitive to difference between expected values (location hypothesis) and shapes of the distributions (scale hypothesis). Its significance level is less that 0.05. It does not require the special conditions for saving the data. The algorithm effectively solve the change-point and is more sensitive than alternative Kolmogorov–Smirnov when the size sample is small (less that 40).

The experiments with samples from normal, lognormal, uniform, and gamma distribution with parameters describing different degrees of overlapping shows that p-statistics is more stable, sensitive and monotonic than Kolmogorov–Smirnov statistics. The Kolmogorov–Smirnov statistics demonstrates non-monotonic behavior due to the sensitiveness to outliers.

The Kolmogorov–Smirnov statistics allow to detect the change-point in data stream, but the p-statistics has better accuracy and robustness, because it is very effective both for shifted samples drawn from the distributions with different means and for samples with large overlapping. The main feature of the p-statistics is the monotonicity depending on the degree of overlapping between the samples (the more overlapping the more p-statistics, and vice versa) and a sharp jump at the change-point.

The future scope of the work is to apply the test to real data obtained during COVID-19 pandemic, decrease its computational complexity, and extend it to multivariate time series.

References

1. Fong, S.J., Li, D., Dey, N., Crespo, R.G., Herrera-Viedma, E.: Composite Monte Carlo decision making under high uncertainty of novel coronavirus epidemic using hybridized deep learning and fuzzy rule induction. Appl. Soft Comput. 106282 (2020)
2. Elghamrawy, S.M., Hassanien, A.E.: Diagnosis and prediction model for COVID19 patients response to treatment based on convolutional neural networks and whale optimization algorithm using CT image. medRxiv 2020.04.16.20063990; (2020). https://doi.org/10.1101/2020.04.16.20063990
3. Fong, S.J., Li, D., Dey, N., Crespo, R.G., Herrera-Viedma, E.: Finding an accurate early forecasting model from small dataset: a case of 2019-ncov novel coronavirus outbreak. Int. J. Interact. Multimedia Artif. Intell. 6(1), 132–140 (2020). https://doi.org/10.9781/ijimai.2020.02.002
4. Elmousalami, H.H., Hassanien, A.E.: Day level forecasting for coronavirus disease (COVID-19) spread: analysis, modeling and recommendations. arXiv preprint arXiv:2003.07778 (2020)
5. Rajinikanth, V., Dey, N., Raj, A.N.J., Hassanien, A.E., Santosh, K.C., Sri Madhava Raja, N.: Harmony-search and otsu based system for coronavirus disease (COVID-19) detection using lung CT scan images. arXiv preprint arXiv:2004.03431 (2020)
6. Shao, X., Zhang, X.: Testing for change points in time series. J. Am. Stat. Assoc. 105(491), 1228–1240 (2010). https://doi.org/10.1198/jasa.2010.tm10103
7. Tran, D., Gaber, M.M., Sattler, K.: Change detection in streaming data in the era of big data: models and issues. SIGKDD Explorations 16, 30–38 (2014)
8. Zhang, W., James, N.A., Matteson, D.S.: Pruning and nonparametric multiple change point detection. In: 2017 IEEE international conference on data mining workshops (ICDMW), New Orleans, LA, pp. 288–295 (2017)
9. Padilla, O.H.M., Athey, A., Reinhart, A., Scott, J.G.: Sequential nonparametric tests for a change in distribution: an application to detecting radiological anomalies. J. Am Statist. Assoc. 114(526), 514–528 (2019). https://doi.org/10.1080/01621459.2018.1476245
10. Padilla, O.H.M., Yu, Y., Wang, D., Rinaldo, A.: Optimal nonparametric change point detection and localization. arXiv preprint arXiv:1905.10019 (2019)
11. Smirnov, N.V.: Estimate of difference between empirical distribution curves in two independent samples. Byull Mosk Gos Univ. 2(2), 3–14 (1939)
12. Smirnov, N.V.: On the deviations of an empirical distribution curve. Mat. Sb 6(1), 3–26 (1939)
13. Dixon, W.G.: A criterion for testing the hypothesis that two samples are from the same population. Ann. Math. Stat. 11, 199–204 (1940)
14. Wald, A., Wolfowitz, J.: On a test whether two samples ate from the same population. Ann. Math. Stat. 11, 147–162 (1940)
15. Mathisen, H.C.: A method of testing the hypothesis that two samples are from the same population. Ann. Math. Stat. 14, 188–194 (1943)
16. Wilcoxon, F.: Individual comparisons by ranking methods. Biometrika 1, 80–83 (1945)
17. Mann, H.B., Whitney, D.R.: On a test of whether one of the random variables is stochastically larger than other. Ann. Math. Stat. 18, 50–60 (1947)
18. Wilks, S.S.: A combinatorial test for the problem of two samples from continuous distributions. Proc. Fourth Berkeley Symp. Math. Stat. Prob. 1, 707–717 (1961)
19. Pitman, E.J.G.: Significance tests which may be applied to samples from any populations. J. Royal Stat. Soc. Ser. A. 4, 119–130 (1937)

20. Lehmann, E.L.: Consistency and unbiasedness of certain nonparametric tests. Ann. Math. Stat. **22**, 165–179 (1947)
21. Rosenblatt, M.: Limit theorems associated with variants of the von Mises statistic. Ann. Math. Stat. **23**, 617–623 (1952)
22. Dwass, M.: Modified randomization tests for nonparametric hypotheses. Ann. Math. Stat. **28**, 181–187 (1957)
23. Fisz, M.: On a result be M. Rosenblatt concerning the Mises-Smirnov Test Ann. Math. Stat. **31**, 427–429 (1960)
24. Barnard, G.A.: Comment on "The spectral analysis of point processes" by M.S. Bartlett. J. Royal Stat. Soc. Ser. B **25**, 294 (1963)
25. Birnbaum, Z.W.: Computers and unconventional test-statistics. In: Prochan, F., Serfling, R.J. (eds.) Reliability and Biometry, pp. 441–458. SIAM, Philadelphia, PA (1974)
26. Jockel, K.-H.: Finite sample properties and asymptotic efficiency of Monte Carlo tests. Ann. Stat. **14**, 336–347 (1986)
27. Allen, D.L.: Hypothesis testing using L1-distance bootstrap. Am. Stat. **51**, 145–150 (1997)
28. Efron, B., Tibshirani, R.J.: An Introduction to the Bootstrap. Vol. 57 of Monographs on Statistics and Applied Probability. Chapman-Hall, New York (1993)
29. Dufour, J.-M., Farhat, A.: Exact nonparametric two-sample homogeneity tests for possibly discrete distributions. Center for interuniversity research in quantitative economics (CIREQ). Preprint 2001–23. California Press, pp. 707–717 (2001)
30. Hill, B.M.: Posterior distribution of percentiles: bayes' theorem for sampling from a population. J. Am. Stat. Assoc. **63**, 677–691 (1968)
31. Madreimov, I., Petunin, Yu.I: Characterization of a uniform distribution using order statistics. Teor. Ver. Mat. Statist. **27**, 96–102 (1982)
32. Andrushkiw, R.I., et al.: Construction of the bulk of general population in the case of exchangeable sample values. In: Proceedings of the International Conference of Mathematics and Engineering Techniques in Medicine and Biological Science (METMBS'03), Las Vegas, Nevada, USA, pp 486–489 (2003)
33. Klyushin, D.A., Petunin, Yu.I: A nonparametric test for the equivalence of populations based on a measure of proximity of samples. Ukrainian Math. J. **55**(2), 181–198 (2003)
34. Andrushkiw, R.I., Klyushin, D.A., Petunin, Yu.I.: Proximity measure between samples with repetition factor greater than one. CAMS Research Report: 0708–12, New Jersey Institute of Technology (2008)
35. Klyushin, D.A., Lyashko, S.I., Zub, S.S.: A(n) Assumption in machine learning. In: Computational Linguistics and Intelligent Systems, Lviv: Lviv Politechnic Publishing House, 2019. Vol 2: Proceedings of the 3nd International Conference, COLINS 2019, Workshop, Kharkiv, Ukraine, April 18–19, pp. 32–38 (2019)
36. Matveichuk, S.A., Petunin, Yu.I: Generalization of Bernoulli schemes that arise in order statistics. I. Ukrainian Math. J. **42**(4), 459–466 (1990)
37. Matveichuk, S.A., Petunin, Yu.I: Generalization of Bernoulli schemes that arise in order statistics II. Ukrainian Math. J. **43**(6), 728–734 (1991)
38. Johnson, N., Kotz, S.: Some generalizations of Bernoulli and Polya-Eggenberger contagion models. Statist. Paper **32**, 1–17 (1991)

Visualization and Prediction of Trends of Covid-19 Pandemic During Early Outbreak in India Using DNN and SVR

Mahua Nandy Pal, Shuvankar Roy, Supriya Kundu, and Sasmita Subhadarsinee Choudhury

Abstract First known case of Covid-19 was found out in Wuhan, China in December, 2019. The virus itself is a novel virus, its harshness is unpredictable, its transmission ability is extremely powerful and its incubation period is compara-tively larger. Covid-19 pandemic affected world health and socio-economy severely. So, it is required to know earlier whether the condition is continuing to get worse or how to scale up medical facilities like tracing, testing, treatment, quarantine etc. to fight against it. Early outbreak data for Novel Corona virus attack in India has been considered for this work. The trend of confirmed cases, recovery cases and deceased cases using deep neural network (DNN) and support vector regression (SVR) using Gaussian and exponential kernel functions are modeled. A comparative view of the prediction analysis is also considered.

Keywords DNN · Leaky ReLu · SVR · Exponential kernel · Gaussian kernel

1 Introduction

COVID-19 is essentially a severe acute respiratory syndrome virus with its origin in the Wuhan Province of China. At the end of 2019, the novel corona virus was identified as the origin of a number of pneumonia cases in Wuhan. Initially it was

M. N. Pal (✉) · S. Roy · S. Kundu · S. S. Choudhury
Computer Science and Engineering Department, MCKV Institute of Engineering, 243, G.T. Road (N), Howrah 711204, India
e-mail: mahua.nandy@gmail.com

S. Roy
e-mail: shuvankarroy2@gmail.com

S. Kundu
e-mail: supriya.kundu.1999@gmail.com

S. S. Choudhury
e-mail: sasmitachoudhury74@gmail.com

© The Editor(s) (if applicable) and The Author(s), under exclusive license to Springer Nature Switzerland AG 2020
A.-E. Hassanien et al. (eds.), *Big Data Analytics and Artificial Intelligence Against COVID-19: Innovation Vision and Approach*, Studies in Big Data 78, https://doi.org/10.1007/978-3-030-55258-9_4

51

considered as an epidemic throughout China but later a number of cases throughout the world appeared. Thousands of people were suffering seriously from COVID-19, and the curse began to grow exponentially in different places worldwide. In February 2020 World Health Organization (WHO) declared Corona Virus as a pandemic with its spread in more than 168 countries in the world. The situation has been devastating since then with increasing number of deaths in countries like Italy, Spain, USA etc. with world class medical facilities. In India the number of infected cases has crossed 3000 at the time of writing this article. The Virus do not have any proper medicine or vaccination till date and in order to reduce the spread of COVID-19, The Government of India had declared entire country under complete lockdown excluding the essential services in order to combat this deadly Virus. The coronavirus causes a range of symptoms such as pneumonia, fever, inhalation difficulty, and lung contamination. These viruses are common in animals worldwide, but very few cases had been known to affect humans before its outbreak in late 2019. WHO renamed it as novel coronavirus that affected the lower respiratory tract of people with pneumonia in Wuhan, China on 29th December of 2019. WHO mentioned the disease as coronavirus disease (COVID-19).Infection preventive and control (IPC) measures that may reduce the risk of exposure include the following: use of face masks; covering coughs and sneezes with tissues that are then safely disposed of; regular hand washing with soap or disinfection with hand sanitizer containing at least 60% alcohol (if soap and water are not available); avoidance of contact with infected people and maintaining an appropriate distance as much as possible; and refraining from touching eyes, nose, and mouth with unwashed hands.

Researchers are currently deficient of adequate data to predict the rapid growth trend of this pandemic using machine learning tools. But predicting enables us in understanding possible consequences which may affect enormously the socio-economical growth. Visualizing and forecasting the pandemic behavior with AI tools and data analysis enable us to prevent heavier health crisis and socio-economic devastation. This may be considered as the motivation of this work.

As per the knowledge no works have been published yet which either represents SVR analysis of Covid-19 data or DNN model trained on growth values of available data. The contribution of the work is that with minimal training samples quite encouraging prediction results have been achieved. The DNN model we proposed here is a simple model which takes less training time and is less prone to overfitting.

Following sections are arranged as follows. Section 2 represents literature survey, Sect. 3 discusses deep neural network architecture and support vector regression, Sect. 4 is dataset description, Sect. 5 is the representation of the early outbreak scenario of India with respect to the World at that time. Sections 6 and 7 are the representations and predictions using DNN and SVR models, Sect. 8 is error computation and Sect. 9 is discussion about the work. Section 10 concludes the chapter.

2 Literature Survey

A meeting of WHO Emergency Committee under the International Health Regulations (IHR) (2005) [1] about the epidemic of novel coronavirus 2019 in China, took place on 30th January, 20. According to them, China rapidly recognized the virus and shared its sequence; hence, other countries could diagnose it to save themselves. According to the mathematical model proposed in the research paper in The Lancet [2], the growth of epidemic spreading rate will decrease down if the transmission rate of the communicable infections diminished to 0.25. A composite Monte-Carlo model (CMCM) is projected in [3] which supports future predictions using non-deterministic data distributions from a deterministic model. Some factors are non-deterministic and contribute to high uncertainty such as gathering of people and some factors are deterministic such as historical data. They claimed that these characteristics are characterized most effectively in probabilistic distribution as non-deterministic variables to the MC model. Second, the sensitivity values obtained from the MC simulation is utilized as remedial feedback to the rules that are produced from a fuzzy rule induction (FRI) system. According to [4], with limited training samples, finding a forecasting model is a huge challenge in the field of machine learning. For this, three generally used methods have been used in the past, (1) augmenting the existing data, (2) using a panel selection to pick the most efficient model from several models, and (3) fine-tuning the parameters of an individual model for maximum achievable accuracy. A methodology that holds these data mining strategies is proposed in [4]. Reference [5] suggests AI-driven tools to forecast the nature of spread of COVID-19 outbreaks. AI driven tools are likely to have active learning-based cross-population train/test models that utilize multitudinal and multi-modal data. The recent trend is to explore the utilization of deep learning architecture in different fields of research. References [6, 7] is a representation of application of deep convolutional neural network. Reference [8] is a reference which represents a well-established CNN architecture capable of extracting features in biomedical applications. In general, deep learning techniques require large amount of training data. They are extremely computationally exhaustive and the training phase is very time consuming with expensive GPUs. Covid-19 patient response to treatment based on Convolutional Neural Networks and Whale Optimization has been discussed in [9]. Detection of affected images from lung CT scan images is presented in [10].

3 Preliminaries

3.1 Deep Neural Network (DNN)

Artificial neural networks having multiple number of layers is called deep neural network. A fully connected (FC) neural network layer is said to be a dense layer. It accepts the input from each of the previous units and produces outputs for all the

Table 1 DNN architecture

Layer	(Type)	Output shape	Param#
Input_1	(Input layer)	[(None), 1]	0
Dense_l1	(Dense)	(None, 160)	320
LRelu_l1	(Leaky ReLu)	(None, 160)	0
Dense_l2	(Dense)	(None, 320)	51,520
LRelu_l2	(Leaky ReLu)	(None, 320)	0
Dense_l3	(Dense)	(None, 160)	51,360
LRelu_l3	(Leaky ReLu)	(None, 160)	0
Dense_l4	(Dense)	(None, 80)	12880
LRelu_l4	(Leaky ReLu)	(None, 80)	0
Dense_l5	(Dense)	(None, 1)	81
Output	(Leaky ReLu)	(None, 1)	0

Total params: 116,161

Trainable params: 116,161

Non trainable params: 0

output units. Activation function helps in learning the patterns of characteristic of data. In this model Leaky ReLu has been used as nonlinear activation function which is capable of learning the nonlinear trend of data. It is defined as,

$$f(x) = \max(\alpha x, x) \tag{1}$$

Here α is a hyper parameter set to 0.3.

In this paper, a DNN architecture is proposed, which consists of only four layers of dense and Leaky ReLu. In comparison with different well-established deep architecture, this model is quite light weight with less number of trainable parameters and takes less time to be trained. As a result, the proposed architecture is less prone to over-fitting also. There are 116,161 trainable parameters as a whole. Table 1 represents the model of DNN where layer wise detailed technical architecture of the network is given. Input and output shape mapping is visible properly from Fig. 1.

3.2 Support Vector Regression (SVR)

Support vector machine (SVM) is a popular machine learning tool for classification and regression. Specifying kernel functions allow facilitating higher dimension transformation of input data. In this work, two kernel functions have been explored to implement support vector regressor (SVR). Kernel functions shift data representation to a transformed coordinate system in the higher dimension feature space.

Gaussian kernel is represented by,

Fig. 1 DNN model

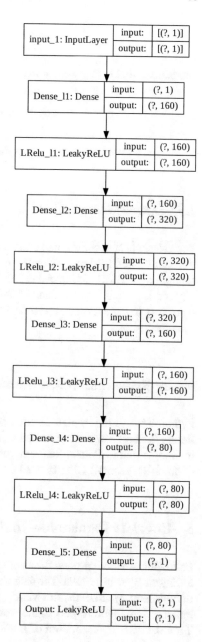

$$k(x, y) = \exp\left(-\frac{||x - y||^2}{2\sigma^2}\right) \tag{2}$$

and exponential is represented by,

$$k(x, y) = \exp\left(-\frac{||x - y||}{2\sigma^2}\right) \tag{3}$$

The parameter σ should be optimized in an application-oriented way.

3.3 Dataset Description

The dataset [11] is contributed and updated on daily basis by Johns Hopkins University Center for Systems Science and Engineering (JHU CSSE). This dataset is supported by ESRI Living Atlas Team and the Johns Hopkins University Applied Physics Lab (JHU APL). Johns Hopkins University is currently using a GitHub repository to store its data. It is in 2019 Novel Coronavirus COVID-19 (2019-nCoV) Data Repository.

4 Implementation Requirements

Python 3.6.8 is the implementation software requirement. Google's deep learning library TensorFlow has been used to implement the work. Code has been executed in Google online Colab cloud environment (Tesla K80 GPU, 12 GB VRAM) with 4* Intel(R) Xeon(R) CPU @ 2.20 GHz, 13.51 GB RAM, 358.27 GB HDD.

5 Covid-19 Pandemic—India with Respect to World

Following are the representations of Covid-19 confirmed cases, deaths and recovery during early stage in India. The data visualization has been considered for the duration of 30th January, 2020 to 30th March, 2020. Figures 2, 3 and 4 are the data representation of India with respect to the world during the same duration and Figs. 5, 6 and 7 are the data representation of India with respect to the most affected countries at that stipulated duration.

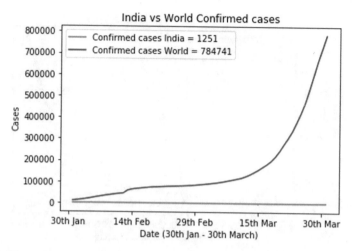

Fig. 2 Confirmed case data visualization during an early outbreak stage of Covid-19 in India with respect to the then world data

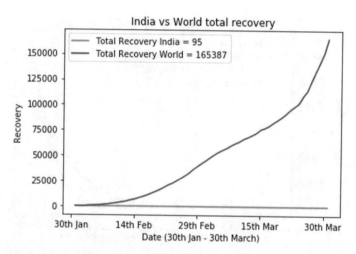

Fig. 3 Recovery data visualization during an early outbreak stage of Covid-19 in India with respect to the then world data

6 Representation and Prediction with DNN Model

The period of early outbreak of covid-19 in India during 30th January to 30th March, 2020 has been considered. DNN was trained with consecutive growth values instead of using the time series data itself. The trained DNN predicts next 15 days confirmed cases, recovery cases and death cases data. Figures 8, 9 and 10 represent DNN training data plots whereas Figs. 11, 12 and 13 represent DNN prediction data plots. Prediction

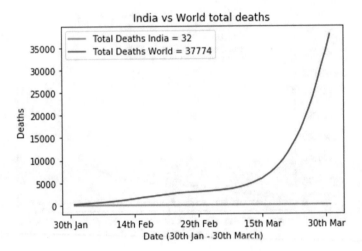

Fig. 4 Death data visualization during an early outbreak stage of Covid-19 in India with respect to the then world data

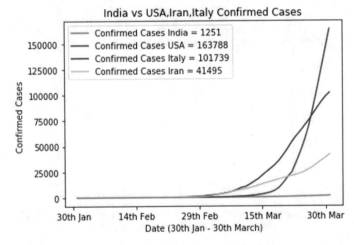

Fig. 5 Confirmed case data visualization during an early outbreak stage of Covid-19 in India with respect to the then most affected countries of the world data

error representation has been done graphically by plotting absolute prediction error as well as by computing the average absolute prediction error percentage (Table 2).

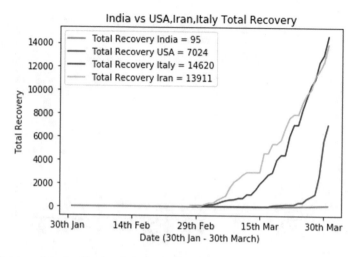

Fig. 6 Recovery data visualization during an early outbreak stage of Covid-19 in India with respect to the then most affected countries of the world data

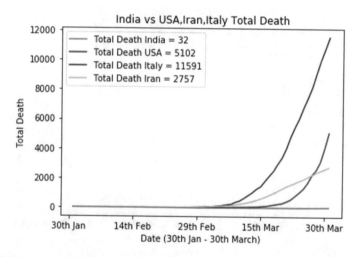

Fig. 7 Death data visualization during an early outbreak stage of Covid-19 in India with respect to the then most affected countries of the world

7 Representation and Prediction with SVR Model

Work experimentation has been done using SVR with Gaussian and exponential kernels. Figures 14, 15 and 16 represent mapping of data up to 30th March, 2020. Figures 17, 18 and 19 are prediction representations of next 15 days respectively (Tables 3, 4 and 5).

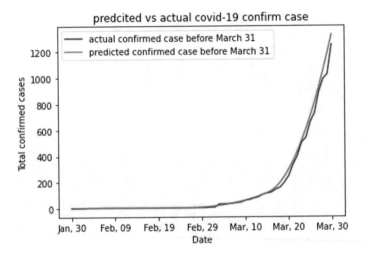

Fig. 8 DNN Confirmed case training data plot

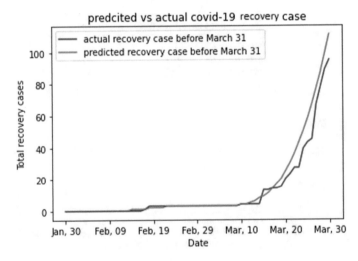

Fig. 9 DNN Recovery case training data plot

8 Error Computation with SVR and DNN Model

Errors incurred by previously discussed three variations of prediction models have been compared. Absolute prediction error (APE) is defined as,

$$APE = |Val_{Pred} - Val_{Obs}| \tag{4}$$

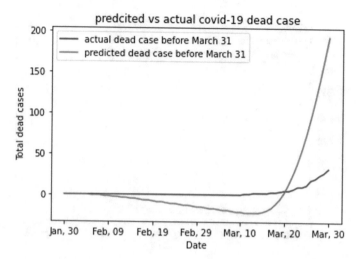

Fig. 10 DNN death case training data plot

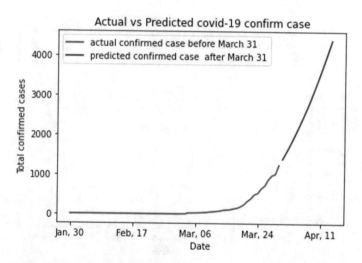

Fig. 11 DNN confirmed case prediction data plot

These comparative error plots are helping in proper visualization of the day wise error trend. These three plots are shown in Fig. 20.

To ascertain the observation from day wise APE plots, average of absolute prediction error percentages (AAPEP) have been computed which is defined as,

$$AAPEP = \frac{\sum_{i=1}^{n}\left(\frac{|Val_{Pred}-Val_{Obs}|}{Val_{Obs}}\right) \times 100}{n} \qquad (5)$$

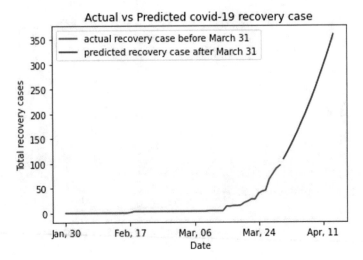

Fig. 12 DNN recovery case prediction data plot

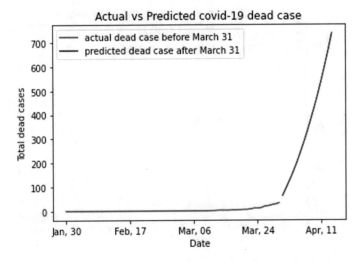

Fig. 13 DNN death case prediction data plot

where n is no. of actual prediction observation.

In Fig. 21, AAPEP values obtained from three models for three different types of data are presented.

Table 2 Actual and predicted cases of Covid-19 for next 15 days by DNN

Date	Actual confirmed cases	DNN prediction-confirmed cases	Actual deceased cases	DNN prediction-deceased cases	Actual recovery cases	DNN prediction-recovery cases
31st Mar, 20	1397	1403	35	108	123	62
1st April, 20	1998	1563	58	121	148	94
2nd April, 20	2543	1732	72	135	191	127
3rd April, 20	2567	1909	72	150	192	162
4th April, 20	3082	2095	86	165	229	200
5th April, 20	3588	2289	99	182	229	241
6th April, 20	4778	2491	136	198	375	284
7th April, 20	5311	2702	150	216	421	330
8th April, 20	5916	2921	178	234	506	378
9th April, 20	6725	3148	226	253	620	430
10th April, 20	7598	3383	246	273	774	484
11th April, 20	8446	3626	288	293	969	542
12th April, 20	9205	3877	331	314	1080	604
13th April, 20	10453	4137	358	336	1181	668
14th April, 20	11487	4405	393	359	1359	737

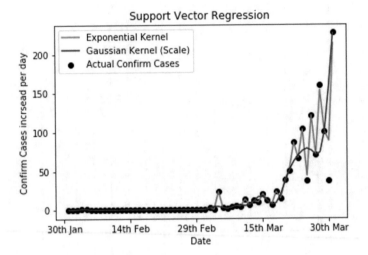

Fig. 14 SVR confirmed case training data plot

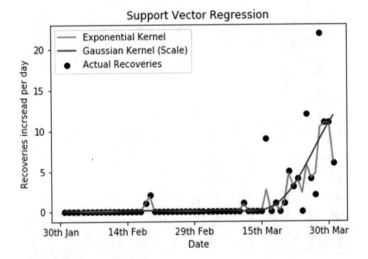

Fig. 15 SVR recovery case training data plot

9   Discussion

The recent Covid-19 pandemic behaviour and its dynamic nature with rapid and wide probability of change in trend are tried to visualize with respect to India in this work. It is very important to forecast as it is associated with threatening of life and social economy. Support vector regression using two different kernel functions and DNN model are used for representation of the growth of available data. Prediction of future data and prediction error is visualized, too, using those models. Average absolute

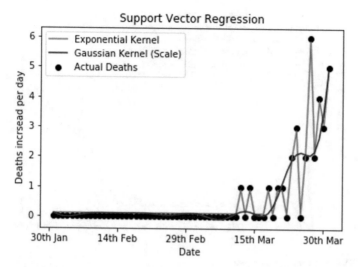

Fig. 16 SVR death case training data plot

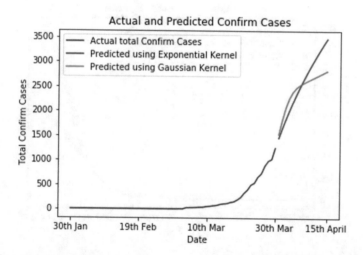

Fig. 17 SVR confirmed case test data plot

prediction error in confirmed case, recovery case and death case prediction for DNN and two models of SVR are as shown in Table 6. DNN is most effective in predicting confirmed cases whereas, Gaussian kernel effectively represents forecasting of death and recovery cases. As per overall observation, we can say that, DNN is the most efficient option among three in forecasting confirmed cases and decreased cases but the model is comparatively less efficient compared to others while predicting recovery cases. Train data availability during the early outburst period in India was not sufficient for learning the trend exactly for a DNN. But it is tried to capture the

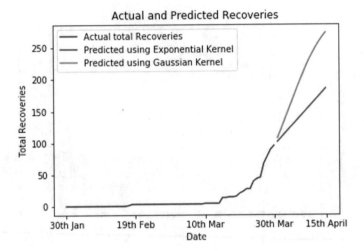

Fig. 18 SVR recovery test data plot

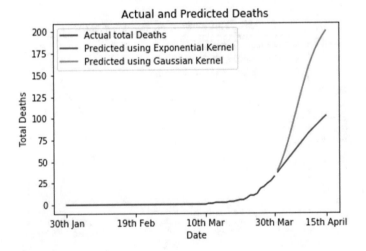

Fig. 19 SVR death test data plot

trend by executing training of DNN on growth data, which is least available in case of death data during the period considered. This is the reason why the model failed to learn the death trend properly and the error percentage is high in death case. This may be considered as the limitation of the work.

Table 3 Actual and predicted confirmed cases of Covid-19 by SVR using Gaussian and exponential kernel functions

Date	Actual confirmed case	Gaussian kernel prediction	Exponential kernel prediction
31st March, 20	1397	1529	1454
1st April, 20	1998	1816	1646
2nd April, 20	2543	2668	1829
3rd April, 20	2567	2259	2003
4th April, 20	3082	2389	2169
5th April, 20	3588	2473	2327
6th April, 20	4778	2305	2478
7th April, 20	5311	2573	2622
8th April, 20	5916	2610	2759
9th April, 20	6725	2645	2891
10th April, 20	7598	2680	3017
11th April, 20	8446	2715	3138
12th April, 20	9205	2750	3254
13th April, 20	10453	2785	3366
14th April, 20	11487	2820	3473

Table 4 Actual and predicted deceased cases of Covid-19 by SVR using Gaussian and exponential kernel functions

Date	Actual deceased cases	Gaussian kernel prediction	Exponential kernel prediction
31st March, 20	35	39	37
1st April, 20	58	48	42
2nd April, 20	72	59	47
3rd April, 20	72	72	52
4th April, 20	86	86	57
5th April, 20	99	101	62
6th April, 20	136	116	67
7th April, 20	150	131	72
8th April, 20	178	145	77
9th April, 20	226	158	82
10th April, 20	246	169	86
11th April, 20	288	179	90
12th April, 20	331	187	94
13th April, 20	358	194	98
14th April, 20	393	200	102

Table 5 Actual and predicted recovery cases of Covid-19 by SVR using Gaussian and exponential kernel functions

Date	Actual recovery cases	Gaussian kernel prediction	Exponential kernel prediction
31st March, 20	123	107	101
1st April, 20	148	120	107
2nd April, 20	191	134	113
3rd April, 20	192	148	119
4th April, 20	229	162	125
5th April, 20	229	176	131
6th April, 20	375	190	137
7th April, 20	421	203	143
8th April, 20	506	216	149
9th April, 20	620	228	155
10th April, 20	774	239	161
11th April, 20	969	249	167
12th April, 20	1080	258	173
13th April, 20	1181	266	179
14th April, 20	1359	273	185

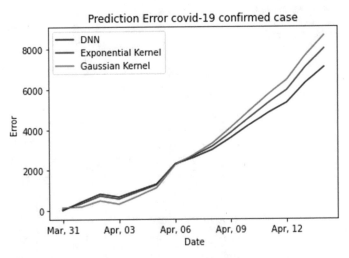

Fig. 20 Absolute prediction error (APE) plots for DNN, support vector regression with Gaussian and exponential kernels

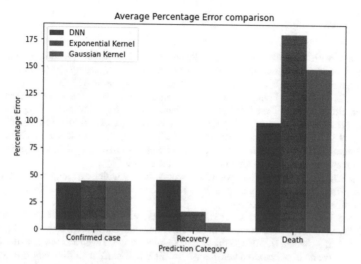

Fig. 21 Average absolute prediction error percentage (AAPEP) plots for DNN, support vector regression with Gaussian and exponential kernels

Table 6 Average APE (absolute prediction error) for three models

Date	Average absolute prediction error		
	Confirmed cases	Recovery cases	Death cases
DNN	42.7506	45.9664	99.3057
SVR (Gaussian)	44.6309	7.1762	7.1762
SVR (exponential)	44.7340	16.7569	16.7569

10 Conclusion and Future Work

Considering general population, at this moment there is no vaccination available for preventing COVID-19. The best prevention to subside this pandemic is to avoid being exposed to the virus. Forecasting its behaviour is necessary to analyze whether it is continuing or getting to be worse day by day or the chain of pandemic outbreak should soon be collapsed. It will be helpful for timely decision making and remedial action.

According to the above analysis DNN prediction performance minimizes error in confirmed cases predictions whereas SVR with Gaussian kernel exhibit minimal error in recovery and death cases prediction. DNN would have performed better if more training samples might be available.

The future scope of this work is to properly analyse the training set representation to the model so that the model learning becomes efficient with limited data available and can frame the trend prediction more powerfully.

References

1. World Health Organization (WHO): Statement on the Second Meeting of the International Health Regulations (2005) Emergency Committee Regarding the Outbreak of Novel Coronavirus (2019-nCoV). 30 January 2020. Geneva, Switzerland (2020)
2. Wu, J.T., Leung, K., Leung, G.M.: Nowcasting and forecasting the potential domestic and international spread of the 2019-nCoV outbreak originating in Wuhan, China: a modelling study, The Lancet (January 31)1–9 (2020). https://doi.org/10.1016/S0140-6736(20)30260-9
3. Fong, S.J., Li, G., Dey, N., Crespo, R.G., Viedma, E.H.: Composite Monte Carlo decision making under high uncertainty of novel coronavirus epidemic using hybridized deep learning and fuzzy rule induction. Appl. Soft Comput. 106282 (2020)
4. Fong, S.J., Li, G., Dey, N., Crespo, R.G., Viedma, E.H.: Finding an accurate early forecasting model from small dataset: a case of 2019-nCoV novel coronavirus outbreak. Int. J. Interact. Multim. Artif. Intell. **6**, 1 (2020)
5. Santosh, K.C.: AI-driven tools for coronavirus outbreak: need of active learning and cross-population train/test models on multitudinal/multimodal data. J. Med. Syst. **44**, 93 (2020)
6. Fu, H., Xu, Y., Wong, D.W.K.: Retinal vessel segmentation via deep learning network and fully connected conditional random fields. In: 2016 IEEE Symposium on Biomedical Imaging
7. Liskowski, P., Krawice, K.: Segmenting retinal blood vessels with deep neural networks. IEEE Trans. Med. Imaging **35**(11), 2369–2380 (2016)
8. Ronneberger, O., Fischer, P., Brox, T.: U-net: convolutional networks for biomedical image segmentation (2015). arXiv:1505.04597 [cs.CV]
9. ELGhamrawy, S.M., Hassanien, A.E.: Diagnosis and prediction model for COVID19 patients response to treatment based on convolutional neural networks and whale optimization algorithm using CT image. medRxiv 2020.04.16.20063990 (2020). https://doi.org/10.1101/2020.04.16.20063990
10. Rajinikanth, V., Dey, N., Joseph Raj, A.N., Hassanien, A.E., Santosh, K.C., Sri Madhava Raja, N.: Harmony-search and Otsu based system for coronavirus disease (COVID-19) detection using lung CT scan images (2020). arXiv preprint arXiv:2004.03431
11. Novel Coronavirus COVID-19 (2019-nCoV) Data Repository by Johns Hopkins CSSE. https://github.com/CSSEGISandData/COVID-19

Diagnosis and Predictions of COVID-19

The Detection of COVID-19 in CT Medical Images: A Deep Learning Approach

Nour Eldeen M. Khalifa, Mohamed Hamed N. Taha, Aboul Ella Hassanien, and Sarah Hamed N. Taha

Abstract The COVID-19 coronavirus is one of the latest viruses that hit the earth in the new century. It was declared as a pandemic by the World Health Organization in 2020. In this chapter, a model for the detection of COVID-19 virus from CT chest medical images will be presented. The proposed model is based on Generative Adversarial Networks (GAN), and a fine-tuned deep transfer learning model. GAN is used to generate more images from the available dataset. While deep transfer models are used to classify the COVID-19 virus from the normal class. The original dataset consists of 746 images. The is divided into two parts; 90% for the training and validation phase, while 10% for the testing phase. The 90% then is divided into 80% percent for the training and 20% percent for the validation after using GAN as image augmenter. The proposed GAN architecture raises the number of images in the training and validation phase to be 10 times larger than the original dataset. The deep transfer models which are selected for experimental trials are Resnet50, Shufflenet, and Mobilenet. They were selected as they include a medium number of layers on their architectures if they are com-pared with large deep transfer models such as DenseNet, and Inception-ResNet. This will reflect on the performance of the proposed model in terms of reducing training time, memory and CPU usage. The

N. E. M. Khalifa (✉) · M. H. N. Taha · A. E. Hassanien
Faculty of Computers and Artificial Intelligence, Cairo University, Giza, Egypt
e-mail: nourmahmoud@cu.edu.eg
URL: http://www.egyptscience.net

M. H. N. Taha
e-mail: mnasrtaha@cu.edu.eg

A. E. Hassanien
e-mail: aboitcairo@cu.edu.eg

S. H. N. Taha
Forensic Medicine and Clinical Toxicology Department, Faculty of Medicine, Cairo University, Giza, Egypt
e-mail: snasrtaha@cu.edu.eg

N. E. M. Khalifa · M. H. N. Taha · A. E. Hassanien
Scientific Research Group in Egypt (SRGE), Giza, Egypt

A.-E. Hassanien et al. (eds.), *Big Data Analytics and Artificial Intelligence Against COVID-19: Innovation Vision and Approach*, Studies in Big Data 78,
https://doi.org/10.1007/978-3-030-55258-9_5

experimental trials show that Shufflenet is selected to be the optimal deep transfer learning in the proposed model as it achieves the highest possible for testing accuracy and performance metrics. Shufflenet achieves an overall testing accuracy with 84.9, and 85.33% in all performance metrics which include recall, precision, and F1 score.

Keywords Coronavirus · COVID-19 CT images · Medical images · Generative adversarial networks · GAN · Deep transfer learning

1   Introduction

The coronavirus disease 2019 (COVID-19) is caused by severe acute respiratory syndrome coronavirus 2 (SARS-CoV-2/2019-nCoV) [1, 2] and is considered one of the newest and most widespread viruses on the earth which was announced in December 2019. In March 2020 the World Health Organization has declared this new virus as a pandemic, meaning that the virus had spread globally and affected the entire world. COVID-19's clinical symptoms range from asymptomatic to acute respiratory distress syndrome and multiorgan dysfunction. The common clinical features of this viral infection are similar to other respiratory infections which makes it indistinguishable. In several patients, the disease can progress pneumonia and respiratory failure [3]. The X-ray on the chest in cases of COVID 19 typically reveals bilateral infiltrations which may be normal in early illness. Computed tomography (CT) is considered a more sensitive and specific imaging tool that can show lung infiltration, ground-glass opacities and subsegmental consolidation in asymptomatic patients and patients with no clinical evidence of lower respiratory tract involvement. In suspicious cases with negative molecular testing, CT scans were used to diagnose COVID-19; most of these patients had positive molecular results on repeated testing [3–5]. Here is the role of Artificial Intelligence and machine learning techniques would help doctors to detect and diagnose COVID 19 accurately and speedily. Over the last decade, various techniques in machine learning were developed and improved rapidly.

These techniques were used to improve the accuracy and time for diagnosis by CAD systems. Artificial intelligence (AI) has made tremendous progress in the area of analysis of medical images. Artificial intelligence including deep-learning systems for medical imaging has been developed especially in the extraction of image characteristics and including shape and spatial relation features.

Learning from a large number of training samples is the most important capability that AI models heavily rely on [6]. Deep learning algorithms achieved impressive and dependable results for computer vision tasks. To achieve high accuracy, huge datasets are needed by these algorithms for training. However, over-fitting is the main concern with deep learning algorithms when they are trained on small datasets, due to generalization lack. This issue is likely to occur with medical images. For supervised learning algorithms, the process of medical image annotation is a time-consuming issue since images would need to be annotated manually by experts [7].

Convolutional Neural Networks have achieved remarkable accuracy and performance in various applications through training on huge-scale annotated training data. Unfortunately, obtaining such huge annotated medical images is challenging. Classical Data Augmentation (DA) techniques such as rotation are geometric/intensity trans-formations of original images for accurate diagnosis [8]. Generative Adversarial Networks learn deep representations from data without the need for annotated training data. Learning is achieved through deriving backpropagation signals through a competitive process involving a pair of networks [9].

In this chapter, a model that is based on Generative Adversarial Networks and fine-tuned deep transfer learning model, is used for the detection of covid-19 from CT chest medical images. GAN is used to increase the number of images in the dataset by generating more images from the available dataset. Deep transfer models are used to differentiate between the COVID-19 virus and the normal class. The remaining of this chapter is organized as follows. In Sect. 2, related work and scope work will be explored. In Sect. 3, an overview of Generative Adversarial Networks and Deep Transfer Learning will be presented. The dataset used in the proposed model is discussed in Sect. 4. In Sect. 5, the proposed model's architecture will be presented while Sect. 6 discusses our outcomes and discussion of the chapter. Finally, Sect. 7 provides conclusions and directions for further research.

2 Related Works

The coronavirus (Covid-19) draws other researchers 'attention to better explore the effects of this infectious disease [2]. One of those ways of investigation is the detection of pneumonia from X-ray chest images. There are numerous datasets for chest X-rays for pneumonia such as [10–12], but in this research, the dataset in [12] has been selected due to the availability of data and the dataset has been used in many research to compare our work with as it will be presented in the next paragraphs.

Saraiva et al. in [13] presented a classification of images of childhood pneumonia using convolutional neural networks. The authors proposed a deep learning model with 7 convolutional layers and 3 dense layers and achieved 95.30% testing accuracy. Liang and Zheng in [14] presented a transfer learning method with a deep residual network for pediatric pneumonia diagnosis. The authors a deep learning model with 49 convolutional layers and 2 dense layers and achieved 96.70% testing accuracy. Wu et al. in [15] presented a model to predict pneumonia with chest X-ray images based on convolutional deep neural learning networks and random forest, the authors achieved 97% testing accuracy.

Loey et al. in [16] proposed Generative Adversarial Networks with deep transfer learning for coronavirus detection in limited chest x-ray images. The lack of benchmark datasets for covid-19 especially in chest x-rays images was the main for authors. The main idea is to collect all the possible images for covid-19 and use the GAN network to generate more images to help in the detection of the virus from the available x-rays images. The authors claim that Googlenet is selected to be the main deep transfer model as it achieves 100% in testing accuracy and 99.9% in the validation accuracy. Although all of the above works have achieved great accuracy in covid-19 classifications based on the patients' x-rays, medical doctors have proven that covid-19 is probably not detected through x-ray images.

Huang et al. [17] used the convolutional neural network architecture of U-Net and trained it on an annotated dataset of COVID-19. A total of 842 patients (all confirmed to have COVID-19) were collected retrospectively for lung opacity segmentation training and testing, who underwent chest CT scans between 10 January 2020 and 25 January 2020 in Tongji Hospital, Wuhan, China.

Jin et al. [18] built an AI system that has can analyze CT images for the detection of COVID-19 pneumonia features. The system was trained on 1136 training cases (723 positives for COVID-19) from five hospitals. The system sensitivity of was 0.974 and the specificity was 0.922 on the test dataset.

Li et al. [19] developed a 3D deep learning framework COVID-19 detection using chest CT. It can extract both 2D local and 3D global representative features. The framework consists of a RestNet50 as the backbone. It takes a series of CT slices as input and generates features for the corresponding slices. The extracted features from all slices are then combined by a max-pooling operation. The final feature map is fed to a fully connected layer and the softmax activation function to generate a probability score for each type (COVID-19, CAP, and non-pneumonia). The framework archived 90% for sensitivity and 96% for Specificity. The collected dataset has about of 4356 chest CT exams for more than 3300 patients.

Sally et al. [20] has proposed Artificial Intelligence-inspired Model for COVID-19 Diagnosis and Prediction for Patient Response to Treatment (AIMDP). The Model has two function, the Diagnosis Module and Prediction Module. The Diagnosis Module is used for detecting the patients with COVID-19, while the Prediction Module is used for predicting the ability of the patient to respond to treatment based on different factors. The authors claim that the proposed model achieved accuracy 97.14%.

3   Generative Adversarial Networks and Deep Transfer Learning

GANs consist of two different types of networks. Those networks are trained simultaneously. The first network is trained on image generation while the other is used for discrimination. GANs are considered a special type of Deep Learning model. According to [21, 22], GANs have the ability and the power to generate reasonable new images from unlabelled or labelled original images with the capability to be used in various life applications.

Academic and industry fields have focused their attention on adversarial training scheme due to its efficiency and effectiveness in the process of new image generation. GANs have made significant improvements and marvelous performance in many applications. These applications include image synthesis, semantic image editing, image super-resolution, style transfer and classification.

3.1 GAN Architecture

The important aspect of GAN is the min-max two-player zero-sum game. In this game, one player takes advantage of the equivalent loss of the other player. Here, the players correspond to different networks of GAN called discriminator and generator. The discriminator denoted as D, the main objective is to determine whether a sample belongs to a real distribution or fake distribution [23]. On the other hand, the generator denoted as G, generates a fake sample of images to deceive the discriminator.

Discriminator generates the probability of a given sample to be a real sample one. A real sample is likely to have a higher probability value. Fake samples are indicated by the near-zero probability value. The generator may have an optimal solution when the discriminator loses its ability to differentiate real and fake samples when the probability value is near to 0.5 [23]. The general architecture of GAN is shown in Fig. 1. A multi-dimensional random sample z is given as an input to the Generator to generate samples [23].

The Generator: The Generator is a neural network that uses random noise Z for image generation. The images generated from the Generator using noise are recorded as G(z). Gaussian noise is considered the input, which is a random point in latent space. During the training process, the parameter of both neural networks G and D are updated iteratively.

The Discriminator: The Discriminator is a neural network that works on determining whether a given image belongs to a real distribution or not. It receives image X as input and produces the output D (x) [24]. The objective function of a two-person minimax game is illustrated in Eq. 1

$$\min_{G} \max_{D} V(D, G) = E_{x \sim P_{data}(x)}\left[\log(d(x))\right] + E_{z \sim p_g(z)}\left[\log(1 - D(G(z)))\right] \quad (1)$$

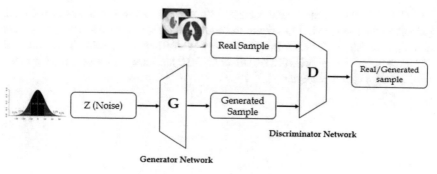

Fig. 1 Graphical representation of the generative adversarial network

The Analysis for time complexity (time performance), any explicit measurements of classification or training time could be a misleading. As the hardware capabilities (CPU, GPU, RAM), in addition to the software libraries (Matlab, Tensorflow) and the size of used dataset may reflect a lot about secondary elements, not on the GAN itself [25]. So the time complexity for GANs could be deceptive due to the large number of parameters that may affect the discrimination and training process.

3.2 Deep Transfer Learning Networks

Deep Learning is considered a branch machine learning that depends on algorithms for data processing and thinking process simulation, or for developing abstractions [26–28]. Deep Learning maps inputs to outputs by using layers of methods to process and analyze hidden patterns in data and visually objects detection [29–31]. Data is passed through each layer of a deep network, with the output of the previous layer providing input for the next layer. The first layer is the input layer in the deep neural network, while the output layer is the final layer in the deep network. All the hidden layers are located between input layers and output layers [26, 32].

Years after, various advances in deep convolutional neural networks further reduced the error rate on the image classification competition tasks. CNN models demonstrated significant improvements in succeeding in the ImageNet Large Scale Visual Recognition Competition (ILSVRC) annual challenges. The Visual Geometry Group at Oxford (VGG) developed the VGG-16 and VGG-19 model for the ILSVRC-2014 competition with a 7.3% Top-5 error rate [33]. The winner of the ILSVRC 2014 competition was GoogleNet with a 6.7% Top-5 error rate [34]. In 2015, Residual Neural Network (ResNet) is the winner ILSVRC 2015 competition with a 3.6% Top-5 error rate [35].

4   Datasets Characteristics

The COVID-19 CT scan images dataset [36] used in this research was created and published by Zhao et al. (https://github.com/UCSD-AI4H/COVID-CT). The dataset contains subfolders for each image category (COVID/NonCOVID). There are 742 CT images and 2 categories (COVID/NonCOVID). Figure 2 presents samples of the used data set in this research.

Fig. 2 Samples of the
COVID-19 CT dataset

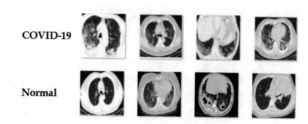

COVID-19

Normal

5 Proposed Model Architecture

The proposed model consists of three main blocks, the first block is responsible for generating a new image from the original data set. The second block is the training and the validation process based on different deep transfer models. The final block is the testing process which calculates the overall testing accuracy with the performance metrics of the proposed model. Figure 3 presents the graphical structure for the proposed model.

In the first block, GAN is used to produce new images that will be used in the second block for the training and the validation. The structure of the proposed GAN architecture is presented in Fig. 4. The proposed GAN architecture consists of three main phases: The first is the generator, the augmentation strategy and the third is the discriminator. The generator network consists of 5 transposed convolutional layers, 4 ReLU layers, 4 batch normalization layers, and Tanh Layer at the end of the model, while the discriminator network consists of 5 convolutional layers, 4 leaky ReLU, and 3 batch normalization layers. All the convolutional and transposed convolutional layers used the same window size of 4*4* pixel. Samples of generated images are presented in Fig. 5.

The second block of the proposed model is the training and the validation process using deep transfer models. Three deep transfer models have been selected for investigation in this research. The three models are Resnet50, Shufflenet, and Mobilenet. Those deep transfer model were selected as the contains a medium number of layers

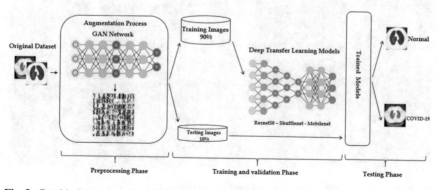

Fig. 3 Graphical representation for the proposed model

Generator Network	Discriminator Network
• Input	• Input
• Transposed Convolution 1	• Convolution 1
• Batch Normalization 1	• Leaky ReLU 1
• ReLU 1	• Convolution 2
• Transposed Convolution 2	• Batch Normalization 2
• Batch Normalization 3	• Leaky ReLU 2
• ReLU 2	• Convolution 3
• Transposed Convolution 3	• Batch Normalization 3
• Batch Normalization 3	• Leaky ReLU 3
• ReLU 3	• Convolution 4
• Transposed Convolution 4	• Batch Normalization 4
• Batch Normalization 4	• Leaky ReLU 4
• ReLU 4	• Convolution 5
• Transposed Convolution 5	
• Tanh	

Fig. 4 GAN proposed architecture

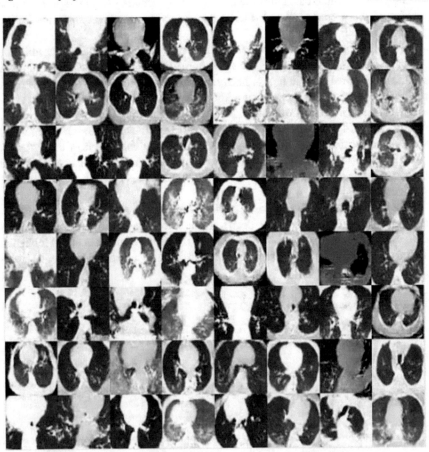

Fig. 5 Samples of GAN generated images for COVID-19 class

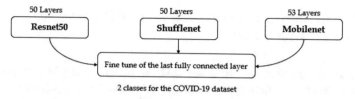

Fig. 6 Selected Deep transfer models with their number of layers

if it is compared with large deep transfer model such as DenseNet [37], and Inception ResNet [38], which consist of 201 and 164 layers. While the selected models only contain 50 layers for Resnet50 [38], 50 layers for Shufflenet [39], and 53 layers for Mobilenet [40] as illustrated in Fig. 6.

The authors of research tried first to build their deep neural networks based on the works presented in [41–43] but the testing accuracy wasn't acceptable. So, the proposed alternative way is to use deep transfer learning models to transfer the learning weights to reduce the training time, mathematical calculations and the consumption of the available hardware resources. This alternative method was adapted in similar research in [44, 45]. The selection of 80% for the training and 20% for validation proved it is efficient in many types of research such as [44, 45].

The selected deep transfer models have been fined tuned in the last fully connected layer to adapt the number of classes in the data set. The number of classes is two (COVID-19, Normal) class.

6 Experimental Results

The proposed model was implemented using a software package (MATLAB). The development was GPU specific. All experiment trials were conducted on a workstation with Intel Core i9 (2 GHz) as a processor and 32 GB of RAM with Titan X GPU. All experiment trials were carried out by dividing the original dataset into two parts. The first part for the training which contains 90% percent of the original dataset while the second part for testing and contains 10% of the original dataset. The 90% percent represents 673 images while 10% represents 73 images from the original dataset.

The 90% percent of the original data was augmented using GAN to be 10 times larger than the original training dataset. The number of images has been raised to 6730 images. The 6730 images were divided into two parts, the first part contains 80% percent of the data which contains 5384 for the training phase. The second part contains 20% percent which contains 1346 for the validation phase. The hyperparameters for the proposed model were set to as following (i) learning rate = 0.001, (ii) mini-batch size: 64, (iii) number of iterations = 30, (iv) early-stopping = 3 epochs, and (v) optimizer: AdaBoost [46].

6.1 Deep Transfer Model's Accuracy and Performance Metrics Without GAN

To measure the effectiveness of using GAN as image augmenters. Experimental trials were conducted directly on the original dataset. Table 1 presents the testing accuracy and performance metrics such as recall, precision, and F1 score [47]. The deep transfer models which are investigated in this research are Resnet50, Shufflenet, and Mobilenet

The testing accuracy and performance metrics which include recall, precision, and F1 score were calculated according to Eqs. (2–5):

$$\text{Testing Accuracy} = \frac{(TN + TP)}{(TN + TP + FN + FP)} \tag{2}$$

$$\text{Precision} = \frac{TP}{(TP + FP)} \tag{3}$$

$$\text{Recall} = \frac{TP}{(TP + FN)} \tag{4}$$

$$\text{F1Score} = 2 * \frac{\text{Precision} * \text{Recall}}{(\text{Precision} + \text{Recall})} \tag{5}$$

where TP is the count of True Positive samples, TN is the count of True Negative samples, FP is the count of False Positive samples, and FN is the count of False Negative samples from a confusion matrix.

Table 1 illustrated that the testing accuracy with other related performance measurements is quite low. The highest accuracy was achieved by Resnet50 and Shufflenet with 80.82%. The performance metrics strengths that Shufflenet achieved better performance measurements than Resnet50. Nevertheless, all the achieved accuracies are quite low. Figure 7 presents the validation accuracy for shufflenet during the training process. The figure reflects that the data is limited to be trained on, as

Table 1 Testing accuracy and performance measurements for deep transfer learning models without GAN

Metric/Model	Resnet50	Shufflenet	Mobilenet
Testing Accuracy	80.82%	80.82%	74.08%
Precision	80.11%	80.78%	74.05%
Recall	80.02%	80.92%	74.92%
F1 Score	80.06%	80.85%	74.48%

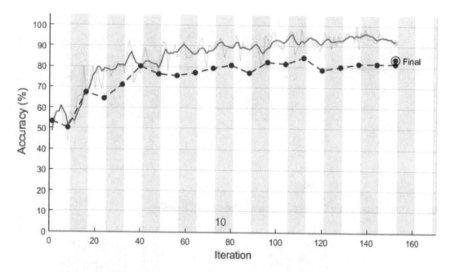

Fig. 7 Validation accuracy progress for the training phase for shufflenet without GAN

the validation accuracy is away below the training accuracy. The need for GAN is mandatory in this case to generate more images.

6.2 Confusion Matrices for Deep Transfer Models with GAN

The confusion matrix illustrates the testing accuracy of every class and the overall testing accuracy for any proposed models. It also helps in deciding the most appropriate deep transfer model that fits the nature of the original dataset. Figures 8, 9, and

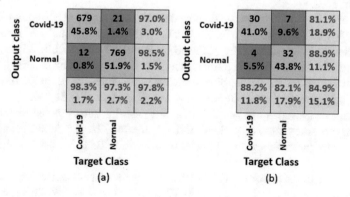

Fig. 8 Confusion matrix for Resnet50 **a** validation, and **b** testing

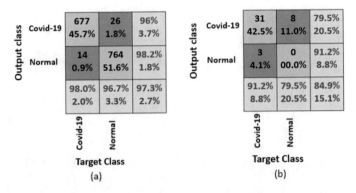

Fig. 9 Confusion matrix for Shufflenet **a** validation, and **b** testing

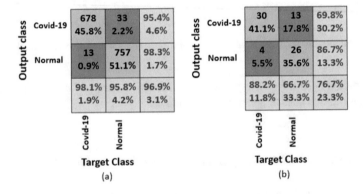

Fig. 10 Confusion matrix for Mobilenet **a** validation, and **b** testing

10 presents the confusion matrices (validation and testing) for Resnet50, Shufflenet, and Mobilenet.

Figures 8, 9, and 10 illustrated that the deep transfer model achieved in validation accuracy 97.8, 97.3, and 96.9% for Resnet50, Shufflenet, and Mobilenet accordingly. The highest validation accuracy achieved by Resnet50 with 97.8%. Moreover, the figures also illustrated that deep transfer models achieved testing accuracy of 84.9, 84.9, and 76.7% for Resnet50, Shufflenet, and Mobilenet accordingly. The highest validation accuracy achieved by Resnet50 and Shufflenet with 84.9%.

Another measurement to test the proposed model accuracy is the measurement of testing accuracy for every class. Table 2 presents the validation accuracy for every class for the different deep transfer models while Table 3 illustrates the testing accuracy.

Table 2 illustrates that on the validation accuracy for every class Resnet50 achieved the highest accuracy possible for Covid-19, and Normal class. While Table 3 illustrates that on the testing accuracy for every class Resnet50 achieved the highest accuracy possible for Covid-19 class with 81.1%. Shufflenet deep transfer model

Table 2 Validation accuracy for every class using different deep transfer models

Accuracy/Model	Resnet50	Shufflenet	Mobilenet
Covid-19	97.0%	96.0%	95.4%
Normal	98.5%	98.2%	98.3%
Total Accuracy	97.8%	97.3%	96.9%

Table 3 Testing accuracy for every class using different deep transfer models

Accuracy/Model	Resnet50	Shufflenet	Mobilenet
Covid-19	81.1%	79.5%	69.3%
Normal	88.9%	91.2%	68.7%
Total Accuracy	84.9%	84.9%	76.7%

achieved the highest accuracy possible for Normal class with 91.2%. As the main target of this research is to detect the Covid-19, so Resent50 will be the optimal model until now. The final decision will be introduced after the investigation of performance metrics in the following subsection. Figure 11 illustrates the progress

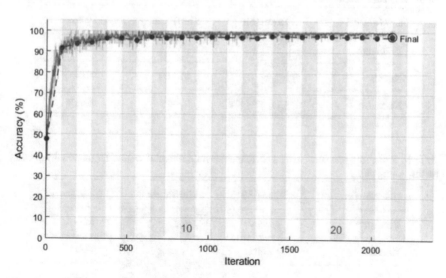

Fig. 11 Validation accuracy progress for the training phase for Shufflenet with GAN

of the validation accuracy for Resent50. Notably, the validation accuracy has been improved when the training was conducted without GAN as presented in Fig. 7.

6.3 Performance Metrics for Deep Transfer Models with GAN

The performance metrics which are investigated in this research are the recall, precision, and F1 score. Table 4 presents the recall, precision, and F1 score metrics for the different deep transfer model using GAN in the validation phase.

Table 4 illustrated that all the deep transfer model achieved competitive results ranging from 96.84 to 98.41% for all the performance metrics in the validation phase. Resent50 achieved the highest percentage in the performance metrics with 98.30% in precision, 98.31% in the recall metric, and 98.30% in the F1 score metric in the validation phase.

Table 5 shows the recall, precision, and F1 score metrics for the different deep transfer model using GAN in the testing phase.

Table 5 illustrates that Resnet50 and Shufflenet achieved a close result in all performance metrics in the testing phase. Shufflenet achieved the highest percentage in the performance metrics with 85.34% on all performance metrics in the testing phase. According to the achieved results in the testing phase for overall testing

Table 4 The recall, precision, and F1 score metrics for different deep transfer models using GAN for the validation phase

Metric/Model	Resnet50	Shufflenet	Mobilenet
Precision	98.30%	97.25%	96.97%
Recall	98.31 %	97.34%	96.84%
F1 Score	98.30 %	97.30%	96.90%

Table 5 The recall, precision, and F1 score metrics for different deep transfer models using GAN for the testing phase

Metric/Model	Resnet50	Shufflenet	Mobilenet
Precision	84.98%	85.33%	78.22%
Recall	85.14%	85.33%	77.45%
F1 Score	85.06%	85.33%	77.83%

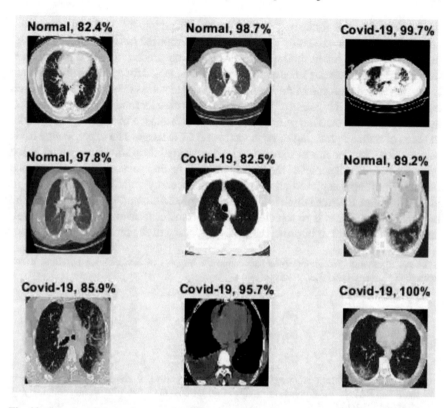

Fig. 12 Samples of testing images with the achieved accuracy

accuracy, accuracy for every class, and the performance metrics Shufflenet is selected to be the optimal deep transfer learning model as it achieved the highest possible testing accuracy and performance metrics. Figure 12 presents samples of testing images with the achieved testing accuracy.

7 Conclusions and Future Works

The COVID-19 coronavirus is one of the latest viruses in the new century. it was declared as a pandemic by the World Health Organization in 2020. In this chapter, a model for the detection of the COVID-19 virus from CT chest medical images is presented. The proposed model was based on Generative Adversarial Networks (GAN), and a fine-tuned deep transfer learning model. GAN has been used to generate more images from the available dataset. While deep transfer models have been used to classify the COVID-19 virus from the normal class. The original data sets consisted of 746 images. The data set has been divided into two parts, 90% for training and validation while 10% for testing. The 90% was divided into 80% percent for training and 20% percent for validation after using GAN. Proposed GAN architecture raised the number of images in the training and validation process to be 10 times larger than the original dataset. The deep transfer models selected for experimental trials are Resnet50, Shufflenet, and Mobilenet. They were selected as they included a medium number of layers if it is compared with a large deep transfer model such as DenseNet, and InceptionResNet. That will reflect on the performance of the proposed model in terms of reducing training time, memory and CPU usage. The experimental trials showed that Shufflenet was selected to be the optimal deep transfer learning in the proposed model as it achieved the highest possible testing accuracy and performance metrics. Shufflenet achieved an overall testing accuracy with 84.9, and 85.33% in all performance metrics which included recall, precision, and F1 score. One of the potential future works is to select deeper deep transfer learning such as DenseNet, and InceptionResNet to improve the testing accuracy of the proposed model.

Acknowledgements We gratefully acknowledge the support of NVIDIA Corporation, which donated the Titan X GPU used in this research.

References

1. Liu, J., et al.: Hydroxychloroquine, a less toxic derivative of chloroquine, is effective in inhibiting SARS-CoV-2 infection in vitro. Cell Discov. **6**(1), 6–9 (2020). https://doi.org/10.1038/s41421-020-0156-0
2. Hageman, J.R.: The coronavirus disease 2019 (COVID-19). Pediatr. Ann. (2020). https://doi.org/10.3928/19382359-20200219-01
3. Singhal, T.: A review of coronavirus disease-2019 (COVID-19). Indian J. Pediatr. **87**(4), 281–286 (2020). https://doi.org/10.1007/s12098-020-03263-6
4. Huang, P., et al.: Use of chest CT in combination with negative RT-PCR assay for the 2019 novel coronavirus but high clinical suspicion. Radiology **295**(1), 22–23 (2020). https://doi.org/10.1148/radiol.2020200330
5. Cinkooglu, A., Bayraktaroglu, S., Savas, R.: Lung changes on chest CT during 2019 novel coronavirus (COVID-19) pneumonia. Eur. J. Breast Heal. **16**(2), 89–90 (2020). https://doi.org/10.5152/ejbh.2020.010420
6. Hosny, A., Parmar, C., Quackenbush, J., Schwartz, L.H., Aerts, H.J.W.L.: Artificial intelligence in radiology. Nat. Rev. Cancer (2018). https://doi.org/10.1038/s41568-018-0016-5
7. Iqbal, T., Ali, H.: Generative adversarial network for medical images (MI-GAN). J. Med. Syst. (2018). https://doi.org/10.1007/s10916-018-1072-9
8. Shorten, C., Khoshgoftaar, T.M.: A survey on image data augmentation for deep learning. J. Big Data (2019). https://doi.org/10.1186/s40537-019-0197-0
9. Yi, X., Walia, E., Babyn, P.: Generative adversarial network in medical imaging: a review. Med. Image Anal. (2019). https://doi.org/10.1016/j.media.2019.101552
10. Oakden-Rayner, L.: CheXNet: an in-depth review. Luke Oakden-Rayner Blog (2019)
11. Irvin, J., et al.: CheXpert: a large chest radiograph dataset with uncertainty labels and expert comparison (2019)
12. Kermany, D., Zhang, K., Goldbaum, M.: Labeled optical coherence tomography (OCT) and chest X-ray images for classification (2018)

13. Saraiva A.A., et al.: Classification of images of childhood pneumonia using convolutional neural networks. In: BIOIMAGING 2019—6th International Conference on Bioimaging, Proceedings; Part 12th International Joint Conference on Biomedical Engineering Systems and Technologies BIOSTEC 2019, pp. 112–119 (2019). https://doi.org/10.5220/000740430 1120119

14. Liang G., Zheng, L.: A transfer learning method with deep residual network for pediatric pneumonia diagnosis. Comput. Methods Programs Biomed. (2020), https://doi.org/10.1016/j. cmpb.2019.06.023

15. Wu, H., Xie, P., Zhang, H., Li, D., Cheng, M.: Predict pneumonia with chest X-ray images based on convolutional deep neural learning networks. J. Intell. Fuzzy Syst. (2020). https://doi. org/10.3233/jifs-191438

16. Loey, M., Smarandache, F., Khalifa, N.E.M.: Within the lack of COVID-19 benchmark dataset : a novel GAN with deep transfer learning for corona-virus detection in chest X-ray images (2020)

17. Huang, L., et al.: Serial quantitative chest CT assessment of COVID-19: deep-learning approach. Radiol. Cardiothorac. Imaging 2(2), e200075 (2020). https://doi.org/10.1148/ryct. 2020200075

18. Jin S., et al.: AI-assisted CT imaging analysis for COVID-19 screening: building and deploying a medical AI system in four weeks. medRxiv p. 2020.03.19.20039354 (2020). https://doi.org/ 10.1101/2020.03.19.20039354

19. Li L., et al.: Artificial intelligence distinguishes COVID-19 from community acquired pneumonia on chest CT. Radiology, p. 200905 (2020). https://doi.org/10.1148/radiol.202020 0905

20. ELGhamrawy S.M., Hassanien, A.E.: Diagnosis and prediction model for COVID19 patients response to treatment based on convolutional neural networks and whale optimization algorithm using CT images. medRxiv p. 2020.04.16.20063990 (2020). https://doi.org/10.1101/2020.04. 16.20063990

21. Sandfort, V., Yan, K., Pickhardt, P.J., Summers, R.M.: Data augmentation using generative adversarial networks (CycleGAN) to improve generalizability in CT segmentation tasks. Sci. Rep. 9(1), 16884 (2019). https://doi.org/10.1038/s41598-019-52737-x

22. Antoniou, A., Storkey, A., Edwards, H.: Data augmentation generative adversarial networks (2017) [Online]. Available: http://arxiv.org/abs/1711.04340

23. Alqahtani, H., Kavakli-Thorne, M., Kumar, G.: Applications of generative adversarial networks (GANs): an updated review. Arch. Comput. Methods Eng. (2019). https://doi.org/10.1007/s11 831-019-09388-y

24. Goodfellow, I.J., et al.: Generative adversarial nets. Adv. Neural Inf. Process. Syst. (2014). https://doi.org/10.3156/jsoft.29.5_177_2

25. Sokolova, M., Lapalme, G.: A systematic analysis of performance measures for classification tasks. Inf. Process. Manag. 45(4), 427–437 (2009). https://doi.org/10.1016/j.ipm.2009.03.002

26. LeCun, Y., Bengio, Y., Hinton, G.: Deep learning. Nature 521(7553), 436–444 (2015). https:// doi.org/10.1038/nature14539

27. Eraslan, G., Avsec, Ž., Gagneur, J., Theis, F.J.: Deep learning: new computational modelling techniques for genomics. Nat. Rev. Genet. 20(7), 389–403 (2019). https://doi.org/10.1038/s41 576-019-0122-6

28. Voulodimos, A., Doulamis, N., Doulamis, A., Protopapadakis, E.: Deep learning for computer vision: a brief review. Comput. Intell. Neurosci. 2018, 7068349 (2018). https://doi.org/10.1155/ 2018/7068349

29. Riordon, J., Sovilj, D., Sanner, S., Sinton, D., Young, E.W.K.: Deep learning with microfluidics for biotechnology. Trends Biotechnol. 37(3), 310–324 (2019). https://doi.org/10.1016/j.tibtech. 2018.08.005

30. You, J., McLeod, R.D., Hu, P.: Predicting drug-target interaction network using deep learning model. Comput. Biol. Chem. 80, 90–101 (2019). https://doi.org/10.1016/j.compbiolchem. 2019.03.016

31. Jaganathan, K., et al.: Predicting splicing from primary sequence with deep learning. Cell **176**(3), 535–548.e24 (2019). https://doi.org/10.1016/j.cell.2018.12.015
32. Cao, C., et al.: Deep learning and its applications in biomedicine. Genomics, Proteomics Bioinf. **16**(1), 17–32 (2018). https://doi.org/10.1016/j.gpb.2017.07.003
33. Liu, S., Deng, W.: Very deep convolutional neural network based image classification using small training sample size. In: 2015 3rd IAPR Asian Conference on Pattern Recognition (ACPR), pp. 730–734 (2015) https://doi.org/10.1109/acpr.2015.7486599
34. Szegedy, C., et al.: Going deeper with convolutions. In: Proceedings of the IEEE Computer Society Conference on Computer Vision and Pattern Recognition, 2015, pp. 1–9. https://doi.org/10.1109/cvpr.2015.7298594
35. He, K., Zhang, X., Ren, S., Sun, J.: Deep residual learning for image recognition. In: 2016 IEEE Conference on Computer Vision and Pattern Recognition (CVPR), 2016, pp. 770–778. https://doi.org/10.1109/CVPR.2016.90
36. Zhao, J. Zhang, Y., He, X., Xie, P.: COVID-CT-dataset: a CT scan dataset about COVID-19. pp. 1–5 (2020)
37. Huang, G., Liu, Z., van der Maaten, L., Weinberger, K.Q.: Densely connected convolutional networks. In: 2017 IEEE Conference on Computer Vision and Pattern Recognition (CVPR), 2017, pp. 2261–2269. https://doi.org/10.1109/cvpr.2017.243
38. Szegedy, C., Ioffe, S., Vanhoucke, V., Alemi, A.A.: Inception-v4, inception-ResNet and the impact of residual connections on learning In: 31st AAAI Conference on Artificial Intelligence, AAAI 2017 (2017)
39. Zhang, X., Zhou, X., Lin, M., Sun, J.: ShuffleNet: an extremely efficient convolutional neural network for mobile devices. In: Proceedings of the IEEE Computer Society Conference on Computer Vision and Pattern Recognition, 2018. https://doi.org/10.1109/cvpr.2018.00716
40. Qin, Z., Zhang, Z., Chen, X., Wang, C., Peng, Y.: Fd-Mobilenet: improved Mobilenet with a fast downsampling strategy. In: Proceedings—International Conference on Image Processing, ICIP, 2018, https://doi.org/10.1109/icip.2018.8451355
41. Khalifa, N.E.M., Taha, M.H.N., Hassanien, A.E., Hemedan, A.A.: Deep bacteria: robust deep learning data augmentation design for limited bacterial colony dataset. Int. J. Reason. Intell. Syst. **11**(3), 256 (2019). https://doi.org/10.1504/IJRIS.2019.102610
42. Khalifa, N.E.M., Taha, M.H.N., Ali, D.E., Slowik, A., Hassanien, A.E.: Artificial intelligence technique for gene expression by tumor RNA-Seq data: a novel optimized deep learning approach. IEEE Access (2020). https://doi.org/10.1109/access.2020.2970210
43. Khalifa, N.E.M., Taha, M.H.N., Hassanien, A.E., Selim, I.M.: Deep Galaxy: classification of Galaxies based on deep convolutional neural networks (2017). arXiv:1709.02245
44. Khalifa, N., Loey, M., Taha, M., Mohamed, H.: Deep transfer learning models for medical diabetic retinopathy detection. Acta Inform. Medica **27**(5), 327 (2019). https://doi.org/10.5455/aim.2019.27.327-332
45. Khalifa, N.E.M., Loey, M., Taha, M.H.N.: Insect pests recognition based on deep transfer learning models. J. Theor. Appl. Inf. Technol. **98**(1), 60–68 (2020)
46. Žižka, J., Dařena, F., Svoboda, A., Žižka, J., Dařena, F., Svoboda, A.: Adaboost. In: Text Mining with Machine Learning (2019)
47. Goutte C., Gaussier, E.: A probabilistic interpretation of precision, recall and F-score, with implication for evaluation. In: Losada D.E., Fernández-Luna J.M. (eds.) Advances in Information Retrieval, pp. 345–359. Berlin, Heidelberg: Springer Berlin Heidelberg (2005)

COVID-19 Data Analysis and Innovative Approach in Prediction of Cases

Abhijeet Kushwaha, Pallavi Vijay Chavan, and Vivek Kumar Singh

Abstract The world went into a standstill when the news of a global pandemic (Coronavirus Disease-19) caused by the Severe Acute Respiratory Syndrome Coronavirus 2 Virus was announced by the World Health Organization. In this chapter, we present a detailed investigation of the spread of COVID-19 in India, its neighboring countries, and other global hotspots. We also analyze the worst-hit states of India with respect to the rise in Confirmed cases and Death cases due to COVID-19 and investigate the growth factor of the same. We then build a Support Vector Machine for Regression analysis of confirmed cases in India and predict the future confirmed cases by analyzing the current growth curve. Our work finally extends to discuss the need for future research to find out the consequences of the COVID-19 crisis in areas of Economy, Agriculture, Health, Education, Secondary sector, and Service Sector.

Keywords COVID-19 · Artificial intelligence · Deep learning · Support vector machine · Regression · Data analysis

1 Introduction

Severe Acute Respiratory Syndrome Coronavirus 2 (SARS-CoV-2) is the virus which causes Coronavirus Disease (COVID-19) in humans. The first human cases of COVID-19 were identified in Wuhan City, China in December 2019. Just like the SARS outbreak in 2003, it is thought that SARS-CoV-2 entered the species barrier and initially affected human bodies, but more likely through an intermediate host,

A. Kushwaha · P. Vijay Chavan (✉) · V. Kumar Singh
Department of Information Technology, Ramrao Adik Institute of Technology, Nerul, Navi Mumbai, MH, India
e-mail: pallavi.chavan@rait.ac.in

A. Kushwaha
e-mail: arkush1234@gmail.com

V. Kumar Singh
e-mail: vivekkumar.singh@rait.ac.in

A.-E. Hassanien et al. (eds.), *Big Data Analytics and Artificial Intelligence Against COVID-19: Innovation Vision and Approach*, Studies in Big Data 78, https://doi.org/10.1007/978-3-030-55258-9_6

that is another animal species more likely to be handled by humans—this could be a domestic animal, a wild animal, or a domesticated wild animal and, as of yet, has not been identified [1]. The spread of COVID-19 has brought all global superpowers and developing nations to a standstill, as the infection has shown an exponential rate of spread. To make matters worse, we are still in the process of understanding the virus and finding vaccines to stop the spread. Until we do find a vaccine, social distancing and home quarantine is the only way to stop the spread. This has led to a complete nationwide lockdown in many countries including developing countries like India, which has had very adverse effects on the country's economy, healthcare facility and administration. Thus, COVID-19 has presented itself as an unconventional situation for the world to deal with, and therefore, it becomes all the more important to do a comprehensive analysis of the data for COVID-19 cases. Before we begin our analysis and prediction on the current COVID-19 crisis in the world, it is important to understand the following key terms: Coronavirus, COVID-19 and SARS-CoV-2. It is also important to understand why COVID-19 escalated exponentially across the world, and why it has been declared as a Pandemic by the World Health Organization.

Data about COVID-19 and its impact is released every day. However, to make sense of the data, to clean the data and to develop prediction models of a high accuracy is the big challenge. These challenges can be overcome by fields of Big Data, Deep Learning and Artificial Intelligence. We take these factors as a motivation to contribute this chapter and to bring out the novel approach of data analysis of COVID-19. This chapter contributes the analysis through different factors like state wise analysis in India, analysis of confirmed cases across India and abroad and the prediction model to predict the possible future cases of COVID-19.

The organization of the chapter is as follows: The chapter begins with the introduction in first section. Second section describes the state- of- art information of COVID-19. Section 3 presents an intelligent data Analysis of COVID-19. This section includes identifying and plotting global hotspots, analysis of spread in India and the comparison with neighboring countries. Section 4 describes the Prediction of future COVID-19 cases in India. Section 5 concludes the chapter with future scope of research with COVID-19 in healthcare. The chapter at the end includes sufficient references for the literature of the domain of healthcare and COVIDE0-19.

2 State-of-Art

The rapid spread of Corona virus, globally, has brought a lot of data that can be analyzed to know the nature of its advancement. Every day, every moment data is changing thus it is very challenging task for the researchers to deal with such big data. This is important for health care industries to analyze this data with the help of some big data algorithms, so that they come up with a solution. Scientist and researches are trying their best to utilize machine learning algorithms to track current progress of corona virus.

According to Ramgopal [2], it is found that in health sector vast amount of data is produced every day e.g. web of things. These stores require undertakings at many layers for better analysis of data stream. Author has presented a critical analysis of health care data. It is proposed to use high statistical analysis of big data to extract some hidden important information. Li et al. [3] picked official data and analyses transmission process of COVID-19. Authors have used both forward prediction and backward interference to analyze the data for better preparation by the affected countries. As work reported in [4], authors have used Susceptible-Infected-Removed (SIR) model. The data was collected on day basis from Jan 2020 for most affected countries by COVID-19. Simon et al. [5], presented a case study of novel Corona virus epidemic using Composite Monte-Carlo. The performance is further enhanced by GROOMS model. The results show a better prediction model for this epidemic forecast.

Various researchers used machine learning models to predict the spread of COVID-19. Similar work is done on Brazilian stats by Mathew's et al. [6]. The researchers used autoregressive integrated moving average, cubist, random forest (RF), Ridge regression and support vector regression for analyzing data.

Bhapkar et al. [7] proposed a graph based spread of COVID-19. Based on pandemic nature authors have divided graphs in four part. Relative analysis shows its hazardous nature. A very useful survey on forecasting methods used for COVID-19 pandemic is presented by Parikshit et al. [8]. Authors have presented analysis of various prediction models considering Day by Day data, data sources, prediction algorithms and all parameters. The day by day transforming nature of corona virus is still a challenge.

Authors in [9]. proposes an accurate forecasting model based on small dataset for COVID-19 cases. This model is able to forecast accurately the epidemic fate. The authors reported the limitations and unavailability of the data for accurate early forecasting. The most important challenge to the machine learning is discussed in this literature; the challenge is insufficient amount of data available for analysis. The model proposed in this literature is based on polynomial neural network and the corrective feedback. The predicted error is lowest with this model and the forecasting is at acceptable level.

3　COVID-19 Intelligent Data Analysis

In this section, we analyze COVID-19 data with respect to the neighboring countries viz. Pakistan, China, Afghanistan, Nepal, Bhutan, Sri Lanka and Bangladesh. In the next segment of analysis, COVID-19 spread in India with respect to major Global Hotspots is presented. The importance of this section is to clearly indicate the understanding about the trend of spread of COVID-19 on a global level. Based on this trend, an understanding of COVID-19 spread in India across the states is presented. This intelligent analysis helps to determine the states with highest confirmed cases, highest Mortality rate and highest Recovery rates.

World Map of Coronavirus

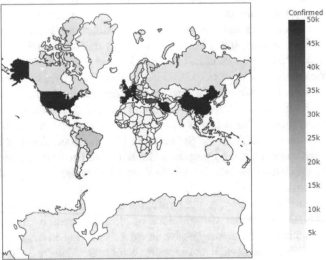

Fig. 1 World map of Coronavirus spread on 9th April 2020

3.1 Identifying and Plotting Global Hotspots

This section plots a choropleth map to visualize the global hotspots of confirmed cases of COVID-19 across the world. The data about confirmed COVID-19 cases throughout the world has been obtained from the data repository on GitHub by Johns Hopkins CSSE [10]. This dataset contains confirmed cases from the world till April 9, 2020. The choropleth map is shown in Fig. 1. It is obtained by using plotly library in Python in Jupyter Notebook. The choropleth map plots the confirmed COVID-19 cases across the world, where the darker hues of blue indicate a higher number of confirmed cases in a region in contrast to the lighter hues of blue that indicate lesser number of Confirmed cases respectively.

3.2 Analysis of COVID-19 Spread in India

Using the same dataset, analysis of COVID-19 spreading in different states of India is presented here. This analysis is plotted using pandas, numpy and matplotlib. The India's data is extracted first from the combined data of multiple countries by setting 'Country/Region' in the dataset equal to 'India'. In the next step, 'Date' column entries are converted to date time using pandas for an effective work using Date entries. The grouping all the data belonging to India date wise by aggregating the entries of 'Confirmed', 'Recovered' and 'Death' cases. Figure 1 is the plot of date wise Distribution of number of active cases in India. An increase or decrease in the

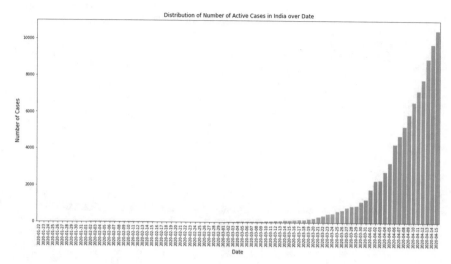

Fig. 2 Distribution of number of Active COVID-19 cases in India

count of the active cases of COVID-19 will be an indication of whether the number of Death cases or Recovered cases are increasing or decreasing.

From Fig. 2 it is observed that the count of Active cases of COVID-19 in India is increasing. This is an indication that the number of closed cases (sum of Death cases and Recovered cases) is less with respect to the daily Confirmed cases. This graph indicates rapid spread of COVID-19 in India.

Now, we plot a graph of the overall count of Confirmed cases, Death cases and Recovered cases of COVID-19 in India, and analyze the reason of a rise in the number of Confirmed cases and number of Closed cases. Figure 3 indicates a sudden increase in the number of Confirmed cases after being flat and steady for a long time earlier. Also, the number of Recovered cases initially is represented as a flat curve, but they eventually start rising which is a positive sign. The number of Death cases isn't rising as fast as the number of Confirmed cases and is mostly steady, which indicates that there have been less deaths per number of Confirmed cases. Also, as the number of Confirmed cases rises faster than both the number of Recovered cases and the number of Deaths combined, this validates the fact that the number of Active cases are rising. From Fig. 3 it is concluded that the number of closed cases is rising because of an increase in the number of Recovered cases, and not because of an increase in Death cases.

The density plot of Recovered cases and Death cases is shown in Fig. 4. From this figure it is concluded that the density of Recovered cases over a section is greater than the density of Death cases.

The recovery rate and mortality rate of the total Confirmed cases of COVID-19 cases in India is analyzed using following:

Recovery rate = (Number of Recovered cases/Number of Confirmed cases) ∗ 100

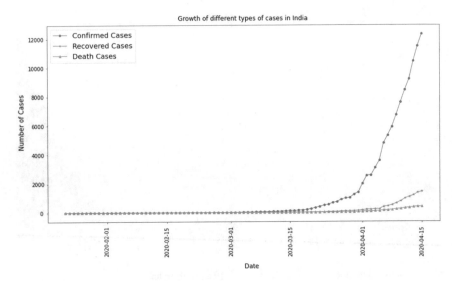

Fig. 3 Confirmed cases, recovered cases and death cases in India

Mortality rate $=$ (Number of Death cases/Number of Confirmed cases) $* 100$

The left graph and right graph in Fig. 5 depicts Recovery rate and Mortality rate of COVID-19 cases observed in India respectively. We can see that initially, the Recovery rate started rising while the mortality rate was still constant for Confirmed COVID-19 cases in India. However, with time, the recovery rate has significantly dropped while the mortality rate has significantly risen, which becomes a matter of concern for India.

The growth factor for the Confirmed cases, Recovered cases and Death cases is given below:

Growth factor of Confirmed cases $=$ New Confirmed cases of a day/New Confirmed cases of Previous day.

Growth factor of Recovered cases $=$ New Recovered cases of a day/New Recovered cases of Previous day.

Growth factor of Death cases $=$ New Death cases of a day/New Death cases of Previous day.

A growth factor above 1 indicates an increase in corresponding cases, while a growth factor above 1 is a positive sign if it is trending downwards. A growth factor constantly above 1 suggests exponential growth, while a constant growth factor of 1 suggests no change of any kind. Figure 6 represents a growth factor.

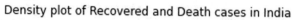

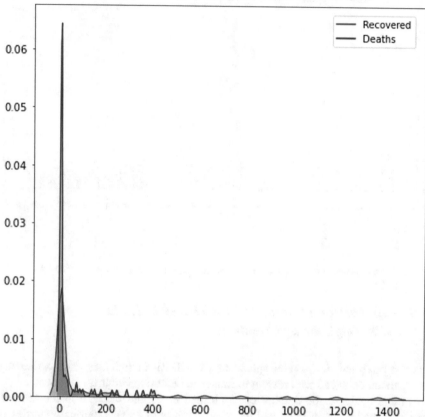

Fig. 4 Density plot for recovered cases and death cases of COVID-19 in India

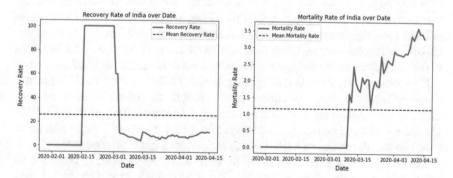

Fig. 5 Recovery rate and mortality rate due to COVID-19 in India

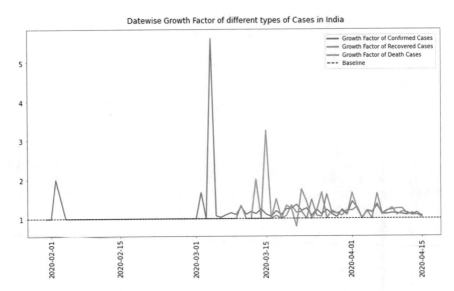

Fig. 6 Growth factor of confirmed cases, recovered cases and death cases of COVID-19 in India

3.3   Comparison of Spread of COVID-19 in India with Neighboring Countries

Having analyzed the general spread of COVID-19 in India, in this section the comparison of spread with respect to India's neighboring countries is shown.

In this analysis, the number of Confirmed cases and increase in the number of Confirmed cases in India and its comparison with its neighboring countries is presented. The logarithmic scale is chosen for an effective visualization of data and shown in Fig. 7. From this figure, it is observed that China is the most affected neighbor of India, as the spread of COVID-19 began from China. After China, cases in India rose, then stayed constant, and then rose again very fast. We also see that initially there were no cases Confirmed in Pakistan for a long time, until the last week of February when confirmed cases in Pakistan started rising. Rise of Confirmed cases in Nepal started very late and is increasing. It is also infer that after a sudden shoot in Confirmed cases in China, the curve is now constantly flat, which indicates that only China in the neighboring countries has managed to contain the spread of COVID-19. Thus, a flat and constant curve is what the countries would have to aim for to conclude that the spread of COVID-19 in their regions has been contained.

Let us now analyze the trend in the number of Recovered cases of India and its neighboring countries. It is evident from Fig. 8 as China started with the recovery very early, and the rising curve suggests that China has seen a significant amount of Recovery of its Confirmed COVID-19 citizens After China, India and Pakistan have seen a significant rise in the amount of Recovered cases, followed by Bangladesh, Sri Lanka and Bhutan.

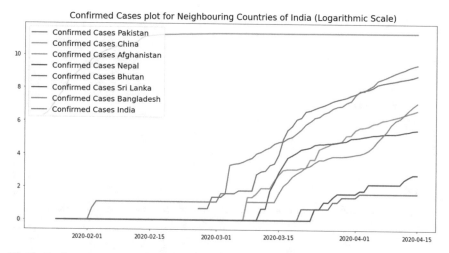

Fig. 7 Confirmed cases plot of India and its neighboring countries in Logarithmic scale

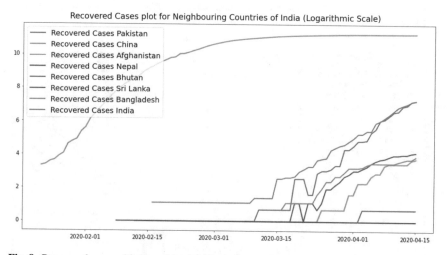

Fig. 8 Recovered cases of India and its neighboring countries

Following Fig. 9 shows the analysis of daily increase in Recovered cases of COVID-19 in neighboring countries. Figure 10 is an analysis of the trend in the number of Death cases of India and neighboring countries.

From Fig. 10, it is evident that China has the highest number of Death cases of all India's neighboring countries, however the curve has become constant suggesting that China has contained the spread of COVID-19. India, Pakistan, Bangladesh, Afghanistan and Sri Lanka have seen a rise in the number of Death cases due to COVID-19. However, until April 15, 2020 when the above data was graphed, Bhutan and Nepal have seen no death cases for COVID-19.

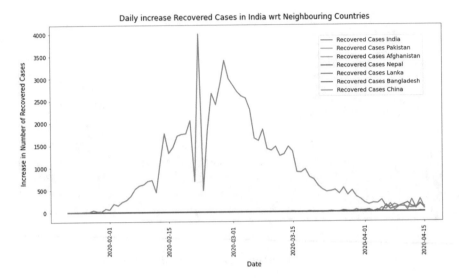

Fig. 9 Daily increase in the number of recovered cases of COVID-19 in India and neighboring countries

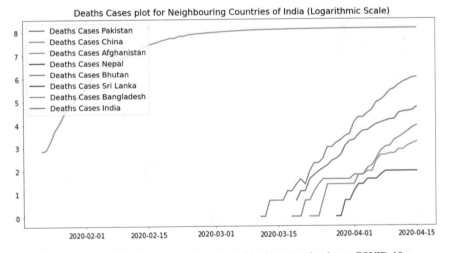

Fig. 10 Comparison of death cases in India and neighboring countries due to COVID-19

3.4 Comparison of COVID-19 Spread in India with Global Hotspots

This section investigates the trends of Confirmed cases, Recovered cases and Death cases due to COVID-19 in India and other global hotspots like Spain, Italy, USA,

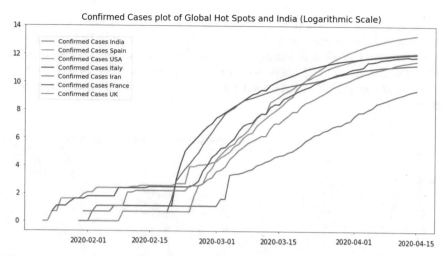

Fig. 11 Comparison of confirmed cases in India and other global hotspots (logarithmic scale)

Iran, France and the United Kingdom's. Figure 11 is the investigation of the number of Confirmed cases in India and its comparison with the global hotspots.

From Fig. 11 it is concluded that India has lowest number of Confirmed cases with respect to other global hotspots. In Fig. 12, the number of Confirmed cases in other countries had increased and are now decreasing, but the daily increase in number of Confirmed cases in USA is still rising and is the highest.

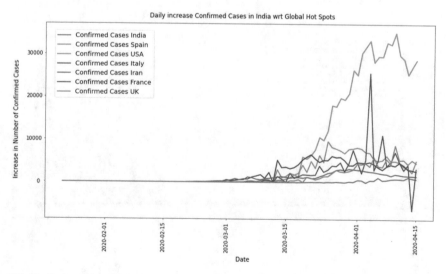

Fig. 12 Comparison of daily increase in number of confirmed cases in India and global hotspots due to COVID-19

At this point, we plot the number of Recovered cases in India and in global hotspots, and the increase in daily number of Recovered cases in India and global hotpots. From Fig. 13, it is concluded that the number of Recovered cases in India and other global hotspots have been rising. We also observe in Fig. 14 that the daily increase in the number of Recovered cases was constant at first, and then started increasing.

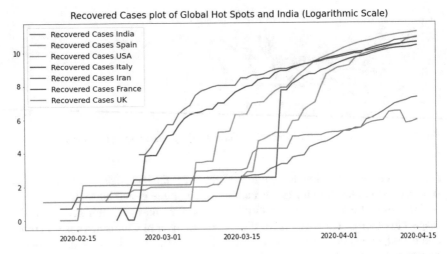

Fig. 13 Comparison of number of recovered cases in India and global hotspots due to COVID-19

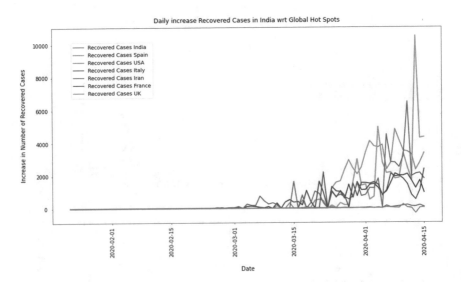

Fig. 14 Comparison of daily increase in number of recovered cases

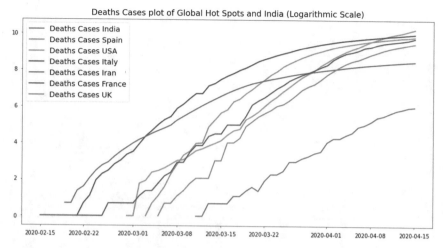

Fig. 15 Daily death cases in India and global hotspots

In the next segment of analysis, we plot the number of Death cases in India and in global hotspots, and the increase in daily number of Death cases in India and global hotpots.

From Fig. 15 it is observed that the number of Deaths in all the major hotspots started rising very fast, while in India, the number of death cases started rising comparatively late. However, we can start to notice that the curves of all the plotted countries are flattening, which indicates a slow rise in Death cases.

From Fig. 16 it is concluded that the increase in daily Death cases in India has been nearly constant when compared to other global hotspots, whose graph is highly rising.

3.5   Comparison of COVID-19 Spread in the States of India

This section analyses and evaluates the spread in the states of India. The dataset used for plotting all graphs in this section is obtained from the following two sources: The Ministry of Health and Family Welfare, Government of India [11] and the world wide web, covid19india [12]. The tools used are pandas for Data Analysis, numpy for Computing and matplotlib and seaborn for plotting the results.

The state's data is extracted from the combined data of multiple states by setting "State/Union Territory" in the dataset equal to that corresponding state or Union Territory. We then convert the 'Date' column entries to *datetime* using pandas for an effective work using Date entries. Finally, we group all the data belonging to states, date wise by aggregating the entries of 'Confirmed', 'Recovered' and 'Death' cases.

Following States are considered for the analysis: Assam, Arunachal Pradesh, Andhra Pradesh, Rajasthan, Bihar, Kerala, Chhattisgarh, Madhya Pradesh, Gujarat,

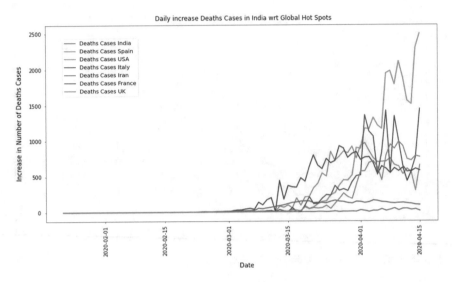

Fig. 16 Increase in daily death cases in India and global hotspots

Haryana, Telangana, Himachal Pradesh, Jharkhand, Karnataka, Nagaland, Manipur, Meghalaya, Mizoram, Odisha, West Bengal, Punjab, Sikkim, Uttar Pradesh, Tamil Nadu, Maharashtra, Tripura, Uttarakhand, Goa. Following Union Territories are considered for the analysis: The Government of NCT of Delhi, Daman & Diu, Dadra and Nagar Haveli, Puducherry, Andaman and Nicobar Islands, Chandigarh, Jammu and Kashmir, Ladakh and Lakshadweep.

The analysis of the number of Confirmed cases of COVID-19 in all states of India is presented in Fig. 17. In this figure, it is observed that the five regions (State/UT) with the highest number of COVID-19 cases are Maharashtra, Delhi, Tamil Nadu, Rajasthan and Madhya Pradesh respectively in descending order. Therefore, we compare and contrast these five regions in further analysis of the number of Confirmed cases in India.

The number of Recovered cases of COVID-19 in all states of India is shown in Fig. 18.

Analyzing Fig. 18, we can conclude that the five regions (State/UT) with the highest number of Recovered COVID-19 cases are Maharashtra, Kerala, Rajasthan, Telangana and Tamil Nadu respectively in descending order. Therefore, we compare and contrast these five regions during analysis of the number of Recovered cases in India.

The analysis of the number of Death cases of COVID-19 in all states of India is shown in Fig. 19. Analyzing this figure, we can conclude that the five regions (State/UT) with the highest number of Death in COVID-19 cases are Maharashtra, Madhya Pradesh, Gujarat, Delhi and Telangana respectively in descending order. Therefore, we will compare and contrast these five regions during analysis of the number of Death cases in India.

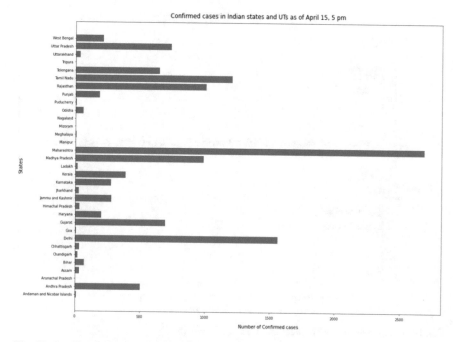

Fig. 17 Confirmed cases of Indian States and UTs as of April 15

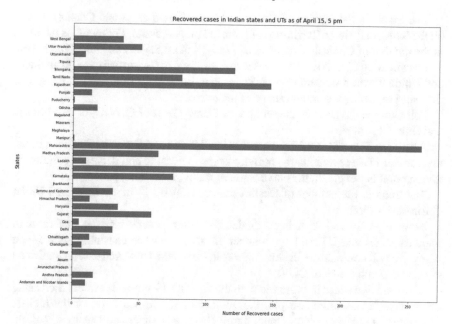

Fig. 18 Recovered cases of Indian States and UTs as of April 15

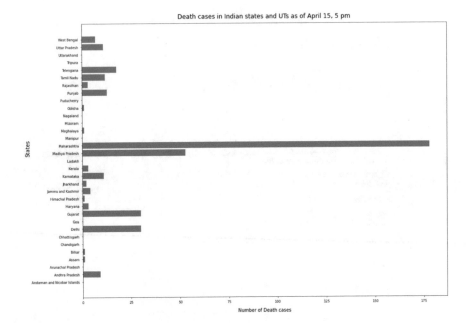

Fig. 19 Death cases of Indian States and UTs as of April 15

The trends in the number of Confirmed cases, Cured cases and Deaths cases of all the States and Union Territories of India are plotted ahead. Following is the trend in the number of Confirmed cases of COVID-19 in all States and Union Territories.

Investigating Figs. 20 and 21, we see that the trend in Confirmed cases in all States and Union Territories seem to be fuzzy at first, however after a point in the graph, they start repeating a common shape of the curve.

Following is the trend in the number of Cured Cases of COVID-19 in all States and Union Territories.

Analyzing Figs. 22 and 23, we see that in all States and Union territories in India, the number of Recovered cases initially keeps increasing and decreasing, however after a point in the graph, the curve starts repeating a common pattern.

The trend in the number of Death Cases of COVID-19 in all States and Union Territories is plotted.

From Figs. 24 and 25 it is concluded that after a quick increase in Deaths in majority states and UTs, a large number of which now see constant rise in Death cases. We will now analyze the five highest states in terms of Cured cases, Confirmed cases and Death Cases of COVID-19.

There are five states in India where in the CIVOD-19 spread is rapidly increasing every day. At this point, we plot the number of Confirmed cases of the highest five states, viz. Maharashtra, Delhi, Tamil Nadu, Rajasthan and Madhya Pradesh. Figure 26 is the representation of confirmed cases in these five regions. Figure 27 represents the number of Recovered cases in highest five regions and Fig. 28

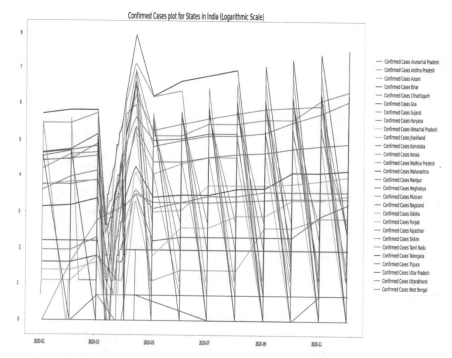

Fig. 20 Confirmed cases of all Indian states as of April 15 (Logarithmic scale)

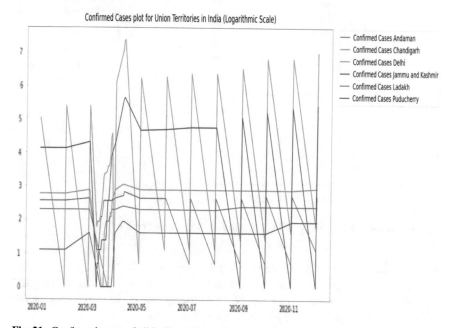

Fig. 21 Confirmed cases of all Indian UTs as of April 15 (Logarithmic scale)

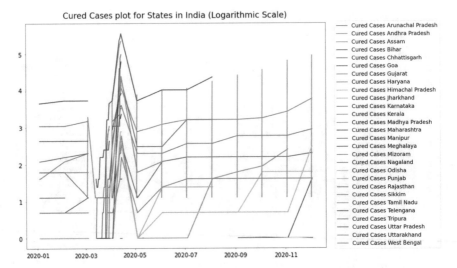

Fig. 22 Cured cases of all Indian states as of April 15 (Logarithmic scale)

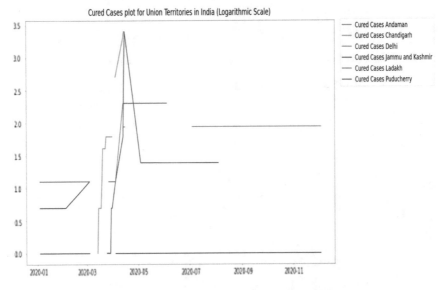

Fig. 23 Cured cases of all Indian UTs as of April 15 (Logarithmic scale)

represents the number of death cases in top five regions.

Finally, the Mortality and Recovery rates of the top 5 regions of India are analyzed and plotted. Figure 29 indicates a plot of the Mortality rate in the top five regions of India. Figure 30 represents the plot of recovery rate in top five regions.

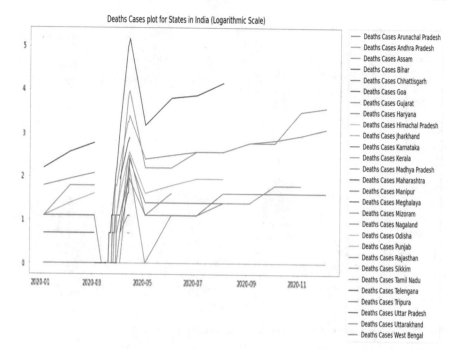

Fig. 24 Death cases of all Indian states as of April 15 (Logarithmic scale)

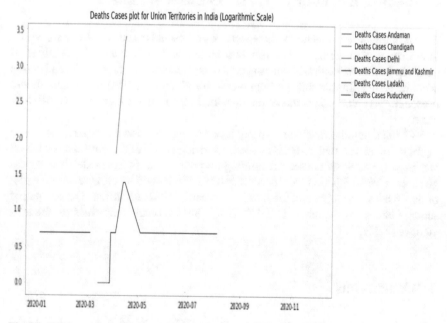

Fig. 25 Death cases of all Indian UTs as of April 15 (Logarithmic scale)

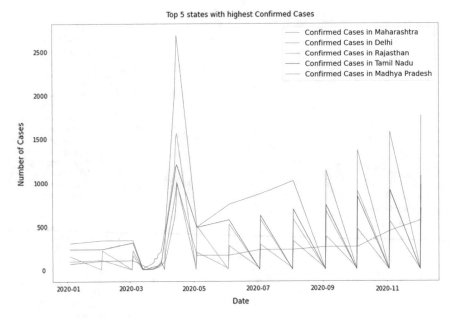

Fig. 26 Confirmed cases of five highest Indian regions as of April 15

4 Prediction of Future COVID-19 Cases in India

The art of prediction depends on how well we understand the current scenario, whose future we want to predict. We devoted the complete Sect. 3 to analyze the different trends in data visualization by looking at as many perspectives as possible, and derive accurate results. In this chapter, Support Vector Machine (SVM) Regression model is used for prediction. This model predicts the future possible number of COVID-19 cases.

SVM is a popular machine learning tool for classification and regression. SVM regressor of polynomial kernel is created with a degree of 10. The same dataset which was used for analysis is used for training purpose and to fit the model. The model gives Root Mean Square Error for SVR as 431.6616564645887. Figure 31 is the plot of data used for training and the fitted curve using SVM regression. The R-squared score obtained for the model is 0.942. Below are the prediction values for the next 10 days (Table 1).

5 Conclusions

With this study, we aimed to investigate the COVID-19 crisis using the official datasets available in the public domain, and the very effective Data Visualization

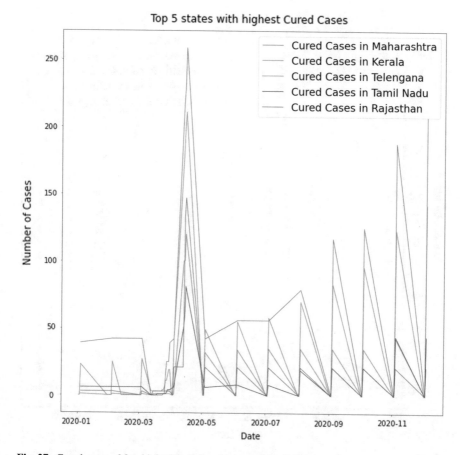

Fig. 27 Cured cases of five highest Indian regions as of April 15

and Machine learning tools. We investigated the spread of COVID-19 using a choropleth map, then went on to investigate the spread throughout the world, in India, in the neighboring countries of India, and in the world's major hotspots of COVID-19 spread. With the help of this study, we were able to visualize and draw conclusions towards the patterns of spread of COVID-19, along with visualizing the rise in mortality rates, recovery rates, growth factors, density plots and predict the number of Future cases with fair accuracy. Data Analytics tools and Intelligent models have made it possible for us to model and visualize the spread of COVID-19. With the help of the predicted values of Confirmed cases, the government and all officials can work towards equipping themselves with all the healthcare requirements like drugs, equipment, and quarantine spaces beforehand. The world going into a complete lockdown has impacted the economy, and therefore all the interlinked services like Agriculture, Service sector, and Industrial Production. More research can be conducted on

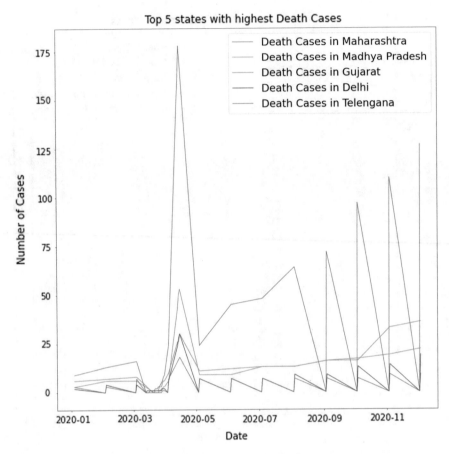

Fig. 28 Death cases of five highest Indian regions as of April 15

these individual matters to realize the impact of the COVID-19 on the world after the COVID-19 crisis.

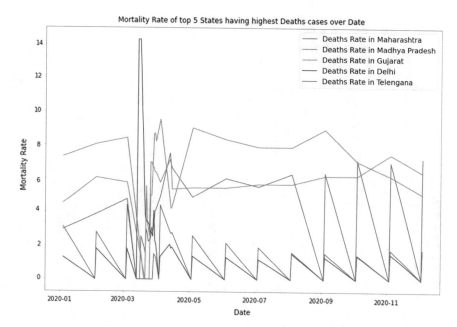

Fig. 29 Highest mortality rates of the top five regions in India

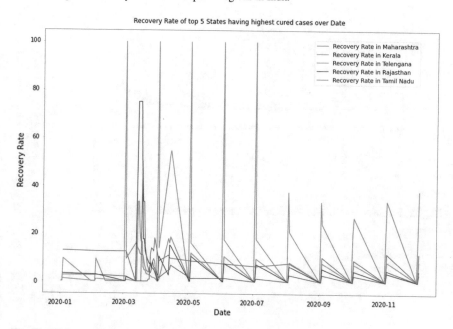

Fig. 30 Highest recovery rates of the top five regions in India

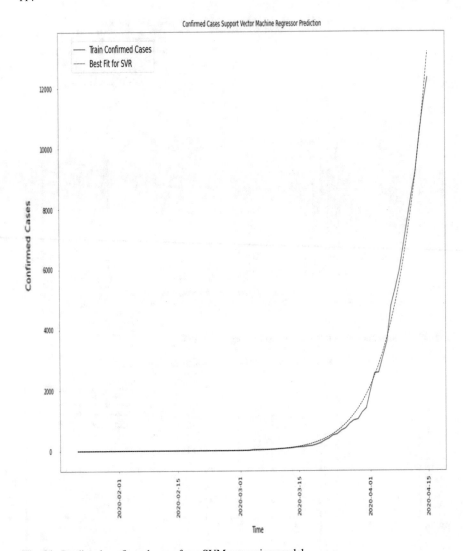

Fig. 31 Predicted confirmed cases from SVM regression model

Table 1 Predicted values of future confirmed cases in India

Sr. No	Date	SVM predictions
1	2020-04-16	14,848.68537
2	2020-04-17	16,690.76385
3	2020-04-18	18,736.04939
4	2020-04-19	21,004.22921
5	2020-04-20	23,516.63986
6	2020-04-21	26,296.38409
7	2020-04-22	29,368.45403
8	2020-04-23	32,759.86395
9	2020-04-24	36,499.78771
10	2020-04-25	40,619.70376

References

1. who.int. 2020. [online] Available at: https://www.who.int/news-room/q-a-detail/q-a-coronavir uses. Accessed 19 Apr 2020
2. Kashyap, R.: Big data analytics challenges and solutions, big data analytics for intelligent healthcare management, a volume in advances in ubiquitous sensing applications for healthcare, Elsevier, pp 19–41 (2019)
3. Bora, D.J.: Big data analytics in healthcare: a critical analysis, big data analytics for intelligent healthcare management, a volume in advances in ubiquitous sensing applications for healthcare,pp. 43–57. Elsevier (2019)
4. Li, L., Yang, Z., Dang, Z., Meng, C., Huang, J., Meng, H., Wang, D., Chen, G., Zhang, J., Peng, H., Shao, Y.: Propagation analysis and prediction of the COVID-19. Infect. Dis. Model. **5**, 282–292 (2020)
5. Ahmetolan, S., Bilge, A.H., Demirci, A., Peker-Dobie, A., Ergonul, O.: What can we estimate from fatality and infectious case data? A case study of Covid-19 pandemic (2020). arXiv preprint arXiv:2004.13178
6. Fong, S.J., Li, G., Dey, N., Crespo, R.G., Herrera-Viedma, E.: Composite monte carlo decision making under high uncertainty of novel coronavirus epidemic using hybridized deep learning and fuzzy rule induction. Appl. Soft Comput. 106282 (2020)
7. Ribeiro, M.H.D.M., da Silva, R.G., Mariani, V.C., dos Santos Coelho, L.: Short-term forecasting COVID-19 cumulative confirmed cases: Perspectives for Brazil, Chaos, Solitons & Fractals, 109853 (2020)
8. Bhapkar, H.R., Mahalle, P., Dhotre, P.S.: Virus graph and COVID-19 pandemic: a graph theory approach, Preprints, 2020040507 (2020)
9. Fong, S., Li, G., Dey, N., Crespo, R.G., Herrera-Viedma, E.: Finding an accurate early forecasting model from small dataset: a case of 2019-nCoV novel coronavirus outbreak. Int. J. Interact. Multimedia Artif. Intell. **6**, 132–140 (2020)
10. GitHub (2020) Cssegisanddata/COVID-19 [online] Available at: https://github.com/CSSEGI SandData/COVID-19/blob/master/README.md
11. mohfw.gov.in (2020) [online] Available at: https://www.mohfw.gov.in/
12. covid19india.org. 2020. *COVID-19 Tracker| India.* [online] Available at: https://www.covid1 9india.org/

Detection of COVID-19 Using Chest Radiographs with Intelligent Deployment Architecture

Vedant Bahel and Sofia Pillai

Abstract The outbreak of Coronavirus Disease (COVID-19) has caused a huge disturbance globally. The problem is the unavailability of vaccines and limited resources for its detection. In this paper, authors have carried out a case study of India to analyse the problem faced by the authorities for detecting COVID-19 amongst the suspected cases and have tried to solve the problem using a Deep Neural Network-based approach for analyzing chest x-rays in order to detect the onset/presence of related disease. After obtaining data from available resources, we trained a transfer learning-based CNN model. The model tries to extract the features of the radiographs and thus classifies it into the appropriate class. Heat map filter was used on the images significantly helping the model to perform better. This paper presents the validation of the model on certain test images and shows that the model is reliable to an extent. This paper also demonstrates a general architecture for the deployment of the model as per the considered case study.

Keywords Deep learning · Radiography · Feature extraction · COVID-19 · Heatmap filter · CNN

1 Introduction

Recently, the outbreak of Coronavirus Disease (COVID-19) proved to be disastrous due to the exponentially increasing number of cases worldwide. Not only the confirmed cases are increasing but also the number of deaths across the world seems to increase exponentially. As of early April 2020, around 1.34 million cases have been

V. Bahel (✉)
Department of Information Technology, G H Raisoni College of Engineering, Nagpur 440016, India
e-mail: vbahel@ieee.org

S. Pillai
CoE in AI & ML, Galgotias University, Noida, India
e-mail: pillaisofia@gmail.com

© The Editor(s) (if applicable) and The Author(s), under exclusive license
to Springer Nature Switzerland AG 2020
A.-E. Hassanien et al. (eds.), *Big Data Analytics and Artificial Intelligence Against COVID-19: Innovation Vision and Approach*, Studies in Big Data 78,
https://doi.org/10.1007/978-3-030-55258-9_7

confirmed affected by COVID-19. Out of which 74,782 have been reported dead. There's no vaccine present currently for this virus/disease. One of the major problems associated with this is complexity in the detection of the disease. The symptoms of this disease are cough, cold, and headache. Differentiating this common flu-like symptom with the existence of Coronavirus is difficult. Moreover, as of April 2020, not enough medical facilities are available to conduct tests in order to detect disease on a wider population. The tests which are available are mostly restricted to developed and urban residences. The following case study of India demonstrates the problem in details.

Case Study: Problem Scenario in India

India stands as at the second position in terms of population in the world. Keeping in mind the population of 1.35 billion, the healthcare facilities are not capable enough to deal with a pandemic situation. The number of cases being detected strongly depends upon the number of people being tested or screened. But in India, the testing is only done for people who came from some foreign nations in a period of a month or the ones who have been in contact with them. This makes it difficult to analyze the community spread in the country with a massive population and density [1, 2]. As per the Indian Council of Medical Research (ICMR), until 24th March 2019, only 18 tests were done per million of the population. Whereas countries like Italy got a greater number of confirmed cases because they had conducted around 5000 tests per million of the population until the same time [3]. Figure 1 depicts the number of tests conducted per million of the population by different countries of the world as per the ICMR reports [4].

Recently India imported certain rapid testing kit from China in order to detect COVID-19 amongst the suspects easily. Unfortunately, ICMR had to impose a halt

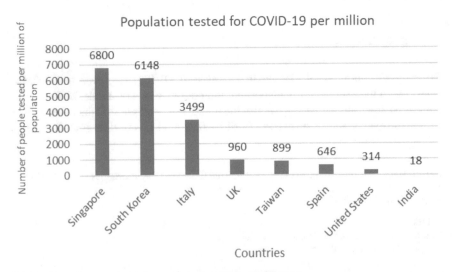

Fig. 1 General comparison of countries as per the test/million rate

on these kits due to the high variation found in the results on 21st April 2020. As per the health ministry of the state of Rajasthan, India, the kits gave an accuracy of only 5.4% [5]. Not only India, but the inaccuracy with the performance of the testing kits have been also reported by various other countries of the world. This showcase that unavailability of better and cost-efficient testing methodology appears as a great barrier for the country to fight back the pandemic.

One of the reasons behind fewer tests being conducted is a lack of medical resources. But the proposed concept can be easily adopted as a proposed test can be carried out at any radiology centres.

Research shows that healthcare as a sector has been lagging on the digital transition as compared to other sectors. Today's response to COVID has accelerated the adoption of virtual and AI tools and their scaling. From the AI bots deployed by various organizations, rapid digital transformation is being employed to counter COVID's exponentially rising hazard. AI promises a large change in the healthcare sector in the future. As per [6], in 2015 in United States, 10% of deaths were caused due to misdiagnosis. In [7], researchers have developed AI-enhanced microscope providing better microbiological diagnosis. Such type of errors is expected to be removed by using the AI-based system. In this paper, authors have implemented a deep learning-based model for detection of COVID-19 through Chest Radiograph. According to a research, 69% of patients being diagnosed by COVID-19 was found with chest abnormalities at the time of admission in the hospital. Even earlier many researchers tried implementing the same concept for detection of general chest related diseases mostly with computational intelligence-based approach. A similar concept can be even used for detection of the disease using MRI, CT Scans or other radiology. Figure 2 shows a sample dataset for the 2 classes that are being classified by the proposed model in this paper. The dataset considered has been taken from the repository at [8]. The classes are as follows:

(i) *Infected*: The first class in the classification model is the infected ones. The infection may be due to the development of SARS or Pneumonia. Some of the features in the x-rays that define the infection are air space consolidation, Broncho vascular thickening, and ground-glass opacities. Although the abnormality in chest radiographs may only be visible after 4–5 days of onset of general symptoms.

(ii) *Un-infected*: The second class of images are the chest radiographs found with no abnormality at the time of scan.

In this paper, various Convolutional Neural Network (CNN) based algorithms are used to achieve the goal. CNN are based on complex neural network architecture with translation invariance characteristics. It uses various types of mathematical concepts related to advance linear operations. For various intelligent tasks like image classification, recognition, tracking and object detection CNNs can be used. This approach is increasingly becoming popular as compared to traditional methods for image classification [9]. A deep learning model learns in all representations in a hierarchical manner as part of the training process. This stands as one of the key advantages to use these algorithms. In addition, the concept can be used in a quick

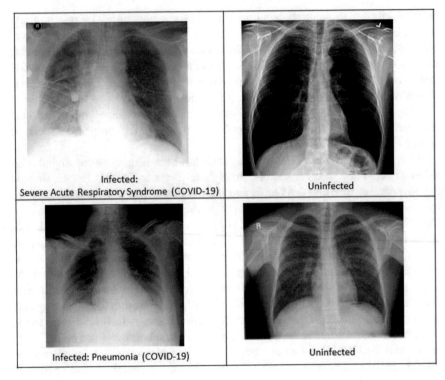

Fig. 2 Sample image dataset for COVID related thoracic diseases

test framework. The paper also presents deployment architecture in order to deploy the model in real time. The main focus of this paper is to devise an architecture for early and easy detection of COVID-19 using heatmap filter approach and deep neural network-based algorithms.

2 Literature Review

Since the outbreak of the disease in various parts of the world, various research organization and healthcare institution has started research in this area to develop methodologies and models that can be used for fighting the disease outbreak. Some researchers and research organizations have also started researching in non-technical fields to fight the pandemic. In [10], authors have studied and analyzed the outcome of this pandemic in the various sectors which might help officials to handle this type of situation better in the future. The paper also highlights the possible reason for the failure of handling the situation. Extended study may also help to derive methodologies to fight against those specific reasons. The paper also highlights the need for additional investigation so as to reach out to the hidden causes. Authors in [11], have presented some of the pathological finding forms one of the infected patients after the biopsy. The result shows that the finding was very similar to that of MERS (Middle Eastern Respiratory Syndrome) or SARS (Severe Acute Respiratory Syndrome). This means that the detection technique of this disease can be somewhere used to de- rive an architecture for detection of COVID-19. In [12], researchers have developed a system to track down the movement of virus across the globe and have tried to identify the cause of the spread from one country to another. The concept used behind the research is related to another machine learning concept named "Pattern Recognition". Baidu launched an infrared technology-based device for contactless analysis of body features in order to detect symptoms related to COVID-19. Some companies or researchers have also developed various chatbots that ask for symptoms of the patient to analyse the suspected case and accordingly guides the patient further steps in the test. This service is remotely accessible, making widespread tests possible.

Some researcher has also used intelligent systems majorly based on Deep Learning for disease detection. CNN is widely used in the field of biomedical or detection and analysis with certain added advanced filters and tuning methods [13]. In [14], authors have used CNN and Whale Opti- misation Algorithm to classify and diagnose COVID-19 using CT images. In [15], the results show that there is a high sensitivity for diagnosis of COVID-19 when chest CT's are considered. Moreover, radiograph-based diagnosis is the easiest way to achieve primary tests in various part of the world where healthcare frameworks are not advanced. In [16], authors have used Composite Monte Carlo Simulation to analyse pandemic situa- tion and forecast the future situation. In [17], authors used data augmentation to use the considerably small amount of data for decision making and forecast of pandemic. Data augmentation increases the significance of the amount of data available for modelling. Considering Pneumonia to be an one of the intermediate state of patient with potentially developing COVID-19 disease, authors in [8] used various algorithms to detect pneumonia from CT Scans. They also used image segmentation to extract the infected region from the images. In [18], researchers have developed a machine learning-based model for the detection of Pneumonia using chest x-rays which in turn may help for the detection of COVID considered in a modelled pipeline. According to the World Health Organization, COVID-19 also opens holes in the lungs like SARS, giving them a "honeycomb- like appearance" [19, 20]. The results in [9] show that the onset of disease causes a significant impact on the lungs causing paving patterns. Such changes can be easily detected using radiographs. In [21], authors concluded that the sensitivity of CT for COVID-19 was found to be 98%. Whereas the sensitivity of RT-PCR (Reverse Transcription Polymerase Chain Reaction), a lab method for detection of abnormal pathogen in the body was found to be only 71%. RT-PCR test is done on respiratory sample. These samples can be obtained via various methods. This includes sputum sample, which is thick mucus or phlegm obtained from lower respiratory tract. Apart from this, nasopharyngeal swap as a sample can also be used for the testing. Nasopharyngeal swap is the method of collecting nasal secretions as the test samples. As per [21], the disadvantages of this test is the associated complexity. Moreover, it suffers from the problems inherent in traditional PCR when it is used as a quantitative method. The problem also includes with the specificity and sensitivity of the test.

3 Proposed Methodology

In this paper, authors implemented multiple models using transfer learning techniques for faster training to optimize the weights of various Deep Convolution Neural Network like Inception V4, VGG 19, ResNet V2 152 and DenseNet on the Chest X-ray dataset. The workflow of the study in this paper has been represented in Fig. 3.

As can be seen from the above figure the process starts with data pre- processing. The dataset used contains certain invalid files which may be certain incorrect x-rays. The size of the dataset is around 300 chest x-rays of infected and uninfected patients each. In some cases, there are CT scans instead of Chest X-rays of the patients which may reduce the accuracy of the model is included in the training. That is why under data pre- processing the removal of just outlier images is must. Later, in the process, authors have applied heat map filters on the images. This helps in increasing the efficiency of feature extraction for the deep learning algorithms. Figure 4 shows some of the training images after applying heat map filter- ing. The use of heatmap over images are being extensively used for revealing pattern from the image data. In [22], the authors used a heatmap for the analysis of genomic data. Heatmaps can also be used for an initial level of classification as they can be used to define a group of separate or overlapping clusters. It also provides a better scope for accuracy and feature scaling by Neural Networks.

Authors split the dataset into ratio of 9:1 i.e. 270 training images and 30 test images for each class. And then the training data was fed into each model.

- *Inception V4*: The inception module first started with Inception V1 which used 1 × 1 dimension reduction layer and a global average pooling layer at the last which helped the module to outperform the previously existing modules. Later the

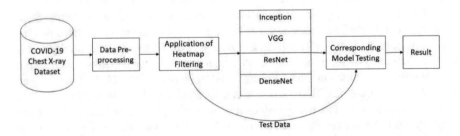

Fig. 3 Layout for proposed architecture

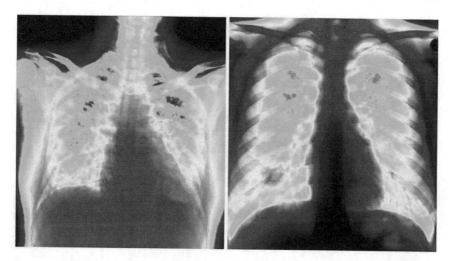

Fig. 4 Heatmap filtered training image sample

inception V4 module was introduced which is trained with memory optimisation with back propagation.

- *VGG 19:* It uses 3×3 convolutional layer which may have already covered the 5×5 or 7×7 layer. It also eradicates the requirement of filter like AlexNet or others. Thus, number of parameters in this case will be fewer providing faster convergence and reduced over-fitting problem.
- *ResNet V2 152:* The core idea behind ResNet is the it's residual connections by adding additive merges. This has made training of deeper model possible.
- *DenseNet:* Instead of using additions, it concatenates output from previous layer making the model more accurate, deeper and efficient to train. This algorithm strengthens the feature propagations. Thus, in turn reducing the number of parameters.

These four algorithms were then trained on the training heat mapped datasets. And the performance graph was found. The graph and the performance of the models are discussed in the next section of this paper.

4 Result and Discussion

In order to decide the algorithm that should be used for the detection of COVID in reals sense, it is very important to compare the individual performances of these algorithms. When these modules were used to train the COVID dataset discussed in this paper the epoch wise performance that was found on the validation dataset is shown in Fig. 5.

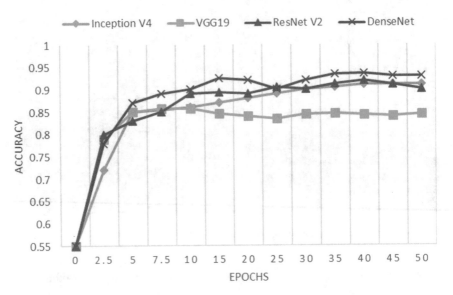

Fig. 5 Accuracy versus Epoch for all the algorithms implemented on the validation dataset

As it can seen, the DenseNet module trained our the COVID dataset out-performs the other implemented algorithms. The maximum accuracy attained by DenseNet algorithm in the process was 0.93. The features of all levels are used in DenseNet classifier making it perform better than other classifier. The results show that the model "DenseNet" though takes more time for training as compared to other algorithm but is worth since its performance over the dataset was found better than the other algorithm. Overall the implemented model showed a high accuracy making it fit to be used for validation in real scenario. If the model is fed with mode amount of dataset the accuracy and performance is expected to increase further. Moreover, introducing new scans for training will also cover some novel cases which may appear to be outlier in the current research.

Table 1 demonstrates the maximum and minimum accuracy attained by all the models considering all epochs.

Table 1 Minimum and Maximum Accuracy for corresponding algorithm

Model name	Minimum accuracy	Maximum accuracy
Inception V4	0.55	0.91
VGG 19	0.50	0.844
ResNet V2	0.55	0.9
DenseNet	0.55	0.93

When the performance of the model is closely observed in term of the metric being accuracy, except VGG 19, the maximum accuracy of the other 3 model seems to be similar. Whereas, initially at a smaller number of epochs, all the algorithm didn't show an acceptable performance metric.

Table 2 shows the validation of model over the sample test date. Heat map filter was also introduced over the test data before feeding it into the model. The algorithm used for validation which is demonstrated here is DenseNet.

5 Deployment Architecture

The model proposed in this paper can be deployed in the Indian scenario as discussed in the case study. Figure 6 describes the deployment architecture.

As it can be seen in the above figure, whenever a person is showing the general symptoms of COVID-19 which are cough, fever and difficulty to breathe, the person can visit the nearest radiology center or clinic. Or in a different scenario, if in case authorities at a rural place wants to screen a suspect in order to detect the presence of COVID-19, the authorities can use this testing method to complete their objective. The radiologist can then take out a chest x-ray of the suspected person. The chest x-ray can be then sent to the model using the mobile phone application installed in one of the devices with the radiologist. The application will send the clicked picture to the model via cloud technology and will also append the image into its dataset along with the predicted label for im- proving the model. The result will be displayed on the same application within seconds of analysis. Figure 7 demonstrates a quick preview of the proposed mobile application in the deployment architecture. At the same time, if the model detects abnormality in the x-ray of the suspected patient, a message will be sent to the nearest governing body. Later the patient can be move towards the main COVID testing centre where he/she can be lab tested with the respiratory specimen to confirm the results. If there is no abnormality found in the x-ray of the patient by the model, the person can be suggested to be in self isolation till the symptoms exists or may ask for additional help if the symptoms keep on prevailing. This process will significantly lead more number tests being conducted in a day. Thus, identifying a greater number of confirmed cases than the conventional methodology being practised.

6 Conclusion

In this paper, authors have studied a scenario of COVID-19 testing in India and have proposed a few CNN models for image classification to detect COVID through Chest X-rays. The objective of this research was to find a way to make detection of COVID-19 possible in areas with relatively lesser medical facilities. The major outcome of this research are as follows:

Table 2 Validation results of test dataset on DenseNet model

Predicted label	Actual label	Image
Infected	Infected	
Infected	Uninfected	
Uninfected	Infected	

(continued)

Table 2 (continued)

Predicted label	Actual label	Image
Uninfected	Uninfected	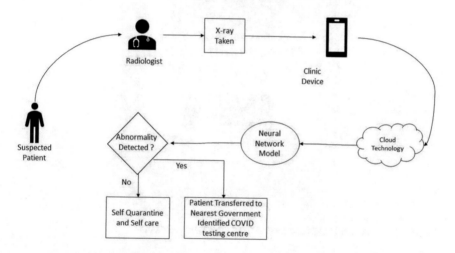

Fig. 6 Model deployment architecture

- The reason for lesser number of cases being found may be directly associated with, lesser number of tests being conducted in India as far as population is considered.
- The reason for this lack of testing methodologies facility and unavailability in rural or semi urban area.
- CNN based DenseNet algorithm seems to outperform the other algorithm implemented of the dataset.
- The use of heatmap filtering over the dataset helped in getting a better performance due to easy feature extraction and scaling.
- The accuracy of the model can be increased further by adding more images into the training data set.

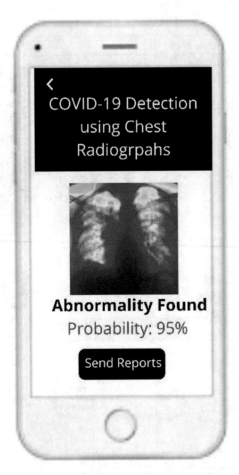

Fig. 7 Mobile application as described in the deployment architecture

The performance of the model proposed in the paper was found optimal for the target set in this research. But in case of COVID, some patients are reported with case where they do not develop any kind of visible abnormality in the chest or thoracic cavity. The abnormality is developed or visible in 2nd or 3rd week from the onset of disease. In such cases the test proposed in this paper may not prove to be reliable. However, such cases are rare to happen and will cause delayed detection in case the described model is considered [23].

There is a need of analysis of this concept in real time as per the proposed deployment architecture to understand the feasibility and performance of the architecture. Authors have also worked on Sensor based belts and mask, to record the physiological data of the suspect that directly gets fed into the database via mobile application as described in the architecture. The performance of the concept is expected to increase if the analysis is done along with the correlation of the sensor data. The sensor data may include pulse rate, presence of Hydrogen Peroxide which acts as biomarker to detect the pathogens and microbes which potentially may act as cause of the disease.

The proposed methods perform better than the traditional methods used for classification. Thus, ensuring a reliable and timely detection and diagnosis of COVID-19 possible. In addition to this, the deployment architecture mentioned in this paper presents a valid set of process to make this test reliable over the set of population. Apart from this the extended version of the same concept can be also used for other disease using some different type of radiological images.

References

1. The Caravan. Public-health experts raise concerns about India's restricted testing for COVID19. March 13, 2020. Accessed at: https://caravanmagazine.in/health/public-health-expertsraise-concerns-about-india-restricted-testing-covid-19)
2. Hindustan Times. India needs a more aggressive testing regimen for coronavirus: Experts. March 15, 2020. Accessed at: https://www.hindustantimes.com/india-news/testing-mustbe-done-on-war-footing/story-4gI2HWQ2WLhVLFOm5rsioM.html)
3. ICMR. Update: COVID-19 (20/03/2020 10:00 AM). March 20, 2020. Accessed at: https://www.icmr.nic.in/sites/default/files/whats_new/ICMR_website_update_20March_1 0AM_IST.pdf
4. Scroll.in Testing is the key to fighting coronavirus—so why does India have such a low testing rate? https://scroll.in/pulse/957380/testing-is-key-to-fighting-coronavirus-so-why-does-india-have-such-a-low-testing-rate
5. https://www.livemint.com/news/india/chinese-rapid-test-kits-come-a-cropper-as-toll-rises-to-640-11587493802859.html
6. Lu, S., Burton, S.: Man vs robots? Future challenges and opportunities within Artificial Intelligence (AI) health care education model. Proc. RAIS Conf. I(6), 7 (2017)
7. Chang, Y.-C., Yamamoto, Y., Matsumoto, H.: Enhancement of callose production by a combination of aluminum and iron in suspension- cultured tobacco (Nicotiana tabacum) cells. Soil Sci. Plant Nutrition 45(2), 337–347 (1999)
8. Cohen, J.P., Morrison, P., Dao, L.: cohen2020covid. ArXiv 2003.11597. Accessed 2020. https://github.com/ieee8023/covid-chestxray-dataset
9. Weston, J., Bengio, S., Usunier, N.: Large scale image annotation: learning to rank with joint word image embeddings. Mach. Learn. 81, 21–35
10. COVID, CDC, and Response Team: Severe Outcomes Among Patients with Coronavirus Disease 2019 (COVID-19)—United States, February 12–March 16, 2020. MMWR Morb Mortal Wkly Rep 69(12), 343–346
11. Xu, Z., Shi, L., Wang, Y., Zhang, J., Huang, L., Zhang, C., Liu, S., et al.: Pathological findings of COVID-19 associated with acute respiratory distress syndrome. The Lancet Respiratory Medicine 8(4), 420–422
12. Wang, Y., Hu, M., Li, Q., Zhang, X.-P., Zhai, G., Yao, N.: Abnormal Respiratory Patterns Classifier may Contribute to Large-scale Screening of People Infected with COVID-19 in an Accurate and Unobtrusive Manner. arXiv preprint arXiv:2002.05534 (2020)
13. Kayalibay, B., Jensen, G., van der Smagt, P.: CNN-Based Segmentation of Medical Imaging Data. arXiv preprint. arXiv:1701.03056 (2017)
14. Ghamrawy, E.L., Sally, M.: Diagnosis and Prediction Model for COVID19 Patients Response to Treatment based on Convolutional Neural Networks and Whale Optimization Algorithm Using CT Images. medRxiv (2020)

15. Ai, T., Yang, Z., Hou, H., Zhan, C., Chen, C., Lv, W., Tao, Q., Sun, Z., Xia, L.: Correlation of chest CT and RT-PCR testing in coronavirus disease 2019(COVID-19) in China: a report of 1014 cases.". Radiology **2020**, 200642 (2020)
16. Fong, S.J., Li, G., Dey, N., Crespo, R.G., Herrera-Viedma, E.: Composite Monte Carlo decision making under high uncertainty of novel coronavirus epidemic using hybridized deep learning and fuzzy rule induction. Appl. Soft Comput. 106282 (2020)
17. Fong, S.J., Li, G., Dey, N., Crespo, R.G., Herrera-Viedma, E.: Finding an Accurate Early Forecasting Model from Small Dataset: A Case of 2019-ncov Novel Coronavirus Outbreak. arXiv preprint arXiv:2003.10776 (2020)
18. Salman, F.M., Abu-Naser, S.S., Alajrami, E., Abu-Nasser, B.S., Ashqar, B.A.M.: COVID-19 Detection using Artificial Intelligence (2020)
19. https://www.nationalgeographic.com/science/2020/02/here-is-what-coronavirus-does-to-the-body/ 20.03.2020
20. Zhang, W.: Imaging changes of severe COVID-19 pneumonia in advanced stage. In: Intensive Care Medicine, 1–3, https://doi.org/10.1007/s00134-020-05990-y (2020)
21. Fang, Y., Zhang, H., Xie, J., Lin, M., Ying, L., Pang, P., Ji, W.: Sensitivity of chest CT for COVID-19: comparison to RT-PCR. Radiology 200432 (2020)
22. Gu, Z., Eils, R., Schlesner, M.: Complex heatmaps reveal patterns and correlations in multidimensional genomic data. Bioinformatics **32**(18), 2847–2849 (2016)
23. VanBerlo, B., Ross, M.: Investigation of Explainable Predictions of COVID-19 Infection from Chest X-rays with Machine Learning

COVID-19 Diagnostics from the Chest X-Ray Image Using Corner-Based Weber Local Descriptor

S. N. Mohammed, A. K. Abdul Hassan, and H. M. Rada

Abstract Corona Virus Disease-2019 (COVID-19) is a novel virus belongs to the corona virus's family. It spreads very quickly and causes many deaths around the world. The early diagnosis of the disease can help in providing the proper therapy and saving the humans' life. However, it founded that the diagnosis of chest radiography can give an indicator of coronavirus. Thus, a Corner-based Weber Local Descriptor (CWLD) for COVID-19 diagnostics based on chest X-Ray image analysis is presented in this article. The histogram of Weber differential excitation and gradient orientation of the local regions surrounding points of interest are proposed to represent the patterns of the chest X-Ray image. Support Vector Machine (SVM) and Deep Belief Network (DBN) classifiers are utilized for CWLD classification. Experimental results on a real chest X-Ray database showed that the gradient orientation gives the desired accuracy which is 100% using DBN classifier and CWLD size equals to 400.

Keywords COVID-19 · Chest X-Ray · Harris corners · Non-maximal suppression · WLD · Support vector machine (SVM) · Deep belief network (DBN)

1 Introduction

The novel Corona Virus Disease-2019 (COVID-19) or the Severe Acute Respiratory Syndrome Corona Virus 2 (SARS-CoV-2), as it is now known, is very fast spreading to the rest of the world from the origin of its manifestation in Wuhan City,

S. N. Mohammed (✉) · H. M. Rada
Department of Computer Science, College of Science, University of Baghdad, Baghdad, Iraq
e-mail: suhailan.mo@sc.uobaghdad.edu.iq

H. M. Rada
e-mail: huda.rada@sc.uobaghdad.edu.iq

A. K. Abdul Hassan
Department of Computer Science, University of Technology, Baghdad, Iraq
e-mail: 110018@uotechnology.edu.iq

© The Editor(s) (if applicable) and The Author(s), under exclusive license
to Springer Nature Switzerland AG 2020
A.-E. Hassanien et al. (eds.), *Big Data Analytics and Artificial Intelligence
Against COVID-19: Innovation Vision and Approach*, Studies in Big Data 78,
https://doi.org/10.1007/978-3-030-55258-9_8

China Province of Hubei [1]. Around 2,418,429 confirmed cases of COVID-19 and 165,739 deaths were reported until 20 April 2020 [2]. This rapid spreading encourages the need for accurate diagnostics method that can be used in hospitals and clinics responsible for the detection of COVID-19 [3, 4].

A suspect case is characterized by sore throat, fever, and cough. In addition, the person may be suspected if he/she has a history of travel to countries with confirmed cases or contact with persons with analogous travel history or those with positive COVID-19 test. Basic diagnosis is conducted by different molecular tests on respiratory samples (for example, nasopharyngeal swab, throat swab, sputum and endotracheal aspirates). The virus can also be found in the stool and blood in extreme cases. However, cases may be asymptomatic or even don't suffer from fever and the test may be negative even the person holds the virus [5].

Computer Tomography (CT) imaging typically reveals penetration, distortion of ground glass and convergence of sub-segments. Computerized tomographic chest screening is commonly abnormal even in those without symptoms or mild disease [6]. In fact, abnormal CT scans have been used as a second diagnose tool to identify the COVID-19 in suspect cases with negative diagnosis in molecular test. It found that many of these patients got positive molecular tests on repeat testing after some time later [7].

The main motivation of the paper is the fact that the corner-based descriptors have not been reported in COVID-19 diagnostics. To fill this research gap, this paper aims at finding the application of WLD within the local regions of points of interest during chest X-Ray analysis. The objective of the paper is to design a COVID-19 diagnostics scheme as a supplementary tool for clinical doctors. The main contributions of this work can be summarized with the following points:

1. Corner based descriptors are proposed to measure the efficiency of such type of features in COVID-19 diagnostics problem.
2. Two different types of classifiers are attempted to classify the extracted descriptors and find the optimal one based on the resulted accuracy.

The remaining of the paper is structured as follows: Sect. 2 shows a literature review for some of recently published works. Section 3 provides the detailed description of the proposed CWLD scheme for COVID-19. Section 4 illustrates the experimental results that are achieved when applying the proposed scheme on real chest X-Ray images. Finally, work conclusions and ideas for future work are presented in Sect. 5.

2 Literature Review

As soon as the disease began to spread, computer science researchers started developing systems that can detect the disease from the X-Ray image of the chest region. Following are some of these published works.

Farid et al. [8] presented a technique for recognizing the COVID-19 in CT images by proposing a Composite Hybrid Feature Extraction (CHFS). The selected features were classified by the Stack Hybrid Classification system (SHC). A total of 51 CT-images collected from Kaggle database website were used for model evaluation. An accuracy of about 96.07% has been achieved when using a Naïve Bayes as a meta-classifier in a hybrid classification.

Xu et al. [9] established an early screening model using deep learning techniques to distinguish COVID-19 pneumonia from Influenza pneumonia using CT images. A 3-dimensional deep learning model has been used to segment the CT image set. The infection type and total confidence score of this CT case were calculated with Noisy-or Bayesian function. The experiments result on a dataset consists of 1710 CT samples, including 357 COVID-19, 390 Influenza-A-viral-pneumonia, and 963 irrelevant-to-infection (ground truth) showed that the overall accuracy of the proposed system was 86.7%.

Zhang et al. [10] developed a deep anomaly detection model for COVID-19 screening. The model consists of three parts: (1) back-bone network (2) classification head, and (3) anomaly detection head. The backbone network is utilized for feature extraction task. The extracted features are then fed into the classification head and anomaly detection head, respectively. The classification head yields a "classification score", and the anomaly detection head yields a "scalar anomaly" score. The final decision is then computed based on minimizing the entropy loss for classification and the deviation loss for anomaly detection. A database consists of 100 chest X-ray images of 70 patients with COVID-19 from the Github repository and 1431 additional 1008 chest X-ray images suffer from other pneumonia from the publicChestX-ray14 dataset. The achieved accuracy was 96.00% for COVID-19 cases and 70.65% for non-COVID-19 cases.

Elghamrawy and Hassanien [11] proposed an Artificial Intelligence-inspired Model for COVID19 Diagnosis and Prediction for Patient Response to Treatment (AIMDP) with two proposed modules: (1) Diagnosis Module (DM) and (2) Prediction Module (PM). DM has been proposed for early detecting the COVID-19 using CT scans. Convolutional Neural Networks (CNNs) has been used for the segmentation of CT image. Whale Optimization Algorithm was used for selecting the most effective features (like age, infection stage, respiratory failure, multi-organ failure and the treatment regimens). Support Vector Machine (SVM) was used for classification. An accuracy of about 97.1% has been reported using 617 CT scans chest which were collected from different resources.

Rajinikanth et al. [12] extracted the infected sections from lung CT scans due to COVID-19 using CT image segmentation. Firstly, threshold filter was applied to eliminate any possible artifacts. After that, the image is enhanced using Harmony-Search-Optimization and Otsu thresholding. Finally, the Region-Of-Interest (ROI) is located from the resulted binary image to identify level of severity by computing the pixel ratio between the lung and infection sections. Radiopedia database was used for evaluation and the results showed that the proposed method can give high priority to CT cases with high level of severity.

Although different methods were proposed, corner based descriptors have not been used in COVID-19 problem yet. By making this fact as a starting point, the proposed work aims at studying the effectiveness of such descriptors in this research issue.

3   The Proposed CWLD Scheme

As depicted in Fig. 1, the proposed CWLD scheme for COVID-19 diagnostics involves contrast enhancement, points of interest localization, WLD extraction and COVID-19 diagnostics stage. The given chest X-Ray image is firstly preprocessed by enhancing the contrast of the different intensity levels. After that, points of interest are detected and reduced in points of interest localization stage. Differential excitation and direction of gradient descriptors are then extracted from each point of interest. SVM and Deep Belief Network (DBN) classifiers are finally attempted to diagnosis the COVID-19 state based on the final descriptors. The detailed descriptions of these stages are presented in the following subsections.

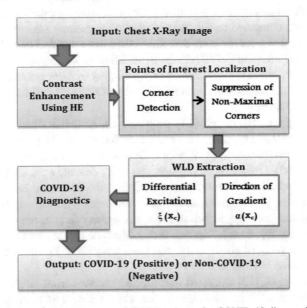

Fig. 1 The general design of the proposed CWLD scheme for COVID-19 diagnostics

3.1 X-Ray Image Contrast Enhancement

Contrast enhancement stage aims at increasing the contrast of X-ray image by spreading its histogram to make full use of available intensities. Histogram Equalization (HE) is adopted for this purpose. HE Increases the local contrast by spreading out the histogram, so that the new histogram is wider and more uniform in term of distribution of each intensity. The following three steps are followed when applying HE on the chest X-Ray image [13, 14]:

1. The probability of each intensity value in the X-Ray image is firstly computed.
2. The accumulated probability is founded using probability values resulted from step 1.
3. The intensity values of X-Ray image pixels are finally remapped to the new range (i.e. [0–255]) by multiplying the accumulated probability with the maximum value of the new range (i.e., 255).

3.2 Points of Interest Localization

This stage aims at defining locations of points of interest in the X-Ray image. To meet this goal, first, all possible corners are detected. After that, the number of detected corners is reduced by suppressing non-maximal corners and selecting the strongest ones only.

3.2.1 Corner Detection

A corner can be defined as the intersection of two edges, it represents a point where the directions of these two edges change, and it is characterized by a region with intensity change in two different directions. The method that is proposed by Chris Harris and Mike Stephens [15] is employed in this work to find corner's coordinates. Harris detects corner by taking into account the differential of the corner score with respect to direction. A shifting window is opened in any direction and the point that gives a large change in the intensity is registered as a corner. The following steps are followed to find Harris corners:

1. Firstly, the x and y derivatives (I_x and I_y) of the contrast enhanced X-Ray image (I) are computed by using Sobel gradient masks (G_x and G_y) as in the following equations:

$$I_x = G_x * I \tag{1}$$

$$I_y = G_y * I \tag{2}$$

where,

$$G_x = \begin{bmatrix} -1 & 0 & +1 \\ -2 & 0 & +2 \\ -1 & 0 & +1 \end{bmatrix} \tag{3}$$

$$G_y = \begin{bmatrix} -1 & -2 & -1 \\ 0 & 0 & 0 \\ +1 & +2 & +1 \end{bmatrix} \tag{4}$$

* represents convolution operation.

2. After that, the products of derivatives at every pixel in the image (I) are calculated using Eqs. 5 and 6.

$$I_x^2 = I_x * I_x \tag{5}$$

$$I_y^2 = I_y * I_y \tag{6}$$

3. Then, the response of the detector (R) at each pixel I(x, y) is computed using Eq. 7.

$$R = det(M) - k(trace(M))^2 \tag{7}$$

where,

$$M = \sum_{x,y} I(x, y) \begin{bmatrix} I_x^2 & I_x I_y \\ I_x I_y & I_y^2 \end{bmatrix} \tag{8}$$

and det(M) is the determinant of the matrix that can be founded using the following equation:

$$det(M) = I_x^2 . I_y^2 - I_x I_y . I_x I_y \tag{9}$$

trace(M) is the sum of diagonal elements and can be computed as:

$$trace(M) = I_x^2 + I_y^2 \tag{10}$$

k is a tunable parameter, it is usually selected from the range [0.04–0.06].

4. Finally, threshold the value of R using threshold value (T) as follows:

$$Decision(R) = \begin{cases} Corner & if\ R > T \\ Non-corner & otherwise \end{cases} \tag{11}$$

3.2.2 Suppression of Non-maximal Corners

In non-maximal suppression, the number of corner points that are generated using Harris method will be reduced to N_{Best} points only. The main reason behind non-maximal suppression step is to reduce the size of CWLD descriptor which in effect speeds up WLD extraction task and increases the efficiency of the resulted model in diagnostics stage. The N_{Best} points are selected using the following steps:

1. For each corner point P(x, y) in the image (I), the fitness value is computed by opening a window of size (5 × 5) around the point and applying the following equation:

$$Fitness(P(x, y)) = \sum_{m=0}^{N_{Ws}} \sum_{n=0}^{N_{Ws}} |I(x, y) - I(x - m, y - n)| \qquad (12)$$

2. The corners are then sorted in ascending order based on their fitness value.
3. The first N_{Best} points which give best fitness values are finally selected and considered as points of interest during WLD extraction stage.

The results of applying Harris corner detection and non-maximal suppression with $N_{Best} = 100$ are shown in Fig. 2 using an example chest X-Ray image.

3.3 WLD Extraction

WLD descriptors, which are introduced by Chen et al. [16] for texture image classification, are used for description the local regions surrounding the selected points of interest. WLD consists of two components: differential excitation and orientation of the gradient. The differential excitation component is the function of the ratio between two terms. The first term is relative intensity differences and the second one is intensity of the current pixel. Orientation of the gradient provides information about the direction of the change in intensity of the current pixel. WLD descriptors are extracted using the following steps:

1. A number of N_{Best} windows with size (N_{Ws} * N_{Ws}) are opened upon the contrast enhanced chest X-Ray image. The positions of these windows are determined based on the coordinates of the final selected points of interest. The coordinates of each point is considered as the centre of the opened window.
2. The differential excitation $\xi(x_c)$ for each pixel within each opened window is computed using the following equation:

$$\xi(x_c) = \arctan\left[\sum_{i=0}^{p-1} \frac{x_i - x_c}{x_c}\right] \qquad (13)$$

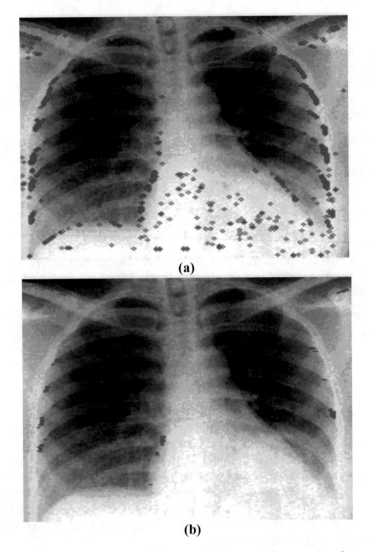

(a)

(b)

Fig. 2 Points of interest localization results, **a** corner detection result, **b** suppression of non-maximal corners

where $x_i(i = 0, 1,..., p - 1)$ denotes the ith neighbour of x_c and p is the number of neighbours.

3. The direction of gradient $\alpha(x_c)$ is computed as:

$$\alpha(x_c) = \tan^{-1}\left[\frac{G_y}{G_x}\right] \qquad (14)$$

where the gradient of the image pixel x_c at location (x, y) is defined as:

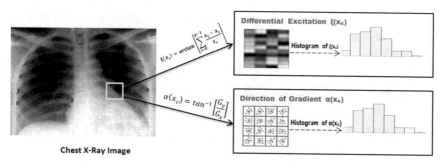

Fig. 3 CWLD extraction process

$$\begin{bmatrix} G_x \\ G_y \end{bmatrix} = \begin{bmatrix} \frac{\partial x_c}{\partial x} \\ \frac{\partial x_c}{\partial y} \end{bmatrix} \tag{15}$$

4. The computed differential excitation and direction of gradients for all pixels are then normalized to be within the range [0–359].
5. For each descriptor, a bin-based histogram is then computed and considered as the WLD descriptor for each corner point. The bin-based histogram is founded by divided the descriptor range [0–359] into equal-size bins (with size = 45). Thus, the size of the resulted histogram (WLD descriptor) for each corner will be equal to 8.
6. Finally, the resulted local WLD are concatenated to form the final CWLD for the given X-Ray image.

Figure 3 demonstrates the process of CWLD extraction process.

3.4 COVID-19 Diagnostics

To determine whether the extracted CWLD is of positive COVID-19 or negative case, two classifiers are utilized which are SVM and DBN. SVM works by building a hyper-plane that separates the positive cases form negative ones [17]. The kernel function of SVM used in the proposed CWLD scheme is the spherical kernel because it is an anisotropic stationary kernel and has positive definite in R^3. Spherical kernel function can be defined as shown in the following equation [18]:

$$k(x, y) = \begin{cases} 1 - \frac{3}{2}\frac{x-y}{\sigma} + \frac{1}{2}\left(\frac{x-y}{\sigma}\right)^3 & if \quad x - y < \sigma \\ 0 & otherwise \end{cases} \tag{16}$$

On the other hand, DBN are formed by the stacked Restricted Boltzmann Machines (RBMs) that perform unsupervised learning. Once a pre-training step is done, network weights are further fine-tuned by propagation the error backward, while the network is treated as a feed-forward net.

4 Experimental Results and Analysis

4.1 Database Description

A dataset contains 51 chest X-Ray images obtained from Kaggle website is used for system evaluation purposes. The dataset involves two classes named positive (with COVID-19) and negative (non-COVID-19). The positive class includes 39 X-Ray images collected from real cases in China, Korea, the USA, Canada, and Taiwan. On the other hand, the negative class includes 12 X-Ray images for patients suffering from MERS, SARS, and ARDS [19].

4.2 Experimental Setup

The proposed CWLD scheme has six tunable parameters: Harris parameter (k), Harris threshold value (T), number of selected corner points (N_{Best}), local window size (N_{Ws}), SVM kernel function sigma (σ), and number of hidden nodes in DBN (H). Based on the extensive experiments, k was obtained as 0.05, T is determined as 10,000,000, the best σ value was chosen as 1.5 and H was within 10 to 12. The effect of N_{Best} and N_{Ws} values on the accuracy of the proposed scheme are studied in the next subsections.

4.3 CWLD Based on Differential Excitation $\xi(x_c)$

The first experiment is conducted using differential excitation as WLD descriptor. Different four values for N_{Ws} and three values of N_{Best} are tested. The achieved accuracy is then computed for each combination of N_{Best} and N_{Ws} values as shown in Tables 1, 2 and 3. Hence, the accuracy is computed using the following equation [20]:

Table 1 Results of using differential excitation descriptor with $N_{Best} = 50$

Classifier	$N_{Ws} = 5$	$N_{Ws} = 9$	$N_{Ws} = 15$	$N_{Ws} = 19$
SVM (%)	94.12	96.08	96.08	96.08
DBN (%)	76.47	88.24	90.02	88.24

Table 2 Results of using differential excitation descriptor with $N_{Best} = 100$

Classifier	$N_{Ws} = 5$	$N_{Ws} = 9$	$N_{Ws} = 15$	$N_{Ws} = 19$
SVM (%)	96.08	92.16	94.12	94.12
DBN (%)	76.47	76.47	76.47	96.08

Table 3 Results of using differential excitation descriptor with $N_{Best} = 150$

Classifier	$N_{Ws} = 5$	$N_{Ws} = 9$	$N_{Ws} = 15$	$N_{Ws} = 19$
SVM (%)	98.04	98.04	98.04	96.08
DBN (%)	76.47	82.35	82.35	92.16

$$Accuracy = \frac{Correct}{Total} \tag{17}$$

where Correct is the number of the samples which are correctly classified into either positive COVID-19 or a negative case, and Total is the total number of samples in the dataset.

As obviously shown in the above tables, the best accuracy is achieved when $N_{Best} = 150$ and $N_{Ws} = 5$ using SVM as a classifier with size of CWLD = N_{Best} (150) × the size of the histogram for each corner (8) = 1200 features.

4.4 CWLD Based on Direction of Gradient $\alpha(x_c)$

Again, as with the differential excitation, four different values for N_{Ws} and three different values for N_{Best} are also attempted and the achieved accuracy is computed as shown in Tables 4, 5 and 6. As it is evident shown in the table, the best accuracy is reached when $N_{Best} = 50$ and $N_{ws} = 9$ using DBN classifier and CWLD size = 400.

Table 4 Results of using direction of gradient descriptor with $N_{Best} = 50$

Classifier	$N_{Ws} = 5$	$N_{Ws} = 9$	$N_{Ws} = 15$	$N_{Ws} = 19$
SVM (%)	96.08	96.08	94.18	94.18
DBN (%)	98.04	100	100	100

Table 5 Results of using direction of gradient descriptor with $N_{Best} = 100$

Classifier	$N_{Ws} = 5$	$N_{Ws} = 9$	$N_{Ws} = 15$	$N_{Ws} = 19$
SVM (%)	96.08	96.08	96.08	96.08
DBN (%)	74.51	74.51	92.16	94.12

Table 6 Results of using direction of gradient descriptor with $N_{Best} = 150$

Classifier	$N_{Ws} = 5$	$N_{Ws} = 9$	$N_{Ws} = 15$	$N_{Ws} = 19$
SVM (%)	96.08	100	100	100
DBN (%)	74.51	76.74	76.74	76.74

Table 7 Results of using combined $\xi(x_c)$ and $\alpha(x_c)$ descriptors with $N_{Best} = 50$

Classifier	$N_{Ws} = 5$	$N_{Ws} = 9$	$N_{Ws} = 15$	$N_{Ws} = 19$
SVM (%)	100	100	100	100
DBN (%)	82.35	86.27	92.16	90.20

Table 8 Results of using combined $\xi(x_c)$ and $\alpha(x_c)$ descriptors with $N_{Best} = 100$

Classifier	$N_{Ws} = 5$	$N_{Ws} = 9$	$N_{Ws} - 15$	$N_{Ws} = 19$
SVM (%)	98.04	96.08	98.04	94.12
DBN (%)	84.31	82.35	86.27	90.20

Table 9 Results of using combined $\xi(x_c)$ and $\alpha(x_c)$ descriptors with $N_{Best} = 150$

Classifier	$N_{Ws} = 5$	$N_{Ws} = 9$	$N_{Ws} = 15$	$N_{Ws} = 19$
SVM (%)	98.04	98.04	98.04	98.04
DBN (%)	80.39	78.43	78.43	78.43

4.5   CWLD Based on Combined $\xi(x_c)$ and $\alpha(x_c)$

The final experiment is conducted to find the effect of combining both differential excitation and direction of gradient on the achieved accuracy for the resulted models of both SVM and DBN classifiers. Tables 7, 8 and 9 show the obtained results for the same N_{Best} and N_{Ws} values used in the previous two experiments. The best accuracy (100%) is achieved when $N_{Best} = 50$ and $N_{Ws} = 5$ using SVM classifier with CWLD size = 800.

4.6   Results Analysis

Figures 4 and 5 illustrate the effect of N_{Best} value on the accuracy of SVM and DBN classifiers, respectively. As shown in Fig. 4, as the value of N_{Best} increases, the accuracy is also increases. This reflects the nature of SVM classifier that can work well with a large descriptor size by finding an optimal hyper-plane that separates the positive cases from the negative ones. In contrast, DBN classifier works in the opposite manner. As shown in Fig. 5, the accuracy decreases as long as the size of

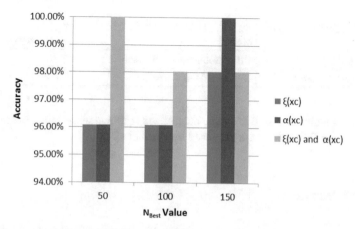

Fig. 4 Effect of N_{Best} value on SVM accuracy

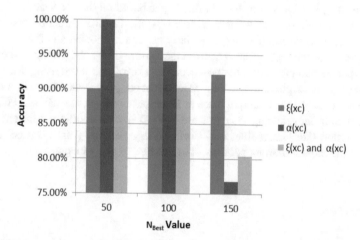

Fig. 5 Effect of N_{Best} value on DBN accuracy

the feature vector increases. This due to the fact that DBN works by finding patterns among the extracted features and this task becomes more complicated as the number of features increase.

4.7 Comparison with Previous Studies

Since the work on this research issue has started in a period not far away from now and the used dataset is newly collected, there are few works that can be used for comparison purpose. Table 10 shows a comparison between the proposed method

Table 10 Results of using combined $\xi(x_c)$ and $\alpha(x_c)$ descriptors with $N_{Best} = 150$

Authors	Method	Accuracy (%)
Farid et al. [8]	CHFS features and SHC classifier	96
The proposed scheme	CWLD and DBN classifier	100

and another study that used the same dataset. As it shown in the table, the proposed scheme outperforms the work proposed by Farid et al. [8].

5 Conclusions

Developing a computer system for COVID-19 diagnostics can improve the early detection rate of the disease and save more humans' life. A scheme for COVID-19 diagnostics has been presented in this paper based on the CT scan of the chest region. The points of interest help in focusing the feature extraction task on the important regions within the image. Weber descriptors showed an effective role in the extraction of the regular patterns from the texture of the chest image. According to the experimental outcomes, the best accuracy (100%) achieved using direction of gradient $\alpha(x_c)$ descriptor and DBN classifier when $N_{Best} = 50$ and $N_{Ws} = 9$. As future work, feature selection techniques such as Principle Component Analysis (PCA) can be used for further reducing the extracted CWLD size. In addition, different image transformation like Gabor filter and Local Binary Patterns (LBP) can be used to highlight the most important patterns in the texture of chest image.

References

1. Singhal, T.: A review of coronavirus disease-2019 (COVID-19). Indian J. Pediatr **87**, 281–286 (2020)
2. Coronavirus Outbreak. https://www.worldometers.info/coronavirus/. Accessed 20 April 2020
3. Li, Y., Xia, L.: Coronavirus disease 2019 (COVID-19): role of chest CT in diagnosis and management. Am. J. Roentgenol. 1–7 (2020)
4. Kooraki, S., Hosseiny, M., Myers, L., Gholamrezanezhad, A.: Coronavirus (COVID-19) outbreak: what the department of radiology should know. J. Am Coll. Radiol. **17**, 1–15 (2020)
5. Jin, Y.H., Cai, L., Cheng, Z.S.: A rapid advice guideline for the diagnosis and treatment of 2019 novel coronavirus (2019-Ncov) Infected Pneumonia (Standard Version). Mil. Med. Res. **7**, 1–23 (2020)
6. Lee, E.Y.P., Ng, M., Khong, P.: COVID-19 pneumonia: what has CT taught Us? Lancet. Infect. Dis. **20**, 384–385 (2020)
7. Huang, P., Liu, T., Huang, L., Liu, H., Lei, M., Xu, W., Hu, X., Chen, J., Liu, B.: Use of chest CT in combination with negative RT-PCR assay for the 2019 novel coronavirus but high clinical suspicion. Radiology **295**, 22–23 (2020)
8. Farid, A.A., Selim, G.I., Khater, H.A.A.: A novel approach of CT images feature analysis and prediction to screen for corona virus disease (COVID-19). Int. J. Sci. Eng. Res. **11**, 11–41 (2020)

9. Xu, X., Jiang, X., MC, Du, P., Li, X., Lv, S., Yu, L., Chen, Y., Su, J., Lang, G., Li, Y., Zhao, H., Xu, K., Ruan, L., Wu, W.: Deep learning system to screen coronavirus disease 2019 Pneumonia. arXiv:2002.09334 [pdf] physics.med-ph cs.LG eess.IV (2019)
10. Zhang, J., Xie, Y., Li, Y., Shen, C., Xia, Y.: COVID-19 screening on chest X-ray images using deep learning based anomaly detection. arXiv:2003.12338 (2020)
11. Elghamrawy, S., Hassanien, A.E.: Diagnosis and Prediction Model for COVID-19 Patient's response to treatment based on convolutional neural networks and whale optimization algorithm using CT images. (2020). medRxiv preprint https://doi.org/10.1101/2020.04.16.20063990
12. Rajinikanth, V., Dey, N., Raj, A.N.J., Hassanien, A.E., Santosh, K.C., Raja, N.S.M.: Harmony-search and otsu based system for coronavirus disease (COVID-19) Detection using lung CT scan images. arXiv preprint arXiv:2004.03431 (2020)
13. Mohammed, S.N., Jabir, A.J., Abbas, Z.A.: Spin-Image Descriptors for Text-Independent Speaker Recognition. In: Saeed, F., Mohammed, F., Gazem, N. (eds) Emerging Trends in Intelligent Computing and Informatics. IRICT 2019. Advances in Intelligent Systems and Computing, vol. 1073. Springer, Cham (2020)
14. Mohammed, S.N., George, L.E.: Illumination—Invariant facial components extraction using adaptive contrast enhancement methods. British J. Appl. Sci. Technol. 12(3), 1–13 (2016)
15. Harris, C., Stephens, M.: A combined corner and edge detector. Proc. Alvey Vision Conf. 23, 1–6 (1988)
16. Chen, J., Shan, S., He, C., Zhao, G., Pietikainen, M., Chen, X., Gao, W.: WLD: a robust local image descriptor. IEEE Trans. Pattern Anal. Mach. Intell. 32, 1705–1720 (2010)
17. Mohammed, S.N., George, L.E., Dawood, H.A.: The effect of classification methods on facial emotion recognition & accuracy. Br. J. Appl. Sci. Technol. 14(4), 1–11 (2016)
18. Boughorbel, S., Tarel, J.P., Fleuret, F., Boujemaa, N.: The GCS kernel for SVM-based image recognition. In: Lecture Notes in Computer Science, Springer, Berlin, Heidelberg (2005)
19. Chest X-Ray database Website. https://www.kaggle.com/bachrr/covid-chest-xray. Accessed 25 Mar 2020
20. Hassan, A.K., Mohammed, S.N.: A novel facial emotion recognition scheme based on graph mining. Defence Technology (In Press) (2019). https://doi.org/10.1016/j.dt.2019.12.006

Why Are Generative Adversarial Networks Vital for Deep Neural Networks? A Case Study on COVID-19 Chest X-Ray Images

M. Y. Shams⊙, O. M. Elzeki⊙, Mohamed Abd Elfattah⊙, T. Medhat⊙, and Aboul Ella Hassanien⊙

Abstract The need to generate large scale datasets from a limited number of determined data is highly required. Deep neural networks (DNN) is one of the most important and effective tools in machine learning (ML) that required large scale datasets. Recently, generative adversarial networks (GAN) is considered as the most potent and effective method for data augmentation. In this chapter, we investigated the importance of using GAN as a preprocessing stage to applied DNN for image data augmentation. Moreover, we present a case study of using GAN networks for a limited COVID-19 X-Ray Chest images. The results indicate that the proposed system based on using GAN-DNN is powerful with minimum loss function for detecting COVID-19 X-Ray Chest images. Stochastic gradient descent (SGD) and Improved Adam (IAdam) optimizers are used during the training process of the COVID-19 X-Ray images, and the evaluation results depend on loss function are determined to ensure the reliability of the proposed GAN architecture.

M. Y. Shams (✉)
Faculty of Artificial Intelligence, Kafrelsheikh University, Kafr Elsheikh 33511, Egypt
e-mail: mahmoud.yasin@ai.kfs.edu.eg

O. M. Elzeki
Faculty of Computers and Information, Mansoura University, Mansoura 35516, Egypt
e-mail: omar_m_elzeki@mans.edu.eg

M. Abd Elfattah
Misr Higher Institute for Commerce and Computers, MET, Mansoura, Egypt
e-mail: mohabdelfatah8@gmail.com

A. E. Hassanien
Faculty of Computers and Artificial Intelligence, Cairo University, Giza, Egypt
e-mail: aboitcairo@fci-cu.edu.eg

T. Medhat
Department of Electrical Engineering, Faculty of Engineering, Kafrelsheikh University, Kafr Elsheikh 33516, Egypt
e-mail: tmedhatm@eng.kfs.edu.eg

© The Editor(s) (if applicable) and The Author(s), under exclusive license to Springer Nature Switzerland AG 2020
A.-E. Hassanien et al. (eds.), *Big Data Analytics and Artificial Intelligence Against COVID-19: Innovation Vision and Approach*, Studies in Big Data 78, https://doi.org/10.1007/978-3-030-55258-9_9

Keywords Deep neural network · Generative adversarial network · Machine learning stochastic gradient descent (SGD) · Improved adam COVID-19 X-ray chest

1 Introduction

Deep Neural Networks (DNN) is inspired by the human biological brain consisting of neurons, synapses, and much more. Artificial neural networks (ANN) are key to building a DNN because they consist of multiple hidden layers stacked. DNN was formulated from hierarchical neural networks to improve the process of classifying supervised patterns [1]. In the process of training DNN, transfer learning is an effective and powerful tool to enable the training of large-scale datasets without over-fitting problem results from the target dataset that is much smaller than the basic dataset [2]. There are many attempts to formulate DNN, for example, multi-layer perceptron (MLP) as well as backpropagation that consists of feed-forward and feedback ANN [3]. DNN can be utilized as a feature extractor and classifier as well. However, to learn one layer of DNN feature vectors at a time, the multiple layers of feature vectors can be used as a starting point for a discriminative that is called the "fine-tuning" phase during which backpropagation through the DNN slightly adjusts the weights found in pre-training [4].

In this chapter, we utilized two different optimizers during the training step for generating COVID-19 X-Ray chest images based on GAN architecture. The first optimizer was the stochastic gradient descent (SGD), and the second was the improved Adam optimizer (IAdam) [5]. The loss function is determined for the two applied optimizers with minimum loss values. The main contribution of this chapter is to enlarge limited datasets to produce augmented COVID-19 X-Ray images with a minimum loss function. On the other hand, we prove the ability of GAN architecture using two both SGD and IAdam optimizers.

The rest of this chapter is organized as background in Sect. 2, which survey using DNN in COVID-19 X-Ray images detection and classifications. Section 3 demonstrates that the proposed methodologies include GAN architecture, SGD, and IAdam optimizers. Finally, the evaluation of experimental results is presented in Sect. 4.

2 Background

At present, researchers in the field of artificial intelligence (AI) are searching and investigating ways to treat this dangerous virus, which grows dramatically and changes a lot of data, which makes it more difficult for researchers to find the appropriate treatment for this virus [6]. The latest report of COVID-19 that updates daily.

AI and machine learning (ML) are considered as the most effective tools that are used to fight COVID-19 virus spread [6]. Rao [7] proposed a conceptual framework of data collection and possible COVID-19 identification. The collected data can be used to assist in the preliminary screening, and early identification of possible COVID-19 infected individuals since the sequence of events suggests that the coronavirus may have been transmitted by the asymptomatic carrier [8]. The incubation period for patient 1 was 19 days, which is long but within the reported range of 0 to 24 days [9].

A survey for Forecasting Coronavirus (COVID-19) Models is proposed by Shinde et al. [10]. This survey illustrates and categorizes several forecasting models available in the literature, challenges of these models, and recommendations for controlling this epidemic.

Pneumonia chest X-Ray detection based on generative adversarial networks (GAN) with a fine-tuned deep transfer learning for a limited dataset for COVID-19 is presented by Khalifa et al. [11]. They used Alexnet, Googlenet, Squeezenet, and Resnet18 were selected as deep transfer learning models with an accuracy reached to 99%. An automated infection detection system based on Computed-Tomography Scan Images of COVID-19 is proposed by Rajinikanth et al. [12] in order to compare the infection based on Infection/Lung pixel ratio.

In this chapter, we attempt to solve some critical issues that are faced by scientists in detecting and classifying COVID-19 X-Ray images. We proposed an algorithm based on Deep Convolutional Neural Networks (DCNN) that classifies the X-Ray image of infected COVID-19 persons. The proposed architecture not only classifies the Infected and uninfected people but also extracts the feature of the X-Ray images that may help extract details for the COVID-19 virus spread. Figure 1 shows the most common and recent types of DNN that is consists of unsupervised, convolutional, recurrent, and recursive neural network.

Fig. 1 The most common types of DNN

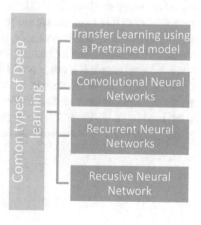

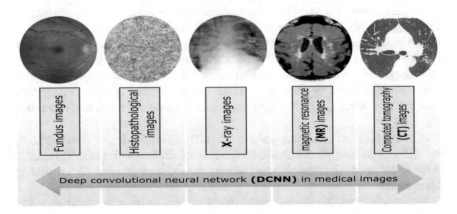

Fig. 2 Examples of DCNN in medical images applications

On the other hand, there are further DNN architecture used, such as deep belief neural networks (DBNN) that are formulated from stacked Restricted Boltzmann machines (RBMs) [13]. Many applications utilized DNN, especially deep convolutional neural networks (DCNN) in medical, healthcare, and biomedical fields, as investigated in Fig. 2.

2.1 Small Data and Augmentation

Generally, some datasets are different in size and shape as well as ways to update and produce them. These datasets in the case they are small in size can be enlarged by using many methods [14]. These methods are called data augmentation. Many researchers in this field are suffering from the problem of searching for data, especially large data. There are methods, such as deep learning methods. In order for these methods to succeed, work efficiently, and to be highly efficient, it is necessary to give them a large database. Thus, people are directed to make augmentation of any data entering any system. Therefore, we will provide a method that benefits researchers to make augmentation of data so that they can deal with it later when it enters into deep learning and solves too many problems such as the problem of overfitting and memo, especially if these databases are imbalanced [15, 16].

2.2 Generative Adversarial Networks

GAN is the network that generally used for data augmentation to estimate generative models via an adversarial process. By which the trained models are simultaneously generated by capturing the data distribution, and the discriminative model for estimating the training data probability [17]. The framework of the GAN can be implemented and summarized, as shown in Fig. 3.

The Generative Adversarial Network (GAN) is a method for the training of generative models, which we briefly describe in the sense of image data. The framework pits two networks against each other: a generative model G that captures the distribution of data and a discriminating model D that distinguishes between samples taken from G and images taken from training data. Adversarial networks have opened up many new directions. Most prominent research in machine learning in the last several years, in the high-dimensional setting (like images), was focused on the discriminative side. At the same time, the need for vast amounts of data has increased as deep learning became common [18, 19].

Another type of data augmentation based on GAN is presented by Radford et al. [18] is called deep convolutional GAN (DCGAN) for unsupervised learning. They replace any pooling layers with stridden convolutions that are called discriminator and the fractional-stride convolutions that are called a generator. Moreover, Makhzani et al. [19] proposed adversarial auto-encoders (AAE) which as an extension to GAN that per-form variational inference for the aggregated posterior of the hidden code vector of the autoencoder with an arbitrary prior distribution. They used AAE for dimensionality reduction of the input features. Information maximizing generative adversarial networks (InfoGAN) is an approach presented by Chen et al. [20]. This approach can learn disentangled representations in a completely unsupervised manner.

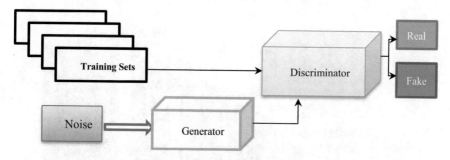

Fig. 3 General framework of generative adversarial network

3   Methodologies

A generated of augmented images are required to improve the architecture of deep neural networks, especially convolutional neural networks (CNN). Due to the limited dataset of the COVID-19 X-Ray images that are maybe imbalance and variable data, we present in this work GAN as an augmentation process. Figure 4 shows the proposed architecture of the generative stage of GAN by which we train CNN to produce augmented images. On the other hand, the discriminator of the GAN architecture takes the 64 × 64 X-Ray COVID-19 image results from the generator and the training sets. This process is typical and inspired by the decoder process in GAN is a discriminator, and the encoder is the generator in the communication channel.

During the augmentation process, two different optimization techniques have been performed, the first is the utilization of SGD optimizer as a preprocessing stage for the GAN entire network, while, the second is based on Adam optimizer. The two optimization techniques are applied to prove the ability of the proposed system to generate and manipulate the COVID-19 X-Ray images. In this section, a brief demonstration of the mentioned optimizers is presented.

3.1   *Stochastic Gradient Decent (SGD) Optimizer*

In SGD in order to minimize the computation time per iteration, an adaptive step size to estimate the most important details of COVID-19 X-Ray images is performed based on the measure of the similarity region in the image content and the transformation model as illustrated by Klein et al. [21]. In this case, the applied images learned by GANs in the training phase can produce a training loss with global minima based

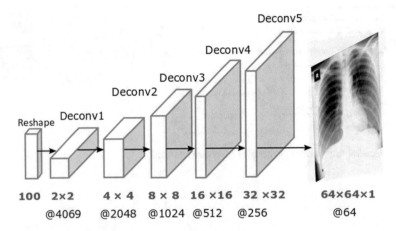

Fig. 4 The proposed generator architecture stage in GAN

on ReLU network. The initialization of SGD produces a sequence of iterations inside a small perturbation region that is around the initial centred weights as investigated by Zou et al. [22]. In this chapter, we present SGD for the trained X-Ray images in normal and COVID-19 cases. The weights are updated on each training images, and there is no need to perform the batch operation as a whole like in GD. The computational time of SGD is lower than traditional GD because the training process does not execute through the whole training set to update the weights. On the other hand, the SGD minimizes loss faster and produce noisy and variation accuracy and loss. In order to overcome the limitation of SGD, we utilized an adaptive momentum estimation (Adam) optimizer as investigated in the forthcoming section.

3.2 Improved Adam Optimizer

The non-convex nature of the optimization problem, as well as the need to design a powerful and reliable deep neural network, are a significant challenge, especially for the systems that require faster performance [23]. Bock et al. [24] proposed an improvement of Adam optimizer based on adaptive step size by changing the weights and momentum to attain the convergence of the applied neural networks. Moreover, Bock and WeiB [25] prove that Adam has a local convergence and posterior boundary for the hyper-parameters of the applied network. Not only, determining the local convergence in Adam helpful for optimization but also the improvement in the speed of convergence is required to achieve the minimum loss function. However, on the other hand, it will require more memory with a high complexity [26]. Therefore, in this work, we used the normalized preserving Adam algorithm presented by Zhang [5], IAdam. To maintain the gradient direction for each weight vector and produce more accurate weight decay with a minimum elapsed time.

3.3 Training and Generating the GAN

For building a GAN model to generate X-ray images, first, we need to build the structures of the network, including the layers of the generator unit and discriminator unit.

Algorithm 1: Build a GAN model to generate X-Ray images

Input ← Dicremenartor_layers **discLay,** generator_layers **genLay,** hyper-parameters **opts,** sample_images **imgSet**	

Output ← **GAN**

1.	Begin
2.	env ← setup(**opts**)
3.	**gen ← NNbuild(genLay)**
4.	**disc ← NNbuild(discLay)**
5.	For e=1: **env.Epoch**
6.	m ← **rnd(num(imgSet))**
7.	For i=1: **env.NBatch**
8.	imgs ← **read(imgSet,m)**
9.	gen ← **train(imgs,nosie)**
10.	// Optimize Generator using Adam optimizer instead of standard SGD
11.	gen ← **adamOptimizer(gen,disc,imgFakes)**
12.	disc ← **train(imgs,nosie,imgFakes)**
13.	// Optimize Generator using IAdam optimizer instead of standard SGD
14.	disc ← **adamOptimizer(gen,disc,imgFakes)**
15.	// Calculate C-Loss & D-Loss
16.	C_loss ← **sigmoid_cross_entropy**(expected,actual)
17.	D_loss ← **sigmoid_cross_entropy**(expected,actual,c_loss)
18.	End for
19.	End for
20.	**GAN ← {gen,disc}**
21.	End

Next, we specify the different values of the hyper-parameters as training options including epochs, iterations, batch size and learning rates. Algorithm 1 represents the pseudocode algorithm for training and building the GAN model to generate X-Ray images based on understanding the given sample image dataset. The algorithm starts by setting up the environment options and training options. Next, the generator and discriminator models are initially constructed with initial weights randomly are setting up. The training process starts using sample images of the given dataset per epoch. During the same epoch, the training process repeats for every batch in the dataset doing the subsequent procedures. These procedures include loading the sample images, training the generator and optimize the learned generator using the Adam optimizer or the standard SGD. Also, these procedures include training the discriminator and optimize its behaviour using the same listed optimizers recently. Finally, the training procedures adjust the weights according to the hybrid activation function that is powered by sigmoid and cross-entropy function. The training process is repetitive for a specified number of iterations. The algorithm is customized and enhanced using the IAdam optimizer.

Table 1 Hyperparameter values of the proposed GAN architecture

Parameter	Value
Batch size	16
Iteration	100
Learning rate	0.001
Optimizer name	SGD and Adam

4 Experimental Results: Discussion and Analysis

Of course, for natural images, GANs do not currently generate very realistic images, but this work has sparked interest in generative models for natural images and has sort of created a new subarea in deep learning, which many research groups today are actively looking for it. So, algorithms that can make and generate data themselves can handle our real-world problems more efficiently.

The main objective of this section is to summarize and provide detailed results of the proposed architectures such that in order to enlarge the training data, we augmented the data using GANs by which the new examples learned from data is generated.

4.1 Dataset Description and Experiments Setup

In this chapter, we used COVID-19 X-ray image collections that were established in [27], which contain 50 images, 25 normal and the other 25 are COVID-19 states. Data sets are enlarged based on the GAN architecture. The images generated are 1000 images that result in a 20-fold GAN increase from 50 images. All experiments were performed using the software package (MATLAB 2020a), using a PC with the following features Core i7, 16-RAM. The hyper-parameters are shown in Table 1 during all experiments.

4.2 Experiments Scenarios

Two different experiments are carried out to compare the proposed approaches. The first experiment is powered by SGD optimizer, while the second experiment based on Improved Adam optimizer. In this chapter, the mean value of the trained images was subtracted from each image fed into GANs. The evaluation is based on two loss function, which is called C-Loss and D-Loss. The C-Loss is the cross-entropy loss and in some cases named as a logarithmic loss. In this type of loss, the predicted probability is compared to the output value (0 or 1), and the result is calculated based on the distance from the expected value. The Cross-entropy for the predicted class prediction is calculated as the average cross-entropy across all examples. Furthermore, the second type of measurement in this chapter is the D-Loss which is the generator loss. Such that each generator tries to maximize this function and attempts to maximize the discriminator's output for its instances.

4.2.1 First Experiment: Optimizing Using SGD Algorithm

Using the standard optimizer SGD generates the loss rates already visualized in Fig. 5 representing the C-loss and D-Loss. Based on the analytical investigation and visual inspection, we noticed the increment of C loss function and on the opposite side D loss decrease. The notice can be justified due to the cross-entropy of the input images which produce an enhancement at the same time in the D loss. The contradiction of loss rate in C loss and D loss leads to optimizer enhancement problem. The histogram of both C loss and D loss is shown in Figs. 6 and 7 respectively. In the histogram, the x-axis represents the loss value, and the y-axis represents the frequency value. Since the total number of iterations was 100 iterations, every frequency is less than

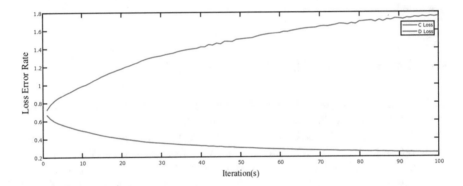

Fig. 5 C-loss versus D-loss in SGD

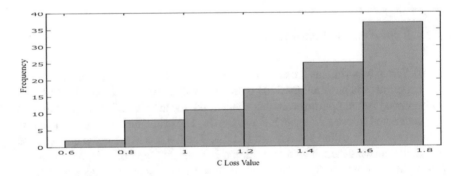

Fig. 6 Histogram of C-loss value

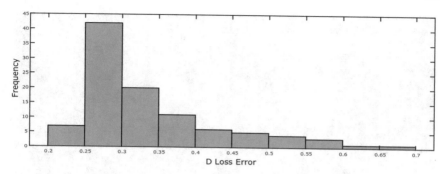

Fig. 7 Histogram of D-loss value

or equal to 100 per loss value. In Fig. 6, the error rates of C loss are binned into six bins each bin has 0.2 as the next step of the previous bin. The binning starts at 0.6 and ends at 1.8. So, the minimum error of C loss is 0.6, and the maximum error of C loss is 1.8. From Fig. 6 the C loss reaches up to 1.6, with a 35 as the frequency, which means C loss is higher using SGD optimizer. On the other hand, the error rates of D loss are binned into ten bins each bin has 0.05 as the next step of the previous bin. The binning starts at 0.2 and ends at 0.7. So, the minimum error of D loss is 0.2, and the maximum error of D loss is 0.7. From Fig. 7, the D loss scored loss rate in [0.25, 0.3) with a 40 as the frequency which leads to the compatibility of the discriminator with SGD optimizer. The first experiment represents the research gab that motivates us to improve using Adam optimizer is helpful for us to determine which optimizer we need. In turn, the second experiment based on Adam optimizer to boost and ensure the accuracy of the proposed architecture. Figure 8 represents a montage of the generated samples for the proposed GAN architecture based on the SGD optimizer.

4.2.2 Second Experiment: Optimizing Using Adam Algorithm

As mentioned in Sect. 3.2, Adam optimizer is utilized for evaluating both C and D losses. Instead of evaluating the gradient of the current position as performed in the SGD, we used Adam optimizer to maintain the gradient direction for each weight vector. Figure 9 represents the comparative analysis of C loss verse the D loss of the proposed GAN using Adam optimizer. After 15 iterations, we noticed the harmony of loss rates where can be considered tightly reduced over iterations progressive. The Adam optimizer enhances the performance through auto-adjusting of the weights over the iteration progress in the early stage of training. The Adam optimizer tolerates the C loss rate almost in the third iteration to be correlated with D loss. In the same manner, histograms are shown in Figs. 10 and 11 for evaluating the error rates verse the frequencies.

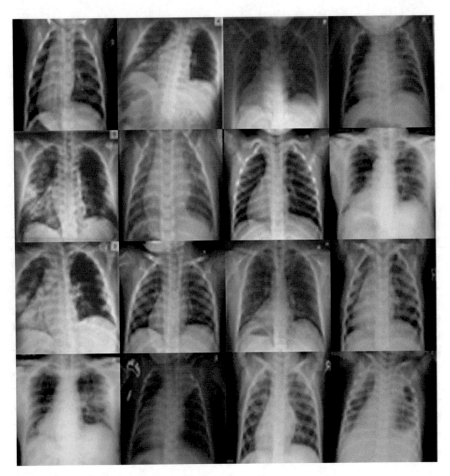

Fig. 8 Sample of generated images using SGD optimizer in GAN architecture

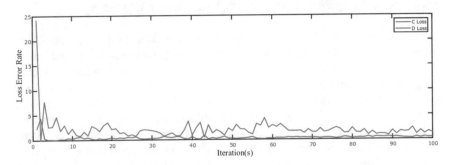

Fig. 9 C-loss vs D-loss in Adam

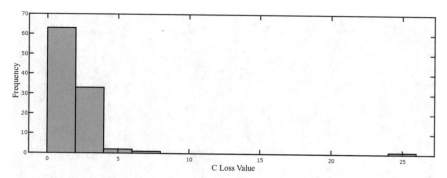

Fig. 10 Histogram of C-loss value

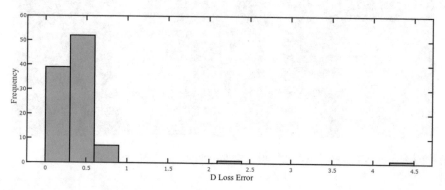

Fig. 11 Histogram of D-loss value

In Fig. 10, the error rates of C loss are binned into five bins each bin has 2.0 as the next step of the previous bin. The binning starts at 0.0 and ends at 26.0. So, the minimum error of C loss is 0.0, and the maximum error of C loss is 26.0. From Fig. 10 the C loss reaches up to 2, with a 65 as the frequency and up to 4 with a 31 as the frequency, which means most of C loss is enclosed between **[0,4)** with 96 as frequent of total 100 using Adam optimizer. On the other hand, the error rates of D loss are binned into five bins each bin has <0.25 as the next step of the previous bin. The binning starts at 0.0 and ends at 4.5. So, the minimum error of D loss is 0.0, and the maximum error of D loss is 4.5.

From Fig. 11, the D loss scored a loss rate in **[0.0, 0.80)** with a 93 as the frequency, which leads to higher compatibility of the discriminator with Adam optimizer. We used the proposed GAN architecture with Adam optimizer to generate montage of the generated samples in Fig. 12. In turn, we can conclude the following points;

- Adam optimizer is better than the SGD optimizer, in enhancing the C-Loss and D-Loss together for X-ray images, especially for COVID-19 according to the case study.

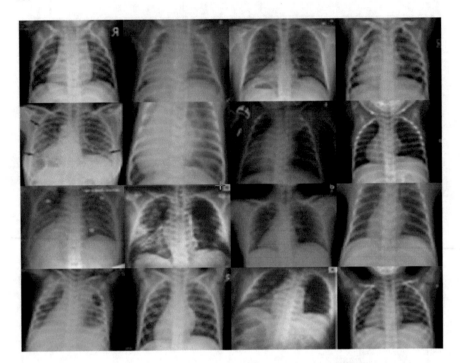

Fig. 12 Sample of generated images using Adam optimizer in GAN architecture

- The pros of Adam optimizer depend on considering the bias, learning rate, and heuristic of the weights verse the learning rate only as SGD behaves.
- We believe that this approach can be generalized to solve and classify other medical classification applications for the improvement of diagnosis.

5 Conclusions

Generative adversarial network (GAN) is proved to be a very effective model for training Generative models. There are several reasons that GANs are essential for deep neural networks DNN: First, a generative model for natural images that evolve to generate more and more realistic looking data, because of the coupling with an adversarial network. Secondly, in principle, when you do not have enough data for understanding a problem, GANs can be used to generate more data rather than using tricks like data augmentation. A GAN architecture is proposed, using two different optimizers. The first is based on the SGD optimizer by which the trained images are evaluated by using both C loss and D loss. An increase of C loss occurred in the SGD optimizer. Therefore, Improved Adam optimizer is utilized as a second experiment used to enhance the results of SGD. The proposed architecture is promising and can be utilized in other medical applications especially in the image processing field. In the future, we plan to use a Region of interest feature extractor instead of the whole image in order to extract more details for medical images.

References

1. Ciregan, D., Meier, U., Schmidhuber, J.: Multi-column deep neural networks for image classification. In: 2012 IEEE Conference on Computer Vision and Pattern Recognition, pp. 3642–3649. IEEE (2012)
2. Yosinski, J., Clune, J., Bengio, Y., Lipson, H.: How transferable are features in deep neural networks?. In: Advances in Neural Information Processing Systems, pp. 3320–3328 (2014)
3. Hinton, G., Deng, L., Yu, D., Dahl, G.E., Mohamed, A.-R., Jaitly, N., Senior, A. et al.: Deep neural networks for acoustic modeling in speech recognition: the shared views of four research groups. IEEE Signal Processing Magazine, Vol. 29, No. 6, pp. 82–97 (2012)
4. Hinton, G.E., Salakhutdinov, R.: Reducing the dimensionality of data with neural networks. Science **313**(5786), 504–507 (2006)
5. Zhang, Z.: Improved Adam optimizer for deep neural networks. In: 2018 IEEE/ACM 26th International Symposium on Quality of Service (IWQoS), pp. 1–2. IEEE (2018)
6. Alimadadi, A., Aryal, S., Manandhar, I., Munroe, P.B., Joe, B., Cheng, X.: Artificial intelligence and machine learning to fight COVID-19, pp. 200–202 (2020)
7. Rao, A.S.S., Vazquez, J.A.: Identification of COVID-19 can be quicker through artificial intelligence framework using a mobile phone–based survey when cities and towns are under quarantine. Infection Control Hospital Epidemiology **41.7**, 826–830 (2020)
8. Bai, Y., Yao, L., Wei, T., Tian, F., Jin, D.-Y., Chen, L., Wang, M.: Presumed asymptomatic carrier transmission of COVID-19. JAMA **323**(14), 1406–1407 (2020)
9. Guan, W.-J., Ni, Z.-Y., Hu, Y., Liang, W.-H., Ou, C.-Q., He, J.-X., Liu, L. et al.: Clinical characteristics of 2019 novel coronavirus infection in China. MedRxiv (2020)
10. Mahalle, P., Kalamkar, A.B., Dey, N., Chaki, J., Shinde, G.R.: Forecasting models for coronavirus (covid-19): a survey of the state-of-the-art (2020)
11. Khalifa, N.E.M., Taha, M.H.N., Hassanien, A.E., Elghamrawy, S.: Detection of coronavirus (COVID-19) associated pneumonia based on generative adversarial networks and a fine-tuned deep transfer learning model using chest X-ray dataset. arXiv preprint: arXiv:2004.01184 (2020)
12. Rajinikanth, V., Dey, N., Raj, A.N.J., Hassanien, A.E., Santosh, K.C., Raja, N.: Harmony-search and otsu based system for coronavirus disease (COVID-19) detection using lung CT scan images. arXiv preprint: arXiv:2004.03431 (2020)
13. Shams, M.Y., Sarhan, S.H., Tolba, A.S.: Adaptive Deep Learning Vector Quantisation for Multimodal Authentication, Vol. 8, No. 3, pp. 702–722 (2017)
14. Mun, S., Park, S., Han, D.K., Ko, H.: Generative adversarial network based acoustic scene training set augmentation and selection using SVM hyper-plane. In: Proc. DCASE, pp. 93–97 (2017)
15. Salehinejad, H., Valaee, S., Dowdell, T., Colak, E., Barfett, J.: Generalization of deep neural networks for chest pathology classification in x-rays using generative adversarial networks. In: 2018 IEEE International Conference on Acoustics, Speech and Signal Processing (ICASSP), pp. 990–994. IEEE (2018)
16. Shamsolmoali, P., Zareapoor, M., Shen, L., Sadka, A.H., Yang, J.: Imbalanced Data Learning by Minority Class Augmentation using Capsule Adversarial Networks. arXiv preprint arXiv: 2004.02182 (2020)
17. Mirza, M., Osindero, S.: Conditional Generative Adversarial Nets. arXiv preprint arXiv:1411.1784 (2014)

18. Radford, A., Metz, L., Chintala, S.: Unsupervised Representation Learning with Deep Convolutional Generative Adversarial Networks. arXiv preprint arXiv:1511.06434 (2015)
19. Makhzani, A., Shlens, J., Jaitly, N., Goodfellow, I., Frey, B.: Adversarial autoencoders. arXiv preprint arXiv:1511.05644 (2015)
20. Chen, X., Duan, Y., Houthooft, R., Schulman, J., Sutskever, I., Abbeel, P.: Infogan: interpretable representation learning by information maximizing generative adversarial nets. In: Advances in Neural Information Processing Systems, pp. 2172–2180 (2016)
21. Klein, S., Pluim, J.P.W., Staring, M., Viergever, M.A.: Adaptive stochastic gradient descent optimization for image registration. Int. J. Comput. Vis. **81**(3), 227 (2009)
22. Zou, D., Cao, Y., Zhou, D., Gu, Q.: Stochastic gradient descent optimizes over-parameterized deep relu networks. arXiv preprint arXiv:1811.08888 (2018)
23. Bello, I., Zoph, B., Vasudevan, V., Le, Q.V.: Neural optimizer search with reinforcement learning. In: Proceedings of the 34th International Conference on Machine Learning, vol. 70, pp. 459–468. JMLR.org (2017)
24. Bock, S., Goppold, J., Weiß, M.: An improvement of the convergence proof of the ADAM-optimizer. arXiv preprint arXiv:1804.10587 (2018)
25. Bock, S., Weiß, M.: A proof of local convergence for the Adam optimizer. In: 2019 International Joint Conference on Neural Networks (IJCNN), pp. 1–8. IEEE (2019)
26. Tato, A., Nkambou, R.: Improving Adam Optimizer (2018)
27. https://github.com/smfai200/Detecting-COVID-19-in-X-ray-images/tree/master/dataset. Accessed in 21 May 2020

Artificial Intelligence (AI) Against COVID-19

Artificial Intelligence Against COVID-19: A Meta-analysis of Current Research

Khalid Raza

Abstract The epidemic of coronavirus disease 2019 (COVID-19) has posed an unprecedented challenge before humankind, with more than 3.2 million confirmed cases and death toll to more than 225 thousand till the end of April, 2020 globally. Currently, one-half of the world is under lockdown and complying with social distancing to arrest its spread. Does the COVID-19 crisis illustrate the necessity for solid artificial intelligence (AI) and machine learning (ML) strategy? AI and ML research groups across the world are extensively working to tackle various aspects of the COVID-19 crisis including epidemiological (e.g. prediction, controlling and forecasting viral dynamics), molecular studies and drug development (e.g. molecular modeling and drug targets identification), medical (e.g. AI-enable diagnostic and treatment), and socio-economical applications (e.g. economical impact forecasting and mitigation). In the last few months, several research papers have been published with AI applications against COVID-19. In this chapter, we performed a meta-analysis of the current state-of-the-art of AI against COVID-19 by using various publication repositories (PubMed, PubMed Central, Scopus, Google Scholar) and preprint servers (bioRxiv, medRxiv, arXiv). This meta-analysis helps the researcher to understand the broad spectrum of AI to combat COVID-19.

Keywords Coronavirus · SARS-CoV-2 · 2019-nCoV · Machine learning · Meta-analysis

1 Introduction

Coronavirus disease 2019 (COVID-19) outbreak has been declared as a pandemic by the WHO on 11th March, 2020. This lethal viral disease has created a public health emergency around the globe, affecting almost 210 countries with more than 3.2 million positive cases, and mortality toll to more than 225 thousand reported

K. Raza (✉)
Department of Computer Science, Jamia Millia Islamia, New Delhi 110025, India
e-mail: kraza@jmi.ac.in

© The Editor(s) (if applicable) and The Author(s), under exclusive license
to Springer Nature Switzerland AG 2020
A.-E. Hassanien et al. (eds.), *Big Data Analytics and Artificial Intelligence*
Against COVID-19: Innovation Vision and Approach, Studies in Big Data 78,
https://doi.org/10.1007/978-3-030-55258-9_10

till the end of April 2020, globally. Although the epic center of this viral disease is Wuhan city of China, it has mostly affected other developed countries including the USA, Spain, Italy, France, UK, Germany, Turkey, Russia, Iran, India, and so on. It has thrown an unprecedented challenge before humankind, leading to shut down half of the world complying social distancing to arrest its spread.

COVID-19 is caused by the severe acute respiratory syndrome coronavirus-2 (SARS-CoV-2), one of the recent and novel strains of coronavirus which is transmitted by inhalation or contact with infected droplets or fomites and whose incubation period ranges from 2 to 14 days [1, 2]. The overall fatality rate of COVID-19 is estimated between 3 and 4% with a major threat to both the elderly population and people with compromised medical conditions. The coronavirus family includes pathogens of both animal species and humans. Scientists and researchers are restlessly working to decode this lethal virus, trying hard to understand its replication, pathogenesis to understand the preference of coronaviruses to switch between species, to identify significant reservoirs of coronaviruses which will dramatically help to prognosticate when and where such viral epidemics may occur. A systematic review that highlights COVID-19 virus genomic composition, pathogenesis, symptomatology, diagnosis and prognosis, mathematical models of viral dynamics can be found in Qazi et al. [1].

Artificial Intelligence (AI) is a powerful tool to fight against COVID-19 pandemic, allowing the application of machine learning, natural language processing, machine vision, and automation and robotics to develop computer-based models for the prediction, pattern recognition, forecasting, explanation, and optimization. AI and data science researchers are scrambling to utilize these methods to predict (epidemic), recognize (diagnose), forecast (future spread dynamics), explain (treat), and optimize (socio-economic impacts) COVID-19 infections. The meta-analysis of current research trends of AI to fight against COVID-19 is not carried out yet. In this paper, we attempt to review recent trends of AI applications to fight against COVID-19 using various indexing and abstracting databases such as PubMed, PubMed Central, Scopus, Google Scholars, and preprints servers such as bioRxiv, medRxiv, and arXiv preprints server. This meta-analysis is not an assessment of the quality of publications, rather a quantitative look at recent publication trends. This meta-analysis will help the COVID-19 researchers to find the areas where AI techniques are prominently applied, and where are the research gaps that need to be addressed.

2   Meta-Analysis

2.1   Journal Database Search

We considered PubMed, PubMed Central (PMC), Scopus, and Google Scholar indexing databases, and bioRxiv, medRxiv, and arXiv preprints server for our meta-analysis of AI against COVID-19 research. The reason for including the preprints

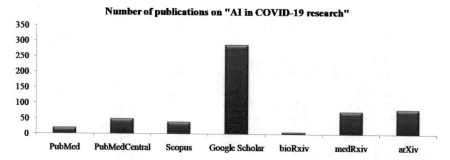

Fig. 1 The number of publications on AI against COVID-19 in various considered journal indexing databases for period 01-01-2020 to 15-04-2020

server in the analysis is that there are several research articles posted on these servers for faster dissemination but are under review with some of the journals. We applied a search strategy with the query string "artificial intelligence" occurring either in the title, abstract or full text, AND keyword either "COVID-19" OR "coronavirus" OR "SARS-COV-2" OR "2019-nCoV" occurring in the title, and publication duration was set from 01/01/2020 to 15/04/2020. This search strategy was applied for all the considered journal indexing databases. As Google Scholar does not provide advance searching facility, therefore we utilized Publish or Perish 7 tool [3] for advance search and filter. The number of publications found in these databases is shown in Fig. 1. Google Scholar has the highest publication (count = 288) among these because it indexes almost all the Journals, Conferences, Pre-Prints including PubMed, PMC, Scopus, bioRxiv, medRxiv arXiv, and others. After manual curation of these publications, we filtered 288 publications showing AI applications in the various aspects of COVID-19 research. Hence, we considered publications found in Google Scholar for our further analysis.

2.2 Publication Profiling

The selected 288 publications showing the application of AI in various aspects of COVID-19 research were profiled based on their application areas. These publications were clustered into 13 groups (or groups) as shown in Table 1 (shown in descending order of the number of publications). The distribution of these publications in percent is shown in Fig. 2 (Pie-chart).

Table 1 Publication profiling in the various aspects of COVID-19 research

S.No.	Application area	Number of publications
1.	Diagnosis and prediction	70
2.	Epidemiology (viral forecasting, control and spread dynamics)	60
3.	Reviews (including advisory, comment, correspondence, editorial, news, guidelines, public awareness)	48
4.	Radiological image analysis	47
5.	Drug design and treatment	22
6.	Governance, economy and affairs	9
7.	Social network analysis	8
8.	Others (health monitoring, surveillance, etc.)	6
9.	Commerce and business	4
10.	Survival and health risk prediction	4
11.	Education and training	4
12.	Text analytics/NLP	3
13.	Molecular and protein disorder	3

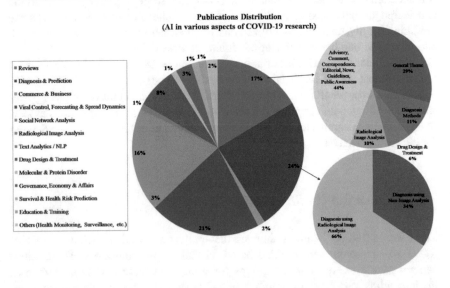

Fig. 2 Distribution of publications on AI application on various aspects of COVID-19 research. The number of reviews and diagnosis and prediction publications is further classified in the subsequent pie chart

3 AI in Various Aspects of COVID-19 Research

AI technologies cannot replace human intelligence, but they are very helpful in COVID-19 patient diagnosis, forecasting, mitigating and controlling the outbreak, disinfecting areas, assisting in the development of therapeutics and treatment, healthcare management, business and commerce, better governance and policymaking, and so on. In this section, some of the prominent areas of applications of AI in COVID-19 research are highlighted.

3.1 *AI in Diagnosis and Prediction of COVID-19*

The laboratory methods to diagnose COVID-19 infection are real-time reverse transcription-polymerase chain reaction (rRT-PCR), isothermal nucleic acid amplification, serology, and radiological images. The rRT-PCR and isothermal nucleic acid amplification are based on nasopharyngeal swab or sputum sample which detects antibodies in response to infection. The serology test is still under the development stage, and recently it has been approved by various authorities (FDA-USA, ICMR-India) as a rapid diagnostic test that gives results in 10–20 min. Further, enzyme-linked immunosorbent assay (ELISA) tests give results in 1–5 h [4]. Radiological images such as x-ray and CT scans are also useful to diagnosis COVID-19 [5]. One of the major challenges of COVID-19 diagnosis is the availability of its testing kits and required reagents. Although rRT-PCR-based diagnosis method is the most commonly available, it is also very sensitive, on the other hand, serological tests measure the amount of proteins/antibodies responding to infection. These diagnosis methods are costly, time-consuming, and available in limited laboratories. Hence, there is a need for an alternative diagnostic method to detect COVID-19 infections faster and at a cheaper cost.

AI and deep learning deemed to be a powerful tool in assisting COVID-19 diagnosis, treatment and decision making. There are several machine learning and deep learning-based models proposed to diagnose COVID-19 cases using clinical symptoms and radiological images. To identify COVID-19 cases faster and automated, an AI-based framework was proposed using a mobile phone-based survey [6]. As far as the diagnosis and prediction is concerned, literature reports a large number of AI-based methods for radiological images such as x-ray [6, 7], CT-scan [8–12], deploying a wide range of machine learning and deep learning. A recent systematic review on the diagnosis and prognosis of COVID-19 can be found in [13–16]. The development of automated AI-based models to detect, diagnose and predict COVID-19 infections for a bigger population is still an open research problem.

3.2   AI in Epidemiology (Viral Forecasting, Control and Spread Dynamics)

Forecasting and prediction of the COVID-19 spread are valuable inputs for government, public health authorities, companies, and people to plan, prepare and manage the pandemic. In order to forecast and predict the spread of COVID-19 disease over time and space, AI techniques can be utilized. A machine learning-based model may be trained with the available outbreak and demographic data to predict its spread. However, due to the lack of data and too much outlier and noisy data, AI-based forecasts of viral spread are not yet very accurate and reliable [17]. Hence, most of the models used to track and forecast COVID-19 outbreak uses epidemiological models, such as SIR (Susceptible, Infected, and Removed) [18, 19], SEIR (Susceptible, Exposed, Infected, and Recovered [20, 21], SIRD (Susceptible, Infected, Recovered, Dead) [22]; extended SIR model incorporating time-varying quarantine protocols such as government-level macro isolation policies and community-level micro inspection measures [23]; ARIMA (Auto-Regressive Integrated Moving Average Model) model [24]. The scope of this section is to focus on AI-based approaches.

Some of the AI-based models reported in the literature are interior search algorithm and multi-layer feedforward ANN to forecast COVID-19 infections [25]; modified stacked auto-encoder for transmission dynamics [26]; non-linear hybrid cellular automata classifier to predict affected, recovered and deaths [27]; agent-based artificial intelligence simulation platform (EnerPol) to predict growth and containment strategy [28]; multi-input deep CNN to predict cumulative number of confirm cases [29]; topological autoencoder to generate similarity map of transmission dynamics [30]; SEIR-SD (with social distancing) model with Differential Evolution as parameter estimator to forecast viral spread dynamics [31]; Polynomial Regression (PR), Support Vector Regression (SVR), Long Short Term Memory (LSTM) network, and deep feedforward neural network to forecast transmission [32]; Bayesian estimation for the logistic growth model to estimate the viral spread [33]; modified SEIR-LSTM model to predict epidemic peaks and sizes [34], and hybridized deep learning and fuzzy rule induction method for epidemic forecasting using incomplete or limited data in early epidemic Composite Monte-Carlo simulation [35]. As more epidemic data are available, the performance of these models will improve. Although, these models play a greater role in clinical diagnosis, optimizing various strategies and critical decision making, however, the next step may be to estimate whether the second wave of COVID-19 will hit China [36] or other suffered country.

3.3   AI in the Molecular Study, Drug Design, and Treatment of COVID-19

Molecular biology and AI have emerged as an interdisciplinary subject of research. Modern molecular biology needs the support of advanced software in tackling complex biological problems, analyzing and interpreting data that remain unresolved in typical laboratory practices. The motivation behind AI research is the hope that their algorithms would provide a fresh outlook on many complex biological problems. Machine learning methods and deep learning, in particular, have been applied for molecular design, simulation, modeling, and drug development. These can contribute to combat the current COVID-19 pandemic, assist in identifying leads for therapies and vaccines, suggesting potential inhibitors, finding structural effects on genetic variation in virus, and so on [37]. Our meta-analysis reported in this article states almost 25 publications showing the application of AI in the molecular study, drug design, and treatment of COVID-19. The random forest machine learning technique has been used to predict infection risk and monitor the evolutionary dynamics of COVID-19 [38]. The data of spike protein sequences of 2666 coronaviruses was used. There were 7 clusters human coronaviruses found namely, 229E, NL63, OC43, HKU1, MERS-CoV, SARS-CoV, and SARS-CoV-2. It was observed that the cluster for SARS-CoV-2 is very close SARS-CoV, hence suggesting that both viruses have the same human receptor [38]. Prediction of protein structures of COVID-19 usually take months by the traditional approach, therefore, Google DeepMind has developed a deep learning system, called AlphaFold [39], which has released predicted protein structures that may serve as valuable information vaccine design [40].

To date, there is no effective and efficient drug exist in order to treat COVID-19 patients, hence an effective and efficient therapeutic is immediately required for the treatment of growing COVID-19 patients globally. Due to the lengthy process of new drug development, drug repurposing is one of the faster solutions adapted to treat COVID-19 infected patients. However, long term drug development objectives are to identify inhibitors aimed to target replication processes associated with this disease, and inhibiting key coronavirus proteins, and what could serve as starting points for drug development [41]. AI has been applied in several studies to develop a therapeutic strategy and drug design for COVID-19. Savioli [42] reports that Heptad Repeat 1 (HR1) domain on the glycosylated spike (S) protein is the region having less mutability, therefore it is an encouraging target for new inhibitors. Savioli [42] trained a Siamese Neural Network (SNN) with a whole 2019-nCoV protein sequence and found knowledge of peptide linkage among virus protein structure. A large number of peptides were tested towards the specific region HR1 of 2019-nCoV exhibiting a good affinity between peptidyl-prolyl cis-transisomerase (PPlase) peptide and HR1 that may open new horizons of research. Chenthamarakshan et al. [43] proposed a deep learning generative model framework, called CogMol, to design drug candidates specific to a given target protein sequence. This model was applied to three 2019-nCoV proteins, namely non-structural protein 9 (NSP9) replicase, main protease, and receptor-binding domain (RBD) of the S protein. Batra et al. [44] applied a machine learning and high-fidelity ensemble docking for rapid screening of possible therapeutic molecules from millions of compounds, based on binding affinity to either S protein at its host receptor region or S protein-human ACE2 interface complex. Beck et al. [45] applied a pre-training deep learning-based drug-target interaction model, known as Molecular Transformer-Drug Target Interaction (MT-DTI), to repurpose drugs and found that atazanavir (an antiviral used to treat HIV) is showing a good inhibitory potency against 2019-nCoV 3C-like proteinase, followed by remdesivir, efavirenz, ritonavir, and dolutegravir. Further, their prediction also shows that several antiviral agents, including Kaletra (lopinavir/ritonavir), may also bind to the replication complex components of 2019-nCoV with acceptable inhibitory potency. Some of the other AI and machine learning assisted drug repurposing was carried out by [46, 47].

The repurposing of known approved drugs, including ritonavir, lopinavir, etc., are not very effective in treating COVID-19. Hence, it is an essential and immediate need to find novel chemical compound against this deadly virus. Tang et al. [48] developed an advanced deep Q-learning network with fragment-based drug design (ADQN-FBDD) to generate potential lead compounds that target 3CL of 2019-nCoV. They reported 47 lead compounds fully generated from the ADQN-FBDD model accessible from the author's molecular library (https://github.com/tbwxmu/2019-nCov). A deep learning-based drug development framework has been developed to produce novel drug-like compounds [49]. Some of the reviews and discussions addressing AI-assisted drug development for COVID-19 can be found in [50, 51].

3.4 AI in Commerce, Business, Governance, Education and Training

The epidemic of COVID-19 has greatly impacted commerce, business, governance, education and training globally. This deadly virus has badly affected the people in particular and society at large. The people have been stacked out of the states and are unable to return to their homes due to lockdown. A country like India where around 73 million people come under the extreme poverty line is the daily wager workers who depend on their daily income. They don't have space to live and not enough food to survive this pandemic. This epidemic has slowed down economic activities around the world. Most of the airports have been sealed, local public transport has been fully suspended, and hence export and import, business and commerce have been impacted. Also, educational institutions, tourism industries, hospitality services, entertainment industries, shopping malls, the textile industry, have been stopped which had badly affected the employment and economy. Global financial markets are already facing serious downfall in trading—pushing the economy into a financial shock.

AI can play a vital role in fighting the economical crisis, commerce, and business, education and training, governance and policymaking in this pandemic situation. E-commerce companies are applying AI for supply chain management [52], planning and procurement, production, and marketing [53]. The integration of AI in e-commerce not only helps in gaining competitive benefits in the online market but also boosts sales and customer satisfaction. AI has potential applications in marketing, including sales forecasting, Chatbots as personal assistants, identifying the trends, AI-powered business market, and improved digital advertising [54, 55].

As far as education and training are concerned, AI-assisted education and training is a growing field, called *Educational Intelligence*. It is defined as *"leveraging data at multiple points across the student lifecycle to make intelligent decisions to positively impact students' outcomes"* [56]. AI technologies are useful to develop and imitate human reasoning and decision-making in the teaching-learning model. AI is employed for adaptive education systems within e-learning, including massive open online courses (MOOCs), educational data mining, and learner analytics [57]. Some of the education intelligence platforms are Questa (https://www.novatia.com/home-questa), Cognii (https://www.cognii.com/), and Kidaptive (https://www.kidaptive.com/) that uses AI help education institutions collect data and increase learning engagement. Other AI-assisted educational and training tools are *Knewton* (https://www.knewton.com/), *Querium* (http://querium.com/), *Century Tech* (https://www.century.tech/) and *Volley* (https://volley.com/). Knewton is an adaptive learning technology that helps in identifying gaps in a student's knowledge and assigns suitable coursework. Querium provides customization tutorials and exercises by using AI. Century Tech platform provides personalized learning plans, reducing workloads for instructors by using cognitive neuroscience and data analytics. Similarly, Volley synthesizes course and quiz results by using AI-based knowledge-engine and helps in finding knowledge gaps among the employees.

4 Conclusion

Coronavirus disease 2019 (COVID-19) epidemic touched almost every corner of the globe. This lethal viral disease has greatly impacted the social life of the people, leading to acute economical, financial, food and health-related crises. It has put an unprecedented challenge before humankind, leading to shut down half of the world's countries complying with the social distancing to arrest its spread. It is caused by the severe acute respiratory syndrome coronavirus-2 (SARS-CoV-2), which is transmitted by inhalation or contact with infected droplets or fomites. The overall fatality rate of COVID-19 is estimated between 3 and 4% with a major threat to both the elderly population and people with compromised medical conditions. Artificial Intelligence (AI) is a powerful tool to fight against COVID-19 pandemic, allowing the application of machine learning, natural language processing, machine vision, and automation and robotics to develop computer-based models for the prediction, pattern recognition, forecasting, explanation and optimization, drug development and understanding the molecular mechanism of SARS-CoV-2 virus. AI and data science researchers are scrambling to utilize these methods to predict (epidemic), recognize (diagnose), forecast (future spread dynamics), explain (treat), and optimize (socio-economic impacts) COVID-19 infections. This article presents a meta-analysis of state-of-the-art AI applications against COVID-19, highlights four major areas of applications: (i) diagnosis and prediction, (ii) epidemiology (viral forecasting, control, and spread dynamics), (iii) molecular study, drug design and treatment and (iv) commerce, business, governance, education and training.

References

1. Qazi, S., Sheikh, K., Faheem, M., Khan, A., Raza, K.: A Coadunation of Biological and Mathematical Perspectives on the Pandemic COVID-19: A Review. Preprints, 2020040007 (2020) (https://doi.org/10.20944/preprints202004.0007.v1)
2. Huang, C., Wang, Y., Cheng, Z.: Clinical features of patients infected with 2019 novel coronavirus in Wuhan, China. Lancet 395(10223), 497–506 (2020). https://doi.org/10.1016/s0140-6736(20)30183-5
3. Harzing, A.W.: Publish or perish, available from https://harzing.com/resources/publish-or-perish (2007)
4. Sheridan, C.: Coronavirus and the race to distribute reliable diagnostics. Nat. Biotechnol. 38(4), 382 (2020)
5. Lee, E.Y., Ng, M.Y., Khong, P.L.: COVID-19 pneumonia: what has CT taught us? Lancet. Infect. Dis. 20(4), 384–385 (2020)
6. Apostolopoulos, I.D., Mpesiana, T.A.: Covid-19: automatic detection from x-ray images utilizing transfer learning with convolutional neural networks. Phys. Eng. Sci. Med. 1 (2020)
7. Narin, A., Kaya, C., Pamuk, Z.: Automatic Detection of Coronavirus Disease (COVID-19) Using X-ray Images and deep convolutional neural networks. arXiv preprint arXiv:2003.10849 (2020)
8. Li, L., Qin, L., Xu, Z., Yin, Y., Wang, X., Kong, B., et al.: Artificial intelligence distinguishes covid-19 from community acquired pneumonia on chest ct. Radiology, 200905 (2020)
9. Zhang, Z., Shen, Y., Wang, H., Zhao, L., Hu, D.: High-resolution computed tomographic imaging disclosing COVID-19 pneumonia: a powerful tool in diagnosis. J. Infect. (2020)
10. Ye, Z., Zhang, Y., Wang, Y., Huang, Z., Song, B.: Chest CT manifestations of new coronavirus disease 2019 (COVID-19): a pictorial review. Eur. Radiol. 1–9 (2020)
11. ELGhamrawy, S.M.: Diagnosis and Prediction Model for COVID19 Patients Response to Treatment based on Convolutional Neural Networks and Whale Optimization Algorithm Using CT Images. medRxiv (2020)
12. Rajinikanth, V., Dey, N., Raj, A.N.J., Hassanien, A.E., Santosh, K.C., Raja, N.: Harmony-Search and Otsu based System for Coronavirus Disease (COVID-19) Detection using Lung CT Scan Images. arXiv preprint arXiv:2004.03431 (2020)
13. Li, Y., Xia, L.: Coronavirus disease 2019 (COVID-19): role of chest CT in diagnosis and management. Am. J. Roentgenol. 1–7 (2020)
14. Salehi, S., Abedi, A., Balakrishnan, S., Gholamrezanezhad, A.: Coronavirus disease 2019 (COVID-19): a systematic review of imaging findings in 919 patients. Am. J. Roentgenol. 1–7 (2020)
15. Wynants, L., Van Calster, B., Bonten, M.M., Collins, G.S., Debray, T.P., De Vos, M., Schuit, E.: Prediction models for diagnosis and prognosis of covid-19 infection: systematic review and critical appraisal. BMJ 369 (2020)
16. Shi, F., Wang, J., Shi, J., Wu, Z., Wang, Q., Tang, Z., Shen, D.: Review of Artificial Intelligence Techniques in Imaging Data Acquisition, Segmentation And Diagnosis for covid-19. arXiv preprint arXiv:2004.02731 (2020)
17. Elmousalami, H.H., Hassanien, A.E.: Day Level Forecasting for Coronavirus Disease (COVID-19) Spread: Analysis, Modeling and Recommendations. arXiv preprint arXiv:2003.07778 (2020)
18. Biswas, K., Khaleque, A., Sen, P.: Covid-19 Spread: Reproduction of Data and Prediction Using a SIR Model on Euclidean Network. arXiv preprint arXiv:2003.07063 (2020)
19. Atkeson, A.: What Will Be the Economic Impact of COVID-19 in the US? Rough Estimates of Disease Scenarios (No. w26867). National Bureau of Economic Research (2020)
20. Prem, K., Liu, Y., Russell, T.W., Kucharski, A.J., Eggo, R.M., Davies, N., Abbott, S.: The effect of control strategies to reduce social mixing on outcomes of the COVID-19 epidemic in Wuhan, China: a modelling study. Lancet Publ. Health (2020)
21. Peng, L., Yang, W., Zhang, D., Zhuge, C., Hong, L.: Epidemic Analysis of COVID-19 in China by Dynamical Modeling. arXiv preprint arXiv:2002.06563 (2020)

22. Fanelli, D., Piazza, F.: Analysis and forecast of COVID-19 spreading in China, Italy and France. Chaos Solitons Fractals **134**, 109761 (2020)
23. Song, P.X., Wang, L., Zhou, Y., He, J., Zhu, B., Wang, F., Eisenberg, M.: An Epidemiological Forecast Model and Software Assessing Interventions on COVID-19 Epidemic in China. medRxiv (2020)
24. Gupta, R., Pal, S.K.: Trend Analysis and Forecasting of COVID-19 Outbreak in India. medRxiv (2020)
25. Rizk-Allah, R.M., Hassanien, A.E.: COVID-19 Forecasting Based on an Improved Interior Search Algorithm and Multi-layer Feed Forward Neural Network. arXiv preprint arXiv:2004.05960 (2020)
26. Hu, Z., Ge, Q., Jin, L., Xiong, M.: Artificial Intelligence Forecasting of Covid-19 in China. arXiv preprint arXiv:2002.07112 (2020)
27. Pokkuluri, K.S.: A Novel Cellular Automata Classifier for COVID-19 Prediction. J. Health Sci. (2020)
28. Abhari, R.S., Marini, M., Chokani, N.: COVID-19 Epidemic in Switzerland: Growth Prediction and Containment Strategy Using Artificial Intelligence and Big Data. medRxiv (2020)
29. Huang, C.J., Chen, Y.H., Ma, Y., Kuo, P.H.: Multiple-Input Deep Convolutional Neural Network Model for COVID-19 Forecasting in China. medRxiv (2020)
30. Hartono, P.: Generating Similarity Map for COVID-19 Transmission Dynamics with Topological Autoencoder. arXiv preprint arXiv:2004.01481 (2020)
31. De Falco, I., Della Cioppa, A., Scafuri, U., Tarantino, E.: Coronavirus Covid-19 Spreading in Italy: Optimizing an Epidemiological Model with Dynamic Social Distancing Through Differential Evolution. arXiv preprint arXiv:2004.00553 (2020)
32. Punn, N.S., Sonbhadra, S.K., Agarwal, S.: COVID-19 Epidemic Analysis using Machine Learning and Deep Learning Algorithms. medRxiv (2020)
33. Bliznashki, S.: A Bayesian Logistic Growth Model for the Spread of COVID-19 in New York. medRxiv (2020)
34. Yang, Z., Zeng, Z., Wang, K., Wong, S.S., Liang, W., Zanin, M., et al.: Modified SEIR and AI Prediction of the Epidemics Trend of COVID-19 in China Under Public Health Interventions. J. Thoracic Dis. **12**(3), 165 (2020)
35. Fong, S.J., Li, G., Dey, N., Crespo, R. G., Herrera-Viedma, E.: Composite Monte Carlo decision making under high uncertainty of novel coronavirus epidemic using hybridized deep learning and fuzzy rule induction. Appl. Soft Comput. 106282 (2020)
36. Jia, Z., Lu, Z.: Modelling COVID-19 transmission: from data to intervention. Lancet Infect. Dis. (2020)
37. Amaro, R.E., Mulholland, A.J.: A community letter regarding sharing bimolecular simulation data for COVID-19. J. Chem. Inf. Model. https://www.doi.org/10.1021/acs.jcim.0c00319 (2020)
38. Qiang, X.L., Xu, P., Fang, G., Liu, W.B., Kou, Z.: Using the spike protein feature to predict infection risk and monitor the evolutionary dynamic of coronavirus. Infect. Dis. Poverty **9**(1), 33 (2020)
39. Senior, A.W., Evans, R., Jumper, J., Kirkpatrick, J., Sifre, L., Green, T., Qin, C., Žídek, A., Nelson, A.W.R., Bridgland, A., Penedones, H., Petersen, S., Simonyan, K., Crossan, S., Kohli, P., Jones, D.T., Silver, D., Kavukcuoglu, K., Hassabis, D.: Improved protein structure prediction using potentials from deep learning. Nature **577**, 706–710
40. Alimadadi, A., Aryal, S., Manandhar, I., Munroe, P.B., Joe, B., Cheng, X.: Artificial intelligence and machine learning to fight COVID-19. Physiol. Genomics **52**(4), 200–202 (2020)
41. Liu, C., Zhou, Q., Li, Y., Garner, L.V., Watkins, S.P., Carter, L.J., Albaiu, D.: Research and development on therapeutic agents and vaccines for COVID-19 and related human coronavirus diseases (2020)
42. Savioli, N.: One-Shot Screening of Potential Peptide Ligands on HR1 Domain in COVID-19 Glycosylated Spike (S) Protein with Deep Siamese Network. arXiv preprint arXiv:2004.02136 (2020)

43. Chenthamarakshan, V., Das, P., Padhi, I., Strobelt, H., Lim, K. W., Hoover, B., Mojsilovic, A.: Target-Specific and Selective Drug Design for COVID-19 Using Deep Generative Models. arXiv preprint arXiv:2004.01215 (2020)

44. Batra, R., Chan, H., Kamath, G., Ramprasad, R., Cherukara, M.J., Sankaranarayanan, S.: Screening of Therapeutic Agents for COVID-19 using Machine Learning and Ensemble Docking Simulations. arXiv preprint arXiv:2004.03766 (2020)

45. Beck, B.R., Shin, B., Choi, Y., Park, S., Kang, K.: Predicting commercially available antiviral drugs that may act on the novel coronavirus (SARS-CoV-2) through a drug-target interaction deep learning model. Comput. Struct. Biotechnol. J. **18**, 784–790 (2020)

46. Mahapatra, S., Nath, P., Chatterjee, M., Das, N., Kalita, D., Roy, P., Satapathi, S.: Repurposing Therapeutics for COVID-19: Rapid Prediction of Commercially Available Drugs Through Machine Learning and Docking. medRxiv (2020)

47. Kim, J., Cha, Y., Kolitz, S., Funt, J., Escalante Chong, R., Barrett, S., Kaufman, H.: Advanced Bioinformatics Rapidly Identifies Existing Therapeutics for Patients with Coronavirus Disease-2019 (COVID-19). ChemRxiv. Preprint (2020)

48. Tang, B., He, F., Liu, D., Fang, M., Wu, Z., Xu, D.: AI-Aided Design of Novel Targeted Covalent Inhibitors Against SARS-CoV-2. bioRxiv (2020)

49. Zhavoronkov, A., Aladinskiy, V., Zhebrak, A., Zagribelnyy, B., Terentiev, V., Bezrukov, D.S., Polykovskiy, D., Shayakhmetov, R., Filimonov, A., Orekhov, P.: Potential COVID-2019 3C-like protease inhibitors designed using generative deep learning approaches. Insilico. Med. Hong Kong Ltd. A **307**, E1 (2020)

50. Ho, D.: Addressing COVID-19 drug development with artificial intelligence. Adv. Intell. Syst. https://doi.org/10.1002/aisy.202000070

51. Ge, Y., Tian, T., Huang, S., Wan, F., Li, J., Li, S., Cheng, L.: A Data-Driven Drug Repositioning Framework Discovered a Potential Therapeutic Agent Targeting COVID-19. bioRxiv (2020)

52. Ivanov, D.: Predicting the impacts of epidemic outbreaks on global supply chains: a simulation-based analysis on the coronavirus outbreak (COVID-19/SARS-CoV-2) case. Transp. Res. Part E Logistics Transp. Rev. **136**, 101922 (2020)

53. Naudé, W.: Artificial intelligence against COVID-19: an early review. Towards Data Sci. (2020)

54. Chaudhary, K.: How AI Can Become a Powerful Marketing Tool to Mitigate Economic Impacts of COVID-19. YourStory. https://yourstory.com/2020/04/ai-powerful-marketing-tool-mitigate-economic-impacts-covid-19. Accessed on 20 April 2020

55. Wu, M.: Can AI Help Us Build a More Resilient Economy in the Face of COVID-19? CMS Wire, 19 March 2020

56. Woolf, M.: Educational Intelligence Should Be in Your Vocabulary. Technology Research, Encoura, 8 Sept 2015. https://encoura.org/educational-intelligence-vocabulary/. Accessed on 20 April 2020 (2015)

57. Colchester, K., Hagras, H., Alghazzawi, D., Aldabbagh, G.: A survey of artificial intelligence techniques employed for adaptive educational systems within e-learning platforms. J. Artif. Intell. Soft Comput. Res. **7**(1), 47–64 (2017)

Insights of Artificial Intelligence to Stop Spread of COVID-19

Abu Sufian, Dharm Singh Jat, and Anuradha Banerjee

Abstract COVID-19, a pandemic that has pushed down human civilization in a severe threat. As viruses of COVID-19 like diseases are transferable from human to human, so it becomes very challenging to stop spreading these pandemics. These challenges are not only limited to the treatment of infected patients but also maintaining systematic social distancing to stop spreading the disease. However, maintaining social distancing is not entirely possible everywhere, like in hospitals, emergency sectors, etc. Some critical issues such as: carefully handling the Intensive Care Unite (ICU), patient care, hygienic practice, and systematic social distancing have become very necessary to slow down the spread of the new virus as appropriate vaccines or drugs are not yet available. In this time of crisis, Artificial Intelligence (AI) could assists in many more ways in addition to assisting diagnosis, drug or vaccine discovery. Therefore, this AI, especially algorithms of machine learning, deep learning, and computer vision along with edge computing and IoT technologies could be smart solutions for such challenges. This chapter brings such solutions through some insights of AI to assist to stop these COVID-19 like pandemics.

Keywords AI · Computer vision · COVID-19 · Deep learning · Edge computing · IoT · Sars-cov-2 pandemic

A. Sufian (✉)
University of Gour Banga, Malda, India
e-mail: sufian.csa@gmail.com

D. S. Jat
Namibia University of Science and Technology, Windhoek, Namibia
e-mail: dsingh@nust.na

A. Banerjee
Kalyani Government Engineering College, Kalyani, India
e-mail: anuradhabanerjee@acm.org

© The Editor(s) (if applicable) and The Author(s), under exclusive license to Springer Nature Switzerland AG 2020
A.-E. Hassanien et al. (eds.), *Big Data Analytics and Artificial Intelligence Against COVID-19: Innovation Vision and Approach*, Studies in Big Data 78, https://doi.org/10.1007/978-3-030-55258-9_11

1   Introduction

A novel influenza corona-virus named 'SARS-CoV-2' is the reason for COVID-19 deceases [1]. Presently over 23 millions people are infected, and over 800 thousands died throughout the world and are increasing this pandemic rapidly. As it was spreading very fast globally since it's first appearance Dec 2019 the World Health Organization(WHO) declared it a 'Pandemic' [2]. To cope with such unexpected pandemic, researchers from all over the world are trying hard to invent vaccines, drugs, equipment, forecasting models, etc. [3–5]. As viruses of COVID-19 like diseases are transferable from human to human, so it becomes very challenging to mitigate [6]. These challenges are not only limited to patient handling, treatment, and care but also maintaining systematic social distancing to stop spreading of COVID-19 [7]. However, maintaining social distancing is not entirely possible everywhere, like in hospitals, emergency sectors, etc. Some critical issues such as: carefully monitoring ICU room, patient care, monitoring hygienic practice and systematic social distancing have become very necessary to slow down the spread of the new virus as appropriate vaccines or drugs are not yet available [8].

Therefore, in this situation, we could be benefited from Artificial Intelligence (AI), as AI could do many more things in addition to assisting to diagnose and drug or vaccine discovery. These days AI has become popular mainly based on the recent success of machine learning, deep learning, and big data, and these are very successful in computer vision tasks [9]. Therefore, these AI techniques along with other technologies such as IoT, edge computing, data science, and sensor network could deliver possible smart solutions for cope with such challenges and stop spreading this deadly COVID-19 like pandemics. This chapter brings some insights thought of AI for assisting to mitigate some challenges mentioned above. This chapter also described brief relevant technical backgrounds and literature review of some current state-of-the-art. The main contribution of the chapter are:

- Describe some selective insights of AI to assist in stopping COVID-19.
- A review of some recent state-of-the-art that related these insights for knowing the recent trends of this area.
- Four critical areas where outbreaks are mostly affected are described with possible solutions through these insights thought of AI.
- Briefly described a possible future scope.

The rest of the chapter is organizing as follows: In Sect. 2, a brief technical background is described. A review of some recent state-of-the-art is done in Sect. 3. In Sect. 4, some insight into AI to stop spreading this kind of pandemic is described. Finally, the conclusion and future scope are mentioned in Sect. 5.

2 Brief Technical Backgrounds

Artificial Intelligence (AI) is one of the greatest inventions despite some drawbacks in the modern era for Information and Communications Technology based intelligent automation. Although the journey had begun in the 1950s, but it has been gaining popularity for the last two decades [10]. The recent development of innovative algorithms, computing devices, and big datasets are the main driving force of this recent progress [9]. This section briefly describes four insights sub-areas of Artificial Intelligence which are relevant to the discussion topic of this chapter as below.

2.1 Deep Learning:

Deep Learning is an Artificial Neural Network-based Machine Learning model under the domain of AI [11]. After the success of a Convolutional Neural Networks(CNN) based model [12] called AlexNet [13], deep learning become a popular machine learning paradigm in modern-era. It was the first successful deep learning-based model in computer vision for the image classification tasks. After that, many improvements come in the domain of this deep learning [14].

Deep learning is a learning model based on multi-layer neural networks that capable of extracting features from data without features engineering. It is trained using a backpropagation algorithm [15] and an optimizer (such as Stochastic Gradient Descent, ReLu, etc.) using a labeled dataset. There are many varieties of learning models such as Convolutional Neural Network (CNN), Recurrent Neural networks(RNN), Long short-term memory (LSTM), Boltzmann Machine, Encoder decoder, Generative Adversarial Neural Networks(GAN), etc [11]. In Fig. 1 a typical CNN based deep learning pipeline is shown, where a trained CNN has used to draw an inference of input X-ray image to find COVID-19 pneumonia or not.

In the time of the COVID-19 crisis, deep learning can assist in many ways [16]. It can classify chest X-ray images to detect COVID-19 pneumonia, such as the study [17] have proposed a Convolutional Neural Network-based model. This model assists screening COVID-19 pneumonia, influenza pneumonia, or no infection in present

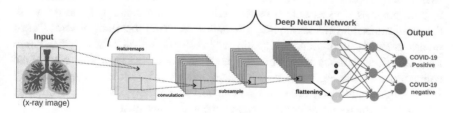

Fig. 1 A typical deep learning model to classify X-ray images to find COVID-19 pneumonia

in a chest X-ray image. In another study [18], a deep learning-based drug selection search have proposed where the model could assist to drug discovery system. A deep learning based forecasting model proposed in a study [19]. This model has tried give a forecast of spreading of COVID-19 pattern and possible resources requirement which are mentioned that study. In addition to these types of works, deep learning can assist in other critical tasks such as patient monitoring and care, social distancing, hygienic practice monitoring, etc. Among them four selective critical areas as mentioned are main focus of this chapter and these are discussed in Sect. 4.

2.2 Computer Vision

Computer Vision is a sub-area of AI which gives powers to a machine to see inside of an image. Computer vision is changing human life by assisting them in various ways. Through computer vision algorithms machine could classify images [20], segmentation of an image [21] and detect objects within an image [22]. With computer vision, we can process thousands of image frames at once and assist humans to their do jobs a better, faster, and automated way. Computer vision has various applications in multiple domains including medical image analysis, self-driving care, remote sensing, crowd management, and many more.

In the COVID-19 outbreak, computer vision could assist many ways including assisting to diagnose, patient monitoring, automated systematic social distance monitoring, etc, to control this pandemic [23]. It can do many remote sensing work using webcam, drone, IoT, etc which made them powerful and widely used for such challenges. Computer Vision with machine learning and deep learning has huge potentialities to mitigate any pandemic or epidemic, some of which are described in section 4.

2.3 IoT or Edge Device

Now we are living in the era of the Internet of Things, in short IoT, as it works at the site of the environment, so it may be called edge device. IoT is a system where many numbers of small to large devices with embedded sensors connected to each other as well as with a server and work as a system. The sensors sense the environment and collect required data and send it for processing or some time it processes locally through edge computing which also described in the next subsection [24]. IoT devices along with wireless sensor networks, 5G networks, edge-cloud computing are reducing human efforts with efficiency [25]. The idea of IoT is highly interdisciplinary in nature because it assembled a wide variety of sensors, computing, protocols, applications, disciplines, etc. in one umbrella called IoT.

IoT is the end device that may work on-site, so it shall assist many ways to cope with this pandemic [26]. With many sensors, IoT can collect all running details within its footprint then transmit with the help of sensor networks. Therefore, COVID-19 related activity also could be easily monitored through IoT and Edge Computing. In a study [27] Li Bai et.al have proposed the IoT-aided diagnosis and treatment of COVID-19. In their IoT-based intelligent diagnosis and treatment assistant program, they mentioned better diagnosis and treatment of COVID-19 patients with different doctors. This chapter mentioned four critical areas for COVID-19 disease which are also get benefit by this technology is discussed in Sect. 4.

2.4 Edge Computing

Computing is the main backbone to make required inference automatically from the data sensed by IoT or edge devices. As edge devices have very limited computing resources, so, cloud computing or sometimes fog computing may be required. But such an edge-cloud scenario, latency, privacy, and security become a huge problem [28]. Therefore, edge computing, a computing methodology where most of the computing will perform near to the devices, has made them powerful and widely used [29, 30]. Edge computing sometimes said it 'fog computing' although technically it is different, but both are pushed computing near to edge devices. A typical Edge-Fog-Cloud hierarchical dependency is shown in Fig. 2.

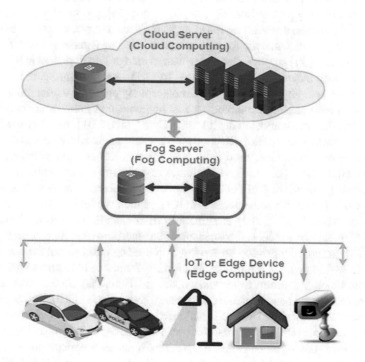

Fig. 2 Cloud, fog and edge computing and relationships

Privacy and security of data of COVID-19 disease as other health data is a very challenging issue. In addition, latency in computing is also a problem. Therefore, to cope with these challenges, edge computing shall be useful [31]. This edge computing along with other AI technique shall assist to mitigate this COVID-19. Some glimpses of these technologies in perspective some critical areas are mentioned in Sect. 4.

3 Review of Some Recent State-of-the-Arts

After the success of AlexNet [13], a lot of machine learning researchers and practitioner has been switched to deep learning areas [14]. This deep learning is very successful in the computer vision area, as a result, many working algorithms and models successively developed [32]. These deep learning and computer vision techniques when merging with edge computing, then many application areas open up such as through drone, IoT, web camera-based applications, etc. Therefore, in this COVID-19 like pandemics, such combined AI techniques would be beneficial. This section reviewed some recent state-of-the-arts works which are related to four critical areas that are mentioned in Sect. 4 through the technologies mentioned in Sect. 2.

In a study Deep Eye-CU (DECU) [33], proposed a pose and motion summarization model in ICU. DECU combines multimodal Hidden Markov Models, extracted frames from multiple sources, and features from multiview multimodal data to monitor the motion of a patient in ICU. The pilot work [34], proposed a non-intrusive computer vision-based system for tracking people's hand hygienic activity in hospitals. This study spatial analytic to analyze human movement patterns to monitor this practice. A study [35] propose a breathing pattern recognition of patient in ICU using computer vision technique. That work used RGB-D camera to the spatial coverage of patients without physical interfering. Another study proposed a pilot model using AI and pervasive sensing technology for autonomous and granular monitoring of patients and the environment in the Intensive Care Unit (ICU) [36]. They used computer vision tasks such as: face detection and recognition, facial action unit detection and expression recognition, head pose detection and recognition, sound and light level detection, and other activity detection. A research multi-view multi-modal systems for sleep monitoring of patients [37]. Sleeping position is very vital for the recovery of a patient for some diseases in ICU, so their model has concentrated this kind of detection in ICU. They used three RGB-D cameras to capture visual data. The Hidden Markov Model and pose recognition algorithm used for processing. The study [38], proposed a privacy-preserving action recognition model for smart hospitals. They first degrade the resolution of video frames to hide privacy then used computer vision algorithms to recognized actions. Here, they used a privet trained model to recognized hand hygienic practice and other actions in ICU. In [39], a work proposed a 3D-Point Cloud-Based Visual Prediction for ICU activities. Their model combines multiple sensors depth data to form a single 3D-point cloud and then used a neural network-based computer vision algorithm. A research work proposed an edge-based deep learning model through IoT for healthcare systems used the cloud to the edge computing model and try to used CNN for classifications [40]. In a study [41], image segmentation technique for Neonatal ICU is described. They used a transfer learning approach to use a trained CNN to process video overhead RGB-D camera. A research study proposed to monitoring patients and visitors based on instance image segmentation [42]. Each instance of ICU is quantified by Mask-RCNN [21] model.

A Pervasive Sensing and Deep Learning-based ICU patient monitoring strategy proposed in [43]. They used many sensors including a camera to capture patient activities and the environment in ICU. A further study used deep learning to understand posture, gesture, facial expression and many more to reduce the burden of nurses and staff. Another research proposed a deep learning-based patient mobilization activity in ICU [44]. Here, the work used 67% data of 98,801 video frames for training a computer vision algorithm. The data are capture in a hospital using seven depth sensors from walls with hiding the privacy of patients. They classified 563 instances in ICU and patient. The study [45], proposed a 3D body pose estimation of a patient from pressure imaging. In that pressure sensor image-based approach they used deep learning to retrieve human poses. In a patent work [46] designed a framework to measure all the major activities in an ICU room. That non-invasive sensor-based works can do Person Localization, Patient Identification, Patient Pose Classification, and Context Detection, Motion Analysis, and Mobility Classification. IRIS [47], an AI model for continuous monitoring and caretaker in the ICU was proposed. That model simultaneously monitors many activities in ICU including ECG electrode, intracranial pressure, etc. Another research proposed an automated hand hygiene monitoring based on CNN [48]. That work used the transfer learning approach to classify region of interest of an image to classify whether a person rubbing his/her hand or doing other actions. A study [49], proposed a model to human activity from video sequence data captured by UAV. In that two-phase model, authors initially trained a CNN to recognized human or non-human which is the first phase. The inference phase, the second phase of the model, detect human and it's activity. The classification of their model maybe in per video frame or entire video sequences.

From this review of the recent state-of-the-art, it could be drawn a conclusion that some critical areas including those four of Sect. 4 of COVID-19 pandemic could be handled in a smart and automated way. Some insights of AI techniques used in the above state-of-arts including those which are mentioned in Sect. 2 could assist to build a resistance to stop spreading COVID-19 pandemic.

4 Some Critical Areas Through AI to Stop Spreading COVID-19

In COVID-19 like pandemics, where vaccine or proper drugs are not available on the right of the moment, stopping the spread is the primary actions that need to be taken. The virus of COVID-19 is 'SARS-CoV-2' which is transferring from human to human through the human droplet. Therefore, finding critical areas and sectors where risk is more to be infected is essential. Mainly the hospital sector, quarantine center, crowded public places are the hot-spot among many. So, interaction with infected persons with non-infected persons needs to be handle carefully and try to be reduced in these hot-spots. Besides that, maintaining systematic social distancing and hygienic practice also becomes necessary. This section brings some AI-based thoughts in mainly four areas which are: monitoring ICU room, patient care, hygienic practice, and monitoring social distancing. These are briefly described in the following subsections in the focus of how AI can assist to mitigate COVID-19 like pandemics in those areas.

4.1 Monitoring Intensive Care Unit (ICU) with AI Technologies

ICU is a critical area that is necessary to treat a severe patient. On the other side, this is one of the hot-spot, may spread this COVID-19 to the important persons who are most essential like doctors and nurses if sufficient protection is not taken. Here, AI can assist to monitor ICU room in a non-intrusive manner, so that physical human interaction may be reduced. Monitoring the ICU room does not mean just a person looking through CCTV or Webcam; instead, it beyond that. There could be many sensors including cameras which would play as a receptor. These receptors shall capture or sensed every running detail in an ICU room, including patient activities. These data will process by an edge computing model with or without the help of for and cloud computing to make inferences. Then according to the inference respective doctors or nurses will decide required actions.

Section 3 mentioned some recent proposed AI techniques for these issues in general. Among them, edge computing-based are most useful [29, 40]. In Fig. 3 an Edge-Fog-Cloud computing-based working model has shown. Here, an ICU room embedded with many IoT or Edge devices, and these devices continuously sense the ICU to collect visual, non-visual data of running environment including activities of patients. These data are processed by an edge, fog, and cloud in tandem based on AI algorithms. These algorithms could be based on machine learning, deep learning including transfer learning which makes many inferences including clustering, classification, object detection and segmentation in image, activity recognition, facial expression recognition, and many more. Based on these inference required actions could be taken. Therefore, through this AI-based practice risk of doctors and nurses are reduces being infected.

Fig. 3 Edge-Fog-Cloud based ICU monitoring

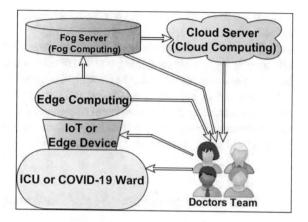

4.2 Patient Care with AI Assistant

Recent progress in robotics technology is very fast. Many intelligent robots are applying as pilot trials, some are already using in real cases including the medical sector [47]. Many studies and experiments are already undergoing that how robots could assist medical practice including robotic surgery [50]. A robot could assist in many ways in this pandemic situation including COVID-19 patient handling, care, etc [51]. Recently a news report mentioned that robots are taking care of COVID-19 patients.[1] With those motivations, we shall see many robots will be in action for such kind of works very soon. Patient care could be done based on AI as ICU monitoring but here robots could be more useful [52]. These robots need to be intelligent enough to assist a doctor or nurses to care for patients of COVID-19 like diseases quickly and safely. AI will play a huge role to make such intelligent robots.

Here, deep learning, computer vision, edge Computing, sensor network, and obviously IoT play major roles to make a robot more intelligent. These AI techniques along with bio-mechanical and electronics technologies together produce intelligent robots. In addition, these IoT enabled robots to have to be visual and voice understanding capabilities so that they can understand and respond to the patient.

4.3 Monitoring Hygienic Practice

For the COVID-19 pandemic, hygienic practice is one of the main steps to stop spreading this infection. According to some studies 'SARS-CoV-2' virus is inactive until it goes to our mouth or nose [3]. So, frequently washing hand and face are effective to mitigate spreading. Nevertheless, as a human being, we sometimes forget to do this practice. So, monitoring is necessary especially in critical areas such as

---

[1] https://www.pri.org/stories/2020-04-08/tommy-robot-nurse-helps-italian-doctors-care-covid-19-patients.

hospitals, clinical, etc. However, human intervention monitoring is hectic and some times it biased. Therefore, AI-based monitoring is a better option for this solution [48]. Here, IoT and sensor network-based computer vision algorithms would be very effective. In a research study [34], a group of researchers has proposed an AI-based hand hygienic practice monitoring model in a hospital. Human action recognition algorithms are in use to process video streams capturing by visual sensors. That model automatically detects movement patterns of human and generate an analytical measurement. These types of AI technologies will assist to monitor hygienic practice which would be very effective to stop infected and spreading COVID-19 like diseases.

4.4 Monitoring Systematic Social Distancing

According to the nature of the 'SARS-CoV-2' virus, social distancing is very necessary to restrict this pandemic [53]. Most of the countries where this pandemic is going on are maintaining it. In order to properly maintain, some countries have declared lockdown. But as expected all people those countries are not obeying it for many reasons. So, respective authorities are trying hard to maintaining this social distancing. Police are patrolling, sometimes, they are using drones (UAV) for observing many areas, quarantine centers, etc. But as usual practice, they are seating in a control room and watching those live video streaming via drones. Therefore, this is hectic as well as accuracy depends on the humans level. As you know as a human we have limitation to do continuous works, so, AI will be very useful in this scenario as it brings intelligence for auto-monitoring.

Computer Vision-based action recognition algorithms [54] could be used to automatically detect such indecent where such necessary social distancing is violating [49]. Here, a drone could capture video streaming and send it to the cloud for processing, from there inference comes to the control room for taking actions. Here, human efforts will be less, and accuracy will be better. In Fig. 4 a possible working pipeline has shown. A drone could be operated from a control room whereas it will capture the video stream and it shall be processed by edge computing before sending it to a cloud server via fog server. The cloud server with the help of the fog server will make inferences then send it to the control room. This AI-assisted auto-generated inference will help respective authorities to maintain social distancing.

5 Conclusion and Future Scope

This chapter tried to bring some insightful thoughts of AI to assists stop spreading COVID-19 like pandemics. Here, a background, as well as a review of the current state-of-the-art are also done. Four critical areas that are most vulnerable to spreading this virus are described with possible AI-based solutions. This chapter also described

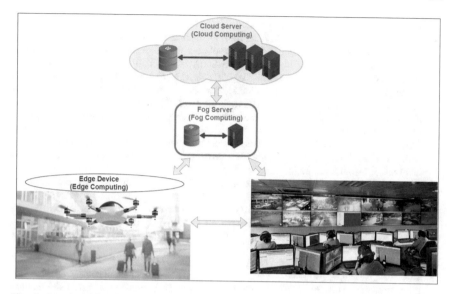

Fig. 4 A typical AI-assisted social distancing monitoring

how IoT, Edge, Fog, and Cloud Computing could work with tandem for remote sensing-based smart solutions to assisting to stop the spread of this COVID-19.

This COVID-19 is not an only pandemic human civilization is facing, the pandemic had in the past, or it may come future. Hopefully, this war-like situation shall be mitigated but it forced the world to think differently. Every associated machineries of this world has to be upgraded to cope with this COVID-19 as well as any future pandemic or epidemic if arises. Many careful measurements have to be taken. Many AI-based techniques need to be invented and adopted in addition to the existing techniques which some of them mentioned in this chapter. Therefore, more interdisciplinary collaborative research involvement will be required to make possible precautionary.

References

1. Guo, Y.-R., Cao, Q.-D., Hong, Z.-S., Tan, Y.-Y., Chen, S.-D., Jin, H.-J., Tan, K.-S., Wang, D.-Y., Yan, Y.: The origin, transmission and clinical therapies on coronavirus disease 2019 (covid-19) outbreak-an update on the status. Mili. Med. Res. **7**(1), 1–10 (2020)
2. World Health Organization et al.: Coronavirus disease 2019 (covid-19): situation report, **74** (2020)
3. Adhikari, S.P., Meng, S., Wu, Y.-J., Mao, Y.-P., Ye, R.-X., Wang, Q.-Z., Sun, C., Sylvia, S., Rozelle, S., Raat, H., et al.: Epidemiology, causes, clinical manifestation and diagnosis, prevention and control of coronavirus disease (covid-19) during the early outbreak period: a

scoping review. Infect. Dis. poverty **9**(1), 1–12 (2020)

4. Fong, S.J., Li, G., Dey, N., Crespo, R.G., Herrera-Viedma, E.: Composite monte carlo decision making under high uncertainty of novel coronavirus epidemic using hybridized deep learning and fuzzy rule induction. arXiv preprint arXiv:2003.09868 (2020)

5. Wong, J., Goh, Q.Y., Tan, Z., Lie, S.A., Tay, Y.C., Ng, S.Y., Soh, C.R.: Preparing for a covid-19 pandemic: a review of operating room outbreak response measures in a large tertiary hospital in singapore. Can. J. Anesth. J. Can. D'anesthésie **1–14**, (2020)

6. Zhou, M., Zhang, X., Jieming, Q.: Coronavirus disease: (covid-19): a clinical update. Front. Med. **1**, 2020 (2019)

7. Wilder-Smith, A., Freedman, D.: Isolation, quarantine, social distancing and community containment: pivotal role for old-style public health measures in the novel coronavirus (2019-ncov) outbreak. J. Travel Med. **27**(2), taaa020 (2020)

8. Lewnard, J.A., Lo, N.C.: Scientific and ethical basis for social-distancing interventions against covid-19. Lancet. Infect, Dis (2020)

9. Haenlein, M., Kaplan, A.: A brief history of artificial intelligence: on the past, present, and future of artificial intelligence. Calif. Manage. Rev. **61**(4), 5–14 (2019)

10. Liu, J., Kong, X., Xia, F., Bai, X., Wang, L., Qing, Q., Lee, I.: Artificial intelligence in the 21st century. IEEE Access **6**, 34403–34421 (2018)

11. Goodfellow, I., Bengio, Y., Courville, A.: Deep Learning. MIT press (2016)

12. Ghosh, A., Sufian, A., Sultana, F., Chakrabarti, A., De, D.: Fundamental concepts of convolutional neural network. In: Recent Trends and Advances in Artificial Intelligence and Internet of Things, pp. 519–567. Springer (2020)

13. Krizhevsky, A., Sutskever, I., Hinton, G.E.: Imagenet classification with deep convolutional neural networks. In: Advances in Neural Information Processing Systems (2012)

14. LeCun, Y., Bengio, Y., Hinton, G.: Deep learning. Nature **521**(7553), 436–444 (2015)

15. Rumelhart, D.E., Hinton, G.E., Williams, R.J.: Learning representations by back-propagating errors. Nature **323**(6088), 533–536 (1986)

16. Sufian, A., Ghosh, A., Sadiq, A.S., Smarandache, F.: A survey on deep transfer learning to edge computing for mitigating the COVID-19 pandemic. J. Sys. Arch. **108**, 101830 (2020)

17. Butt, C., Gill, J., Chun, D., Babu, B.A.: Deep learning system to screen coronavirus disease 2019 pneumonia. Appl, Intell (2020)

18. Beck, B.R., Shin, B., Choi, Y., Park, S., Kang, K.: Predicting commercially available antiviral drugs that may act on the novel coronavirus (sars-cov-2) through a drug-target interaction deep learning model. Comput. Struct. Biotechnol. J. (2020)

19. Grasselli, G., Pesenti, A., Cecconi, M.: Critical care utilization for the covid-19 outbreak in lombardy, italy: early experience and forecast during an emergency response. JAMA (2020)

20. Rawat, W., Wang, Z.: Deep convolutional neural networks for image classification: a comprehensive review. Neural Comput. **29**(9), 2352–2449 (2017)

21. Sultana, F., Sufian, A., Dutta, P.: Evolution of image segmentation using deep convolutional neural network: a survey. Knowl.-Based Syst. **201–202**, 106062 (2020)

22. Sultana, F., Sufian, A., Dutta, P.: A review of object detection models based on convolutional neural network. In: Mandal J., Banerjee S. (eds) Intelligent Computing: Image Processing Based Applications. Advances in Intelligent Systems and Computing, vol 1157. Springer (2020)

23. Ulhaq, A., Khan, A., Gomes, D., Pau, M.: Computer vision for covid-19 control: a survey. arXiv preprint arXiv:2004.09420 (2020)

24. Li, H., Ota, K., Dong, M.: Learning iot in edge: deep learning for the internet of things with edge computing. IEEE Network **32**(1), 96–101 (2018)

25. Gubbi, J., Buyya, R., Marusic, S., Palaniswami, M.: Internet of things (iot): a vision, architectural elements, and future directions. Future Gener. Comput. Syst. **29**(7), 1645–1660 (2013)

26. Ting, D.S.W., Carin, L., Dzau, V., Wong, T.Y.: Digital technology and covid-19. Nat. Med. **1–3**, (2020)

27. Bai, L., Yang, D., Wang, X., Tong, L., Zhu, X., Bai, C., Powell, C.A.: Chinese experts' consensus on the internet of things-aided diagnosis and treatment of coronavirus disease 2019. Clinical eHealth (2020)

28. Mahmud, R., Kotagiri, R., Buyya, R.: Fog computing: a taxonomy, survey and future directions. In: Internet of Everything, pp 103–130. Springer (2018)
29. Shi, W., Cao, J., Zhang, Q., Li, Y., Lanyu, X.: Edge computing: vision and challenges. IEEE Internet of Things J. **3**(5), 637–646 (2016)
30. Satyanarayanan, M.: The emergence of edge computing. Computer **50**(1), 30–39 (2017)
31. Wan, S., Zonghua, G., Ni, Q.: Cognitive computing and wireless communications on the edge for healthcare service robots. Comput. Commun. **149**, 99–106 (2020)
32. Sultana, F., Sufian, A., Dutta, P.: Advancements in image classification using convolutional neural network. In 2018 Fourth International Conference on Research in Computational Intelligence and Communication Networks (ICRCICN), pp. 122–129. IEEE (2018)
33. Torres, C., Fried, J.C., Rose, K., Manjunath, B.S.: Deep eye-cu (decu): summarization of patient motion in the icu. In: European Conference on Computer Vision, pp. 178–194. Springer (2016)
34. Haque, A., Guo, M., Alahi, A., Yeung, S., Luo, Z., Rege, A., Jopling, J., Downing, L., Beninati, W., Singh, A., et al.: Towards vision-based smart hospitals: a system for tracking and monitoring hand hygiene compliance. Preprint arXiv:1708.00163 (2017)
35. Rehouma, H., Noumeir, R., Jouvet, P., Bouachir, W., Essouri, S.: A computer vision method for respiratory monitoring in intensive care environment using rgb-d cameras. In: Seventh International Conference on Image Processing Theory, Tools and Applications (IPTA), pp. 1–6. IEEE (2017)
36. Davoudi, A., Malhotra, K.R., Shickel, B., Siegel, S., Williams, S., Ruppert, M., Bihorac, E., Ozrazgat-Baslanti, T., Tighe, P.J., Bihorac, A., et al.: The intelligent icu pilot study: using artificial intelligence technology for autonomous patient monitoring. arXiv preprint arXiv:1804.10201 (2018)
37. Torres, C., Fried, J.C., Rose, K., Manjunath, B.S.: A multiview multimodal system for monitoring patient sleep. IEEE Trans. Multimedia **20**(11), 3057–3068 (2018)
38. Chou, E., Tan, M., Zou, C., Guo, M., Haque, A., Milstein, A., Fei-Fei, L.: Privacy-preserving action recognition for smart hospitals using low-resolution depth images. arXiv:1811.09950 (2018)
39. Liu, B., Guo, M., Chou, E., Mehra, R., Yeung, S., Downing, N.L., Salipur, F., Jopling, J., Campbell, B., Deru, K., et al.: 3d point cloud-based visual prediction of icu mobility care activities. In: Machine Learning for Healthcare Conference, pp. 17–29 (2018)
40. Azimi, I., Takalo-Mattila, J., Anzanpour, A., Rahmani, A.M., Soininen, J.P., Liljeberg, P.: Empowering healthcare iot systems with hierarchical edge-based deep learning. In: IEEE/ACM International Conference on Connected Health: Applications, Systems and Engineering Technologies (CHASE), pp. 63–68. IEEE (2018)
41. Dossso, Y.S., Bekele, A., Nizami, S., Aubertin, C., Greenwood, K., Harrold, J., Green, J.R.: Segmentation of patient images in the neonatal intensive care unit. In: 2018 IEEE Life Sciences Conference (LSC), pp. 45–48. IEEE (2018)
42. Kumar, R.M., Davoudi, A., Siegel, S., Bihorac, A., Rashidi, P.: Autonomous detection of disruptions in the intensive care unit using deep mask r-cnn. In: Proceedings of the IEEE Conference on Computer Vision and Pattern Recognition Workshops, pp. 1863–1865 (2018)
43. Davoudi, A., Malhotra, K.R., Shickel, B., Siegel, S., Williams, S., Ruppert, M., Bihorac, E., Ozrazgat-Baslanti, T., Tighe, P.J., Bihorac, A., et al.: Intelligent icu for autonomous patient monitoring using pervasive sensing and deep learning. Sci. Rep. **9**(1), 1–13 (2019)
44. Yeung, S., Rinaldo, F., Jopling, J., Liu, B., Mehra, R., Downing, N.L., Guo, M., Bianconi, G.M., Alahi, A., Lee, J., et al.: A computer vision system for deep learning-based detection of patient mobilization activities in the icu. NPJ Digital Med. **2**(1), 1–5 (2019)
45. Casas, L., Navab, N., Demirci, S.: Patient 3d body pose estimation from pressure imaging. Int J. Comput. Assisted Radiol Surgery **14**(3), 517–524 (2019)
46. Saria, S., Ma, A.J., Reiter, A.: Measuring patient mobility in the icu using a novel non-invasive sensor, August 1 2019. US Patent App. 16/339,152
47. Baldassano, S., Roberson, S.W., Balu, R., Scheid, B., Bernabei, J., Pathmanathan, J., Oommen, B., Leri, D., Echauz, J., Gelfand, M.: Iris: a modular platform for continuous monitoring and caretaker notification in the intensive care unit. IEEE J. Biomed, Health Informat (2020)

48. Kim, M., Choi, J., Kim, N.: Fully automated hand hygiene monitoring in Operating Room Using 3d Convolutional Neural Network. arXiv preprint arXiv:2003.09087 (2020)
49. Mliki, H., Bouhlel, F., Hammami, M.: Human activity recognition from uav-captured video sequences. Pattern Recognit. **100**, 107140 (2020)
50. Lee, G.I., Lee, M.R., Green, I., Allaf, M., Marohn, M.R.: Surgeons' physical discomfort and symptoms during robotic surgery: a comprehensive ergonomic survey study. Surg. Endosc. **31**(4), 1697–1706 (2017)
51. Yang, G.-Z., Nelson, B.J., Murphy, R.R., Choset, H., Christensen, H., Collins, S.H., Dario, P., Goldberg, K., Ikuta, K., Jacobstein, N., et al.: Combating covid-19-the role of robotics in managing public health and infectious diseases (2020)
52. Am van Kemenade, M., Hoorn, J.F., Konijn, E.A.: Do you care for robots that care? exploring the opinions of vocational care students on the use of healthcare robots. Robotics **8**(1), 22 (2019)
53. Asian Healthcare Work. Infection control (2020)
54. Zhang, H.-B., Zhang, Y.-X., Zhong, B., Lei, Q., Yang, L., Ji-Xiang, D., Chen, D.-S.: A comprehensive survey of vision-based human action recognition methods. Sensors **19**(5), 1005 (2019)

AI Based Covid19 Analysis-A Pragmatic Approach

Prerana Mukherjee and Sarul Malik

Abstract In this chapter, we provide detailed background about Covid-19. Then, we discuss the recent approaches of AI based techniques to prevent and predict Covid-19. We also detail about the forecasting methods for analyzing the trends of the affected patients all over the world. We highlight the main datasets utilized in the image based Covid analysis. We also provide a detailed discussion on the use cases how AI can be used in different applications for Covid-19 analysis.

1 Introduction

Wuhan, Hubei province in central china is densely crowded city with a population of 11 million, reported the earliest cases of pneumonia of unknown etiology on 17th November 2019. On 7th January, Chinese Centre for Disease Control and Prevention (CCDC) identified the causative agent from the throat swab samples of the patients and thereupon named Severe Acute Respiratory Syndrome Coronavirus 2 (SARS-CoV-2) which was later named as COVID-19 by World Health Organization (WHO).

At present, it has been observed that majority of the patients have developed mild symptoms such as sore throat, high fever and dry cough however fatal complications including severe pneumonia, organ failure, septic shock and Acute respiratory distress syndrome has also been noted during severe stages of disease. The scenario is much more complicated for elderly population with previous record of hypertension, diabetes or respiratory disorders.

S. Malik: Equal Contribution.

P. Mukherjee (✉)
Indian Institute of Information Technology, Sri City, India
e-mail: prerana.m@iiits.in

S. Malik
Shaheed Rajguru College of Applied Sciences for Women,
University of Delhi, New Delhi, India
e-mail: sarulmalik@gmail.com

A.-E. Hassanien et al. (eds.), *Big Data Analytics and Artificial Intelligence
Against COVID-19: Innovation Vision and Approach*, Studies in Big Data 78,
https://doi.org/10.1007/978-3-030-55258-9_12

191

1.1 Motivation and Contributions

For mass prevention and protection different countries have come up with varied measures to counteract this infectious disease. Technology is being used not only for drug discovery but efforts are being done in tracing the patients and detection of Covid-19 using the advances in artificial intelligence techniques. This will ease the job of the health workers in early diagnostics without manual intervention. Even lot of traction has been seen where the data scientists are trying to model the infectious disease and find the short term forecasting of Covid-19. Nowcasting is a term where in absence of any data, one can predict the current levels. However, the AI can work or predict for these tasks if there is some data available, due to the unprecedented crisis of Covid-19 currently no much data is available. In order to mitigate this problem, lot of data scientists and researchers are creating open forums for collaboration for data curation.

Since, it is highly new problem which has emerged and become such a menace to deal with, not many works are trying to bridge the gap of the utilization of AI in dealing with Covid-19 crisis. Through this chapter, we have addressed this knowledge gap by providing holistic information to the readers in terms of (i) understanding the finer details of Covid-19, (ii) Prevention measures and efforts towards treatment being done, (iii) Role of AI in managing the crisis, (iv) Mathematical preliminaries of infectious disease modeling and (v) AI based application case scenarios. We envisage that this amalgamation of technology with real crisis situation and documentation about it will allow more collaborative works. To the best of author's knowledge, this chapter is a unique effort which provides comprehensive knowledge on how advances in AI can be leveraged in Covid-19 disease modeling and diagnostics.

1.2 Section Organization

To this end, in the next few paragraphs, the reader is introduced to the evolution and inception of Covid-19. We believe that in order to appreciate the AI utility in mitigating and fighting the problem of Covid-19, the reader should be familiar with fundamentals of the Covid-19 disease evolution. Therefore, detailed discussion on state of the art work is deferred till the end of this chapter. Then, we go through an in-depth literature survey of the latest works in the three subjective areas including images, big data analytics and drug discovery and the role of AI in each. Lastly, we open the scope of research avenues in dealing with Covid-19.

In Sect. 2, we discuss the global scenario due to Covid-19 crisis and the pathophysiology of Covid-19. In Sect. 4, we outline the guidelines given by WHO to prevent Covid-19. In Sect. 3, we provide transmission details. In Sect. 5, we discuss the diagnostic processes. In Sect. 6, we discuss in detail the treatment processes being done by doctors and pathologists. In Sect. 7, we provide the comprehensive literature review of AI based analysis. In Sect. 7.5 gives the role of mathematical modeling of infectious diseases and subsequently Sect. 8 gives the mathematical preliminaries behind it. In Sect. 9, we discuss the datasets related to Covid-19 image diagnostics. In Sect. 10, we give the application case scenarios for the role of AI in Covid-19 monitoring and diagnostics. Finally, we provide the conclusion in Sect. 11.

2 Global Health Emergency Declared by WHO

WHO declared the outbreak of COVID-19 as Public health emergency on 30th January 2020, however they strongly believed that virus spread could be interrupted by encouraging the countries to detect early case, quarantine them and take measures to treat them effectively. Also, contact tracing is equally mandatory along with promoting social distancing in order to prevent further cases. They also emphasized upon the need of pathogen genome sequencing to understand its pathophysiology and transmission cycle which could pave its way for the early treatment approach globally. Meanwhile, they coordinated upon the policies essential to ensure rapid development and access to potential vaccines development, diagnostics kits, antiviral medicines and other supplementary therapeutics to prepare the low-and middle-income countries to overcome the risk associated with the outbreak. Besides, it was announced worldwide to restrict travel and trade for the time being to further prevent the spread of novel corona virus. The recent update of COVID-19 infected cases and total death incurred along with other essential details is provided on corona virus worldmeter web portal [1].

2.1 Global Scenario

As of 28th March 2020, COVID-19 has affected 210 countries and territories around the world. Currently, it has been reported that more than 3 million are affected by this deadly virus, which has claimed more than nearly 2 lakh lives however more than 9 lakh were able to recover themselves from this life-threatening virus. WHO Director-General Dr. Tedros Adhanom Ghebreyesus in his opening notes stated the severity of COVID-19 (3.4%) against the seasonal flu (less than 1%). The world is coming together to combat the COVID-19 pandemic bringing all the administrators, management groups from across industries and sectors and individuals together to help respond to this global outbreak. The Strategic preparedness and response plan outlines a funding need of at least US $675 million for critical response efforts in countries most in need of help through April 2020 to encounter the current scenario. In order to effectively manage the crisis of COVID-19, EU mobilized 10,000,000 into the research fund to manage infected case along with future preparedness [2]. United kingdom (UK) government has also invested £20,000,000 to develop COVID-19 [3].

In addition, Chinese central bank also invested 150 billion to support the stability of the current market [4]. On similar lines, various countries are cutting their expenses to utilize their funds judiciously to fight battle against the novel coronavirus.

2.2 COVID-19 Pathophysiology

Corona virus (CoVs) belongs to subfamily Orthocoronavirinae of the Coronaviridae family (order Nidovirales) and classifies into four genera of CoVs: (i) Alphacoronavirus (alphaCoV), (ii) Betacoronavirus (betaCoV), (iii) Deltacoronavirus (delta-CoV), and (iv) Gammacoronavirus (gammaCoV) [5]. They are positive-strand RNA viruses genome contains 29891 nucleotides, encoding for 9860 amino acids with a crown-like appearance under an electron microscope due to the presence of spike glycoproteins on the envelope [6].

The Coronaviridae family virus have well established records to cause respiratory, neurological and hepatic diseases in different animal species, including camels, cattle, cats, and bats. Till date, seven human HCoVs (Human coronavirus) have been identified which are potent enough of infecting humans. The earlier HCoVs were identified in the mid-1960s, while others were only detected in the new 21st century. Approximately 2% of the entire population are the active carriers of corona virus who could make a transmission chain to infect numerous if not controlled at the right time. Around 5–10% of the respiratory diseases are the true source of these viruses infection manacles [7]. The genomic isolation of this new HCoVs from Wuhan patients has shown 89% resemblance with bat SARS-like-CoVZXC21 and 82% with that of human SARS-CoV hence, the new virus was called SARS-CoV-2 [8]. Bioinformatics based genomic sequencing has also shown that probably bats and rodents are the gene sources of alpha CoVs and beta CoVs [9]. Despite the fact that, SARS-CoV-2 has resembled bat genome, it is difficult to claim upon its existence species because it's genome is vulnerable to numerous mutations. Thus, SARS-CoV-2 belongs to the betaCoVs category.

Once the virus enters into the host body, its spike protein binds with human angiotensin-converting enzyme 2 (ACE-2) receptors which are present on the surface of the host cell. Next occurs the activation of spike protein of the virus due to the binding of type II transmembrane serine protease (TMPRSS2) to ACE-2 protein which is responsible of its cleavage. Then, this cleaved ACE-2 receptor and activated spike protein assist the viral entry into the host machinery. Host immune system is triggered by the viral entry and inflammatory cascade begins by antigen-presenting cells (APC) which further stimulated B-cell production to facilitated antigen-antibody reaction [10]. Cellular uptake of the corona virus increases by the expression of TMPRSS [11]. ACE-2 receptors are innumerably present in hypertensive and diabetic population hence these groups of individuals are advised to strict government advisories to follow all the essential norms [12].

3 Transmission of SARS-CoV-2

Huanan Seafood Wholesale Market of Wuhan, has been spotted for the first transmission case of this deadly virus from an animal to human communication [13]. Thereafter, a transmission chain was established from human-to-human through both symptomatic as well as asymptomatic transmission. Coughing, Sneezing and physical contact were recognized as most attacking weapons to spread the disease [14]. The primary transmission occurs among the family members and close contact of an infected individual which eventually turns into community spread if concrete measures were not taken timely. Since then, government has uploaded the advisory to maintain social distancing aiming to cut this transmission chain [15]. As per the investigation, it was proclaimed that the incubation time may vary from 2 to 14 days(95% CI, 9.2 to 18) [16]. The doubling rate of case was found to be seven days on an average scale and each patient can transmits the infection to an additional 2.2 individuals [17]. However, with increased investigations and studies over the time there is a fair chance that these results might get change.

4 Prevention

It is well stated that "Prevention is always better than cure". This pandemic will never end until concrete prevention policies are being adopted globally. Careful prevention strategies need to be focused upon the isolation of patients and tracing back their contacts. WHO and other organizations have issued the following guidelines as a preventive measures [18]:

- To restrict close contact with someone manifesting the symptoms of acute respiratory infections.
- To maintain personal hygiene.
- To restrict unprotected contact with farm animals.
- To promote social distancing
- Immuno-compromised individuals, elderly population and children below 10 years of age should avoid public gatherings as much as possible.

Apart from these crucial measures, frequent hand washing is strongly recommended to wash away the lipid envelope of the virus with the soapy lipid layer [19]. Respiratory etiquettes during sneezing and coughing needs to be adopted, following that hand sensitization would vanish the possible chance of infection [20]. One should avoid touching eyes, noses and mouth after interacting with a possible infectious source. Use of mask is the best remedy to protect the transmission through droplets or aerosols however the proper discarding protocol of mask after use is equally essential [21]. Health workers and armed forces are the front line warriors during this pandemic, their protection is the utmost responsibility for the nation. Use of PPEs such as N95 masks, eye googles, gowns, gloves and protective shoe covers are strongly recommended while working in the hospital and other contagious environment [22].

5 Diagnosis

Epidemiological record and medical expression fabricates the ground of clinical diagnostic approach for COVID-19 infection. These approaches has been classified as : (1) Nucleic acid detection; (2) Immunosorbent assay; (3) Imaging technique; and (4) Blood culture. Until now, sign and symptoms of patients infected with covid-19 includes were reported as high fever, dry cough, dyspnea and viral pneumonia. Surprisingly, it was reported that significant transmission has been contributed by people who were asymptomatic [22, 23]. To battle such scenario, auxiliary inspection such as epidemiological record plays a crucial role.

5.1 Nucleic Acid Detection Technology

Initially, blood culturing and high throughput sequencing approach was adopted to identity SARS-CoV-2. Later, it was realized that these methods were time consuming, expensive and requires sophisticated instruments for the analysis [24]. Thereafter, the interest of scientific community was inclined to RT-qPCR due to its high efficiency and feasibility to detect the infected cases. [25]. RT-qPCR detection also showed high sensitivity and specificity for SARS-CoV and MERS-CoV infection [26]. Supplementary to this, RT-PCR was also reported to suffer from long detection hours and inconvenient nucleic acid detection operations.

5.2 Computed Tomography (CT) Scanning

Though RT-PCT is an extremely sensitive technique yet it may result in false negative, hence a combination of CT scan along with RT-PCT would assist to detect those missed cases. It has been recommended to employ high-resolution CT (HRCT) to diagnosis the severity of patients with SARS-CoV-2 at very early stage [27]. Bilateral pulmonary parenchymal ground-glass and consolidative pulmonary opacities is clearly seen in a conventional CT scan [28]. It is evident that Ct has a huge clinical potential to spot the infection cases however at times it is unable to clearly distinguish the SARS-CoVs-2 image from that of other cases of viral pneumonia.

To overcome the limitations of RT-qPCR and CT scanning, point of care testing (POCT) which is based upon the principal of specific antigen-antibody binding showed even better detection rates [29].

6 Treatment

Till date, no specific antiviral treatment or vaccine have foot forward to be competent against covid-19. Majority of health workers are recommending the symptomatic treatment and empathetic supervision. The supportive treatment includes ventilation and use of antiviral against the prevailing infection. Recent studies have reported the effect of choroquine (antimalarial drug) and remdesivir (antiviral drug) as an inhibitor on the growth of SARS-CoV-2 in vitro [30]. Today, numerous countries are anticipating the use of plasma therapy as a promising treatment against COVID-19. The objective of plasma therapy is to provide the defence against corona virus in a struggling patient through the antibodies of recovered patient. Not only this, its potential can be effective to immunise those who are at a high risk of contracting the virus [31].

7 Literature Review of AI Based Analysis

7.1 State-of-the-art in Covid-19 Scenario

In this subsection, we give a brief overview of the state of the art methods and their performance in image based Covid-19 analysis. In [32], authors proposed a joint model for classification and segmentation pipeline with explainable results. They also provided Covid-CS dataset with classification and pixelwise lesion segmentation data. In the classification task, the model has achieved an average sensitivity of 95% and specificity of 93% on the test set. On the segmentation test set, the model achieved a Dice index of 78.3%. In [33], authors have proposed an extension to EfficientNet for detecting Covid-19. The main idea is to reduce the computational cost and the form factor of the models by reducing the number of hyperparameters thus making it suitable to perform mobile processing. It achieved a state of the art results on Covidx dataset with an average accuracy of 93.9%, sensitivity of 96.8% and prediction rate of 100%. The performance gain is while having 28 times fewer parameters than baseline VGG16 and 5 times lesser than Resnet50 architectures.

7.2 Image Processing Based Analysis

In [34], authors proposed an automated Covid19 detection using chest CT scans and its performance analysis. They proposed COVNet to detect and predict the occurrence of Covid-19 and compared it with community acquired pneumonia and non-pneumonia CT scans. The data was acquired over 6 hospitals from Apr, 2016 to Feb, 2020. The thorough performance analysis was given using receiver operator characteristics curves, Area under the curves and precision, recall rates. In [35], authors provided review of al the works which address the detection of Covid-19 using CT scan images and also elaborated the challenges faced during this. However, the deep learning models such as GoogleNet, ResNet are doing the detection accurately it is quite challenging to predict whether the pneumonia caused in the lungs is due to Covid-19 or any other bacterial or fungal infection. In [36], authors provided a review on image processing based techniques for segmentation. It has detailed the entire pipeline of acquisition, analysis, diagnosis and follow-up. In [37], authors investigated Covid-19 CT scans with bedside CXRs in Italy. In [38], authors provided first of its kind open source data repository of Covid-19 frontal view XRays collected via several websites and publications. Apart from Covid-19 it also contains images of Severe acute respiratory syndrome(SARS), Middle East respiratory syndrome (MERS) and acute respiratory distress syndrome (ARDS). In [39], authors have provided the survey of all the medical imaging data available for Covid-19. In [40], authors have provided a generative adversarial network GAN based technique for leveraging the data for augmentation in order to provide more data for generalization. In [41], authors utilized MobileNet for training on 3905 X-Ray images and achieved an accuracy of 99.18%. In [42], authors have proposed an AI inspired model for Covid-19 analysis for patients to respond to treatmet. Here, they have used two modules detection using CNN based techniques and prediction module that utilizes whale optimization algorithm to select the best features of the patient to decide the survival rate. In [43], authors utilized a technique to detect the severity level of infection due to Covid-19. They first extract the lung region and then utilize image enhancement using Harmony search and Otsu based analysis followed by segmentation of the affected area. Once the region of interest is extract based on image based ratio analysis the severity level is determined.

7.3   Data Science Based Forecasting

In [44], authors proposed the forecasting analysis of the Covid-19 spread in the Chinese provinces and cities. They utilized an unsupervised technique using stacked autoencoders to forecast the transmission dynamics of Covid-19. The data was collected across 4 months from Jan, 2020 to Apr, 2020 and a total of 9 groups were formed by clustering techniques. It was predicted that the spread curves would reach a plateau around April. In [45], authors have suggested that Covid-19 cases can be quickly identified by using mobile phone based web survey. In [46], the authors provided a review of AI advances in molecular, medical and epidemiological applications during Covid-19 crisis. They illustrated how AI can be used for non invasive tracking of disease evolution based on multiple data inputs inclusive of e-health records. It is highly effective for promising drug development. In [47], authors utilized autoencoders to predict the epidemic transmission rate, its trajectory, predict severity. In [48], authors provided a conceptual framework that combined block chain and AI to combat Covid-19. They highlighted different use case scenarios in Covid-19 where such a joint framework is usable and the potential impact on them. In [49], authors have proposed a cough sound analysis dataset to do the tracking of the evolution of the patient's condition by just analyzing the cough patterns. This dataset is mainly for the analysis of patients who are under quarantine. In [50], authors provided an approach for early forecasting of Covid-19 based on less data. In [51], authors proposed an approach where composite Monte Carlo based method is used for forecasting in high uncertainty based Covid-19 analysis. They utilized a hybrid architecture of deep learning and fuzzy rule induction.

7.4   Genomics Based Analysis

In [52], authors utilized deep learning based techniques to identify progeny drugs similarity with parent drugs used for Covid-19. Apart from the molecular formation similarity, the arrangement (context) of the functional groups is taken into consideration. In [53], authors utilized deep learning approaches for novel drug discovery by pocket based generator, ligand estimators etc. In [54], authors utilized artificial intelligence for examining the blood samples to test positive cases. In this, they used an ensemble of support vector machine, SMOTEBoost, KNN based approaches. They designed it in 2 stage process first used the AI model to check for influenza cases and then check whether they are also positive for Covid-19. In [55], authors utilized metaheuristic based techniques to identify the ordinary spreaders and super spreaders and developed a fitness function to see the current population based on two additional parameters i.e. travel and isolation. They further leveraged this with Long Short term Memory (LSTM) Networks to optimize the hyperparameters used. In [56], authors proposed network for drug repurposing based on 3 methods: network proximity, diffusion and AI based methods. It is ascertained that the virus can dwell in other tissues like reproductive organs and brain regions.

7.5   Role of Mathematical Modelling in Infectious Diseases

It has been well evident from the fact that how infectious diseases outbreak affected the harmony worldwide [57]. However, advancement in technological ground to battle these epidemics always showed the light of hope in that darkness. Antiviral drugs and vaccines against these deadly viruses have protected generations from devastation [58]. Yet, certain queries of any epidemic situations for instance: how the infection is going to disperse, for how long it will last, how much destructive it will going to be, how about its re-emergence and what type of medications are required to control it at earliest etc. can only be untangled with the development of a mathematics model [59]. A mathematical model is a tool which illuminates from the mechanism of a disease dissemination to its future chain prediction in order to develop substantial approach to struggle across the path [60]. Long back in the year 1854, London has witnessed the first successful mathematical model which was used to eradicate cholera epidemic [61]. Till date, considerable statistical model has been reported for the apprehension of infectious disease eruption [62]. A conventional regression model has always been the prime-most choice for the researchers due to its simplicity and feasibility however it sometimes suffers from a high prediction error due to numerous factors [63]. Hidden Markov model is a well recognized model to ascertain about the kinetics of an infectious disease and could estimate its convulsion from the possible indicators [64]. Susceptible-Infected-Recovered (SIR) model [65] is yet another simple model and profoundly acceptable model used to explain the dynamics of COVID-19 outbreak which is explained in next subsection.

8 Mathematical Preliminaries of Infectious Disease Modeling

Mathematical modeling of infectious diseases help in understanding how the disease will spread and the likely outcomes of an epidemic. A rather specialized domain in AI is machine learning and statistics which governs the mathematical modeling of infectious diseases. The first work was done by statistician Bernoulli in 1766. He gave a model around inoculating against the infectious disease smallpox. There were emergence of other epidemic modeling around 1900s. These models were termed as Suspected-Infected-Recovered (SIR) models. There are two basic types of epidemic models: (i) Stochastic and (ii) Deterministic. Stochastic models can be used when the infectious disease is further dependent on one or more random variables (such as exposure or contact based risk, environmental factors etc). Whereas deterministic models work on the inherent assumption that the epidemic process is deterministic. In this, the population is divided into compartments or subgroups and transition between states take place. The entire model can be defined by set of differential equations.

The generic SIR model [66] can be defined as,

$$N = S(t) + I(t) + R(t) \tag{1}$$

where N denotes the total population divided into three compartments S: suspected cases, I:infected cases, R: recovered cases (due to immunization or death) and t denotes time. The reproduction number or R_0 denotes how transferable the disease is. For e.g. there is an infected person due to which 2 more persons can be contracted with disease then the R_0 becomes 2. It can be computed as the ratio of known spread rates over time. Lets say, the infectious individuals comes in contact with β individual per unit time and all of them get contracted with disease and the mean infecting period of the disease is given by $\frac{1}{\gamma}$ then the reproduction number $R_0 = \frac{\beta}{\gamma}$.

The transition in the SIR model is $S(t) \rightarrow I(t) \rightarrow R(t)$. The three differential equations are given as,

$$\frac{dS}{dt} = -\frac{\beta S I}{N} \tag{2}$$

$$\frac{dI}{dt} = \frac{\beta S I}{N} - \gamma I \tag{3}$$

$$\frac{dR}{dt} = \gamma I \tag{4}$$

The assumption in this model is that every individual is having equal probability of contracting the disease. These differential equations are governed by the law of mass action which states that rate of contract between any two groups will be proportional to size of each individual group that is concerned.

9 Datasets Available

In this section, we highlight the main imagery datasets available for covid-19 detection. Figure 1 gives few examples of Covid-19 and other similar ailments Xray images.

COVID-CS dataset: This is the first dataset to provide the pixel level annotations of the covid-19 infected regions in the lungs (CT scans collected using different scanners). It is named as Covid-19 Classification and Segmentation dataset. There re in total 144 167 CT scan images of 750 patients out of which 400 (175 males and 225 females) are positive cases and rest are negative. Here, community acquired pneumonia cases are not considered. For pixel level annotations, professional labelling is done by senior radiologists. After this step, a total 3,855 pixel level annotations for 200 positive case patients is performed. Rest 200 patients data is used for test purpose. The number of lesion counts varies between 1 to 10 in each CT scan image. The infected patches are uniformly distributed.

Covid-chestxray-dataset[1]: It consists of 123 frontal view Xray images. It has the images of the following viral infections: Severe acute respiratory syndrome (SARS), Acute respiratory distress syndrome (ARDS), COVID-19, Pneumonia. each image file has a file identifier or metadata associated to it which consists of the patient ID, numbber of days for onset of symptoms, sex, age, type of pneumonia, survival rate, view angle, modality, date on which it is taken, location and other file identifiers.

COVIDx dataset[2]: It consists of 13 800 CXR images of 13,725 patient cases which is collected over 3 publicly available datasets. It consists of both non-covid pneumonia (8066 cases) and non pneumonia patients (5538 cases). Also, it contains 183 CXR images from 121 Covid-19 patient cases.

---

[1]https://github.com/ieee8023/covid-chestxray-dataset.
[2]https://github.com/lindawangg/COVID-Net/.

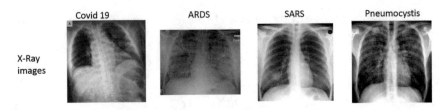

Fig. 1 Some sample images of Covid-chestxray-dataset (Postanterior chest Xray images of different closely related disease of Covid-19

COVID-19 Radiography Database dataset[3]: It contains 219 COVID-19 positive images, which comprises 1341 normal images and 1345 pneumonia patient images. It is a Kaggle challenge dataset.

COVID-19 CT segmentation dataset[4]: It contains 100 axial CT images collected from more than 40 COVID-19 patients basically converted from JPG images (openly accessible). The images are rescaled, normalized and compiled into a single NIFTI file. The segmentation masks consisted of 3 labels namely, ground class opacification (label 1), consolidations (label 2) and pleural effusions (label 3). They were normalized back into Hounsfield Unit scale.

COVID-CT-Dataset[5]: It consists of 275 CT scans positive for 143 COVID-19 cases. This is a unique dataset collected from all medRxiv and bioRxiv preprints available online. The authors used PyMuPDF[6] to preserve the structural information of the images embedded in these preprints. Then they analyzed the captions of the figures in order to identify whether they belong to positive or negative cases. In case the figure had conjoint images they would do a split of CT scan images and then select it. In case it is not evident from the caption about the label of image data they would scan in the relevant text excerpt which would certify the positive/negative label about the image.

10   Case Scenarios: Problem and Solution

These are the following thrust areas where main action needs to be targeted to mitigate the problem of Covid-19.

Forecasting and alert generation: Based on the past data and trends, the system can predict the outbreaks of pandemics [67], potential hotspots, suspected cases, death toll etc. However, such forecasting tasks may require a huge amount of data. With certain amount of uncertainty, it can be extrapolated to get the future course of trends to be followed. Most of the Covid data has been simulated by the Center

---

[3]https://www.kaggle.com/tawsifurrahman/covid19-radiography-database.

[4]http://medicalsegmentation.com/covid19/.

[5]https://github.com/UCSD-AI4H/COVID-CT.

[6]https://github.com/pymupdf/PyMuPDF.

for Systems Science and Engineering (CSSE), Johns Hopkins University[7] where the entire pandemic data including casualties, recoveries and infected cases have been reported worldwide. Several statistical models such exponential smoothing functions, logistic/S-curves or maximum likelihood approaches can be used to build such forecasting models. It helps in finding the convergence rate of the curves such as mortality rate etc.

Covid-19 patient tracing and prediction: AI based approaches can be used for contact tracing of the susceptible patients who might have come in contact with positive patients. Now, using the IMEI number in the phones and GPS live tracking of the people it can be ascertained whether they are following quarantine norms or not. Also, if they are near more people it can be live-traced. Based on the symptoms and travel history of the person, the AI based models can do an early prediction of the disease and the person can take the necessary actions by performing social distancing.

Dashboard Preparation for data: Another important application is to develop dashboard which reflects the data for pandemics or epidemiological spread. One can interactively visualize graphs and bar charts to compare the ongoing trends. Different features can be utilized to visualize the data and see the effect on the spread. Some of the most popular ones which have been trending in data visualization in Covid-19 cases include UpCode,[8] Thebaselab,[9] the BBC,[10] the New York Times,[11] and HealthMap.[12]

Diagnosis of Covid-19: The diagnosis and prognosis of this pandemic can be done either by discovering new drugs at the earliest or by studying the CT scan reports and identify the patients who are suffering with this. AI based techniques particularly resorting to Deep learning based techniques have been very successful. It enables the doctors to do an automated scanning of the reports and generate authenticated and accurate reports of the patients thus reducing manual inspection.

11 Conclusion

In this chapter, we have provided a thorough report on the inception of Covid-19, details on the spread worldwide and the approaches followed by the researchers and scientists to cope with it. Particularly, we focus on the efforts that researchers are taking on AI based solutions can offer. Primarily, we observed that if proper diagnosis is done using AI based imagery techniques and AI based patient tracing is done, then we can perform stringent measures on ensuring quarantine is being

---

[7] https://github.com/CSSEGISandData/COVID-19.

[8] https://www.againstcovid19.com/singapore/dashboard.

[9] https://coronavirus.thebaselab.com/.

[10] https://www.bbc.com/news/world-51235105.

[11] https://www.nytimes.com/interactive/2020/world/coronavirus-maps.html.

[12] https://www.healthmap.org/covid-19/?mod=article_inline.

followed and social distancing is managed. Forecasting and prediction models again can be extremely helpful as it enables to know the epidemiological trends and take the successive measures. We envisage that our holistic study can be helpful and provide a bird's eye view on the problem.

References

1. https://www.worldometers.info/coronavirus/worldwide-graphs/#daily-cases
2. https://ec.europa.eu/info/news/coronavirus-eu-mobilises-eur10-million-for-research-2020-jan-31_en
3. https://www.bbc.com/news/health-51352952
4. https://www.bbc.co.uk/news/business-51347497
5. Perlman, S., Netland, J.: Coronaviruses post-sars: update on replication and pathogenesis. Nat. Rev. Microbiol 7(6), 439–450 (2009)
6. Su, S., Wong, G., Shi, W., Liu, J., Lai, A.C., Zhou, J., Liu, W., Bi, Y., Gao, G.F.: Epidemiology, genetic recombination, and pathogenesis of coronaviruses. Trends Microbiol. 24(6), 490–502 (2016)
7. Sanders, J.M., Monogue, M.L., Jodlowski, T.Z., Cutrell, J.B.: Pharmacologic treatments for coronavirus disease 2019 (covid-19): a review. JAMA (2020)
8. Jiang, S., Du, L., Shi, Z.: An emerging coronavirus causing pneumonia outbreak in wuhan, china: calling for developing therapeutic and prophylactic strategies. Emerg. Micro. Infect. 9(1), 275–277 (2020)
9. Rodhain, F.: Bats and viruses: complex relationships. Bulletin De La Societe De Pathologie Exotique (1990) 108(4), 272 (2015)
10. Boopathi, S., Poma, A.B., Kolandaivel, P.: Novel 2019 coronavirus structure, mechanism of action, antiviral drug promises and rule out against its treatment. J. Biomol Struct Dyn (just-accepted), 1–14 (2020)
11. Kuba, K., Imai, Y., Rao, S., Gao, H., Guo, F., Guan, B., Huan, Y., Yang, P., Zhang, Y., Deng, W., et al.: A crucial role of angiotensin converting enzyme 2 (ace2) in sars coronavirus-induced lung injury. Nat. Med. 11(8), 875–879 (2005)
12. Padda, R.S., Shi, Y., Lo, C.S., Zhang, S.L., Chan, J.S.: Angiotensin-(1–7): a novel peptide to treat hypertension and nephropathy in diabetes? J. Diabetes Metab. 6(10) (2015)
13. https://www.sciencemag.org/news/2020/01/wuhan-seafood-market-may-not-be-source-novel-virus-spreading-globally
14. Rothan, H.A., Byrareddy, S.N.: The epidemiology and pathogenesis of coronavirus disease (covid-19) outbreak. J. Autoimmun. 102433, (2020)
15. https://www.who.int/emergencies/diseases/novel-coronavirus-2019/advice-for-public
16. Li, Q., Guan, X., Wu, P., Wang, X., Zhou, L., Tong, Y., Ren, R., Leung, K.S., Lau, E.H., Wong, J.Y., et al.: Early transmission dynamics in wuhan, china, of novel coronavirus-infected pneumonia. New England J, Med (2020)
17. Bauch, C.T., Lloyd-Smith, J.O., Coffee, M.P., Galvani, A.P.: Dynamically modeling sars and other newly emerging respiratory illnesses: past, present, and future. Epidemiology pp. 791–801 (2005)
18. https://www.ncbi.nlm.nih.gov/books/NBK554776/
19. Organization, W.H., et al.: Rational use of personal protective equipment for coronavirus disease (covid-19): interim guidance, 27 february 2020. World Health Organization, technical report (2020)
20. Machida, M., Nakamura, I., Saito, R., Nakaya, T., Hanibuchi, T., Takamiya, T., Odagiri, Y., Fukushima, N., Kikuchi, H., Kojima, T., et al.: Adoption of personal protective measures by ordinary citizens during the covid-19 outbreak in japan. Int. J. Infect, Dis (2020)

21. Feng, S., Shen, C., Xia, N., Song, W., Fan, M., Cowling, B.J.: Rational use of face masks in the covid-19 pandemic. The Lancet Respiratory Medicine (2020)
22. Cascella, M., Rajnik, M., Cuomo, A., Dulebohn, S.C., Di Napoli, R.: Features, evaluation and treatment coronavirus (covid-19). In: Statpearls [internet]. StatPearls Publishing (2020)
23. Bai, Y., Yao, L., Wei, T., Tian, F., Jin, D.Y., Chen, L., Wang, M.: Presumed asymptomatic carrier transmission of covid-19. Jama (2020)
24. Lillie, P.J., Samson, A., Li, A., Adams, K., Capstick, R., Barlow, G.D., Easom, N., Hamilton, E., Moss, P.J., Evans, A., et al.: Novel coronavirus disease (covid-19): the first two patients in the uk with person to person transmission. J. Infect. (2020)
25. Corman, V.M., Landt, O., Kaiser, M., Molenkamp, R., Meijer, A., Chu, D.K., Bleicker, T., Brünink, S., Schneider, J., Schmidt, M.L., et al.: Detection of 2019 novel coronavirus (2019-ncov) by real-time rt-pcr. Eurosurveillance 25(3), 2000045 (2020)
26. Xie, X., Zhong, Z., Zhao, W., Zheng, C., Wang, F., Liu, J.: Chest ct for typical 2019-ncov pneumonia: relationship to negative rt-pcr testing. Radiology p. 200343 (2020)
27. Xiong, Y., Sun, D., Liu, Y., Fan, Y., Zhao, L., Li, X., Zhu, W.: Clinical and high-resolution ct features of the covid-19 infection: comparison of the initial and follow-up changes. Invest, Radiol (2020)
28. Ooi, G.C., Khong, P.L., Müller, N.L., Yiu, W.C., Zhou, L.J., Ho, J.C., Lam, B., Nicolaou, S., Tsang, K.W.: Severe acute respiratory syndrome: temporal lung changes at thin-section ct in 30 patients. Radiology 230(3), 836–844 (2004)
29. Woo, P.C., Lau, S.K., Wong, B.H., Tsoi, H.w., Fung, A.M., Kao, R.Y., Chan, K.H., Peiris, J.M., Yuen, K.Y.: Differential sensitivities of severe acute respiratory syndrome (sars) coronavirus spike polypeptide enzyme-linked immunosorbent assay (elisa) and sars coronavirus nucleo-capsid protein elisa for serodiagnosis of sars coronavirus pneumonia. J. Clin. Microbiol. 43(7), 3054–3058 (2005)
30. Gautret, P., Lagier, J.C., Parola, P., Meddeb, L., Mailhe, M., Doudier, B., Courjon, J., Giordanengo, V., Vieira, V.E., Dupont, H.T., et al.: Hydroxychloroquine and azithromycin as a treatment of covid-19: results of an open-label non-randomized clinical trial. Int. J. antimicrob. Agents 105949, (2020)
31. Graham, R.L., Donaldson, E.F., Baric, R.S.: A decade after sars: strategies for controlling emerging coronaviruses. Nat. Rev. Microbiol 11(12), 836–848 (2013)
32. Wu, Y.H., Gao, S.H., Mei, J., Xu, J., Fan, D.P., Zhao, C.W., Cheng, M.M.: Jcs: An explainable covid-19 diagnosis system by joint classification and segmentation. arXiv preprint arXiv:2004.07054 (2020)
33. Luz, E., Silva, P.L., Silva, R., Moreira, G.: Towards an efficient deep learning model for covid-19 patterns detection in x-ray images. arXiv preprint arXiv:2004.05717 (2020)
34. Li, L., Qin, L., Xu, Z., Yin, Y., Wang, X., Kong, B., Bai, J., Lu, Y., Fang, Z., Song, Q., et al.: Artificial intelligence distinguishes covid-19 from community acquired pneumonia on chest ct. Radiology p. 200905 (2020)
35. Ilyas, M., Rehman, H., Nait-ali, A.: Detection of covid-19 from chest x-ray images using artificial intelligence: an early review. arXiv preprint arXiv:2004.05436 (2020)
36. Shi, F., Wang, J., Shi, J., Wu, Z., Wang, Q., Tang, Z., He, K., Shi, Y., Shen, D.: Review of artificial intelligence techniques in imaging data acquisition, segmentation and diagnosis for covid-19. arXiv preprint arXiv:2004.02731 (2020)
37. Castiglioni, I., Ippolito, D., Interlenghi, M., Monti, C.B., Salvatore, C., Schiaffino, S., Polidori, A., Gandola, D., Messa, C., Sardanelli, F.: Artificial intelligence applied on chest x-ray can aid in the diagnosis of covid-19 infection: a first experience from lombardy, italy. medRxiv (2020)
38. Cohen, J.P., Morrison, P., Dao, L.: Covid-19 image data collection. arXiv preprint arXiv:2003.11597 (2020)
39. Kalkreuth, R., Kaufmann, P.: Covid-19: a survey on public medical imaging data resources. arXiv preprint arXiv:2004.04569 (2020)
40. Loey, M., Smarandache, F., Khalifa, N.E.M.: Within the lack of covid-19 benchmark dataset: a novel gan with deep transfer learning for corona-virus detection in chest x-ray images (2020)

41. Apostolopoulos, I., Aznaouridis, S., Tzani, M.: Extracting possibly representative covid-19 biomarkers from x-ray images with deep learning approach and image data related to pulmonary diseases. arXiv preprint arXiv:2004.00338 (2020)
42. ELGhamrawy, S.M., et al.: Diagnosis and prediction model for covid19 patients response to treatment based on convolutional neural networks and whale optimization algorithm using ct images. medRxiv (2020)
43. Rajinikanth, V., Dey, N., Raj, A.N.J., Hassanien, A.E., Santosh, K., Raja, N.: Harmony-search and otsu based system for coronavirus disease (covid-19) detection using lung ct scan images. arXiv preprint arXiv:2004.03431 (2020)
44. Hu, Z., Ge, Q., Jin, L., Xiong, M.: Artificial intelligence forecasting of covid-19 in china. arXiv preprint arXiv:2002.07112 (2020)
45. Rao, A.S.S., Vazquez, J.A.: Identification of covid-19 can be quicker through artificial intelligence framework using a mobile phone-based survey in the populations when cities/towns are under quarantine. Inf. Control Hosp. Epidemiol. pp. 1–18 (2020)
46. Bullock, J., Pham, K.H., Lam, C.S.N., Luengo-Oroz, M., et al.: Mapping the landscape of artificial intelligence applications against covid-19. arXiv preprint arXiv:2003.11336 (2020)
47. Hu, Z., Ge, Q., Li, S., Boerwincle, E., Jin, L., Xiong, M.: Forecasting and evaluating intervention of covid-19 in the world. arXiv preprint arXiv:2003.09800 (2020)
48. Nguyen, D., Ding, M., Pathirana, P.N., Seneviratne, A.: Blockchain and ai-based solutions to combat coronavirus (covid-19)-like epidemics: a survey (2020)
49. Subirana, B., Hueto, F., Rajasekaran, P., Laguarta, J., Puig, S., Malvehy, J., Mitja, O., Trilla, A., Moreno, C.I., Valle, J.F.M., et al.: Hi sigma, do i have the coronavirus?: Call for a new artificial intelligence approach to support health care professionals dealing with the covid-19 pandemic. arXiv preprint arXiv:2004.06510 (2020)
50. Fong, S.J., Li, G., Dey, N., Crespo, R.G., Herrera-Viedma, E.: Finding an accurate early forecasting model from small dataset: a case of 2019-ncov novel coronavirus outbreak. arXiv preprint arXiv:2003.10776 (2020)
51. Fong, S.J., Li, G., Dey, N., Crespo, R.G., Herrera-Viedma, E.: Composite monte carlo decision making under high uncertainty of novel coronavirus epidemic using hybridized deep learning and fuzzy rule induction. Appl. Soft Comput. **106282**, (2020)
52. Moskal, M., Beker, W., Roszak, R., Gajewska, E.P., Wołos, A., Molga, K., Szymkuć, S., Grzybowski, B.: Suggestions for second-pass anti-covid-19 drugs based on the artificial intelligence measures of molecular similarity, shape and pharmacophore distribution (2020)
53. Zhavoronkov, A., Aladinskiy, V., Zhebrak, A., Zagribelnyy, B., Terentiev, V., Bezrukov, D.S., Polykovskiy, D., Shayakhmetov, R., Filimonov, A., Orekhov, P., et al.: Potential covid-2019 3c-like protease inhibitors designed using generative deep learning approaches. Ins. Med. Hong Kong Ltd A **307**, E1 (2020)
54. Soares, F., Villavicencio, A., Anzanello, M.J., Fogliatto, F.S., Idiart, M., Stevenson, M.: A novel high specificity covid-19 screening method based on simple blood exams and artificial intelligence. medRxiv (2020)
55. Martínez-Álvarez, F., Asencio-Cortés, G., Torres, J., Gutiérrez-Avilés, D., Melgar-García, L., Pérez-Chacón, R., Rubio-Escudero, C., Riquelme, J., Troncoso, A.: Coronavirus optimization algorithm: a bioinspired metaheuristic based on the covid-19 propagation model. arXiv preprint arXiv:2003.13633 (2020)
56. Gysi, D.M., Valle, Í.D., Zitnik, M., Ameli, A., Gan, X., Varol, O., Sanchez, H., Baron, R.M., Ghiassian, D., Loscalzo, J., et al.: Network medicine framework for identifying drug repurposing opportunities for covid-19. arXiv preprint arXiv:2004.07229 (2020)
57. https://www.who.int/csr/don/archive/year/en/
58. Hota, S., McGeer, A.: Antivirals and the control of influenza outbreaks. Clin. Infect. Dis. **45**(10), 1362–1368 (2007)
59. Siettos, C.I., Russo, L.: Mathematical modeling of infectious disease dynamics. Virulence **4**(4), 295–306 (2013)
60. Aron, J.L.: Mathematical Modeling: The Dynamics of Infection. Theory and Practice, Infectious Disease Epidemiology (2000)

61. McLeod, K.S.: Our sense of snow: the myth of john snow in medical geography. Soc. Sci. Med **50**(7–8), 923–935 (2000)
62. Unkel, S., Farrington, C.P., Garthwaite, P.H., Robertson, C., Andrews, N.: Statistical methods for the prospective detection of infectious disease outbreaks: a review. J. Royal Statist. Soc. Series A (Statist. Soc.) **175**(1), 49–82 (2012)
63. Serfling, R.E.: Methods for current statistical analysis of excess pneumonia-influenza deaths. Public Health Reports **78**(6), 494 (1963)
64. Rath, T.M., Carreras, M., Sebastiani, P.: Automated detection of influenza epidemics with hidden markov models. In: International Symposium on Intelligent Data Analysis. pp. 521–532. Springer (2003)
65. Toda, A.A.: Susceptible-infected-recovered (sir) dynamics of covid-19 and economic impact. arXiv preprint arXiv:2003.11221 (2020)
66. Kermack, W.O., McKendrick, A.G.: A contribution to the mathematical theory of epidemics. In: Proceedings of the Royal Society of London. Series A, Containing Papers of a Mathematical and Physical Character **115**(772), 700–721 (1927)
67. Petropoulos, F., Makridakis, S.: Forecasting the novel coronavirus covid-19. PloS one **15**(3), e0231236 (2020)

Artificial Intelligence and Psychosocial Support During the COVID-19 Outbreak

Poonam Dhaka

Abstract World Health Organization (WHO) declared new coronavirus disease, COVID-19 as a pandemic in January 2020 and stated that support is needed for mental health and psychosocial wellbeing during this pandemic. Machine learning is the subset of artificial intelligence which can provide resources to overcome the current mental health crisis during COVID-19. It provides the opportunity to solve challenges with the ability to learn from experiences automatically. This chapter gives useful insight to assess the feasibility and efficacy of artificial intelligence and psychosocial support during the COVID-19 outbreak. The demographic data of Namibia during the infestation period of COVID-19 spread is presented and analysed by statistical methods about age, citizen and gender. Further in this study, a regression model is developed, which gives the relationship between the independent variable which is the date of infestation and a dependent variable which is the number of patients, and the available data is being used to predict the future value of infected COVID-19 outbreak in a similar environment.

Keywords Artificial intelligence · COVID-19 · Psychosocial support · Mental health

1 Introduction

World Health Organization (WHO) declared new coronavirus disease, COVID-19 as a pandemic in January 2020 [1]. World Health Organization and public health authorities mentioned that this time of crisis is developing stress throughout the world population. World Health Organization stated that support is needed for mental health and psychosocial wellbeing during this pandemic. World Health Organization released a series of messages for the healthcare workers, general population, team

P. Dhaka (✉)
Department of Human Sciences, University of Namibia, Windhoek, Namibia
e-mail: pdhaka@unam.na

© The Editor(s) (if applicable) and The Author(s), under exclusive license
to Springer Nature Switzerland AG 2020
A.-E. Hassanien et al. (eds.), *Big Data Analytics and Artificial Intelligence Against COVID-19: Innovation Vision and Approach*, Studies in Big Data 78,
https://doi.org/10.1007/978-3-030-55258-9_13

leaders, managers in health services, elderly people, care of children, people with severe health conditions and their careers, and for people in self-isolation [1].

Advancement in computing power, machine learning and data collection methods are developing an interest in artificial intelligence (AI). The effective usage of AI into healthcare can improve quality of care. Artificial intelligence can provide resources to overcome the current mental health crisis during COVID-19. There is a lack of mental health professionals in Namibia and other countries [2]. Artificial Intelligence can provide psychosocial support that an individual can access all the time remotely in the present scenario. Artificial intelligence can be helpful to analyse data faster, advise appropriate treatments and monitor the progress of patient's.

The demographic data of Namibia during COVID-19 spread is presented and analysed by statistical methods about age, citizen and gender. Various statistical methods are required with certain assumptions to analyses massive data generated during COVID-19. In industrial revolution 4.0, AI is a pivotal approach to analyse a large amount of data efficiently. This chapter gives useful insight to assess the feasibility and efficacy of artificial intelligence and psychosocial support during the COVID-19 outbreak. Machine learning is a subset of AI, and it provides the opportunity to solve science challenges with the ability to automatically learn from their experiences and increase the speed of data interpretation and analysis. The chapter analyses distribution of infestation in different gender, citizens and age group by Chi-square test for association. Simple linear regression analysis was also conducted to predict the relationship between the two variables [3, 4].

1.1 Motivation

With the speedy progression in technology and its application in the medical field, scientists and medical doctors are now looking forward to cure many disease. Research has been done to develop an image aided examination method using CT scan images to find out the pneumonia infection from the lungs. This study also proposes a method to compute the rate of infection in the lugs using the pixel level ratio of the lung region, which is infected [5]. Another study developed an optimised forecasting model by using a new algorithm called a polynomial neural network with corrective feedback. This algorithm is capable of predicting and has comparatively lowest prediction error. This model is advantageous to produce forecast during COVID-19 outbreak [6]. The proposed model helps to detect COVID-19 positive cases using a light-weight CNN-tailored shallow architecture. This model also needs a few parameters, and it has no false positive and chest X-rays is used to find out COVID-19 infected cases [7].

A study suggests that using Composite Monte Carlo (CMC) simulation, which is enriched by adding deep learning network and fuzzy rule induction is a better way to get stochastic understandings about the epidemic spread. The researchers suggested that instead of merely applying Monte Carlo (MC), deep learning incorporated CMC can be used in combination with fuzzy rule induction so that the decision-makers can get the benefit to forecasting the epidemic in China and the rest of the world [8].

The research proposed a model (Artificial Intelligence Model for COVID-19 Diagnosis and Prediction—AIMDP) using artificial intelligence to diagnose and predict patients infected by COVID-19. Mainly the model has two tasks, firstly the Diagnosis Module (DM), which is responsible for detecting the patient suffering from COVID-19 at an early stage and with accuracy using CT scans. This model also distinguishes it from other viral infections. The DM is based on Convolutional Neural Networks and can process a large number of CT scans in a few seconds. Secondly, the Prediction Module (PM) is for predicting capability of the patient to respond to the treatment based on various factors such as medical condition, age, stage of infection etc. Whale Optimization Algorithm was used in PM to select genuine cases. The results show good performance for both the modules using a large dataset of CT images [9].

As COVID-19 has now attained pandemic status. The WHO has given specific guidelines to manage the problem for both biomedical as well as a psychological aspect. At this stage, preventive action is very crucial but to provide psychosocial support to people suffering from COVID-19 is also essential. According to the researcher best knowledge, a few published literature exists on artificial intelligence and psychosocial support during the COVID-19 outbreak.

Further, the chapter is organised as follows: Sect. 2 gives an update on COVID-19 in Namibia. Recent studies are included in Sect. 3, under the psychosocial support heading. In Sect. 4, some insight is given related to statistical and machine learning methods. Section 5 includes statistical results and discussion. In Sect. 6, linear regression for machine learning is described. Results of regression-machine learning are shown in Sect. 7. Lastly, the conclusion and future scope are mentioned in Sect. 8.

2 Update on COVID-19 in Namibia

The test for COVID-19 was conducted on two traveller's couple who came to Namibia from Madrid Spain and were immediately quarantined on 13th March 2020 when positive results were found, and contact tracing commenced. This was intensified to ensure that all contacts are traced in order to prevent community spread [3].

The President of the Republic of Namibia addressed the country and said, "The health of Namibians is the first priority. Appropriate precautionary measures must be taken" [4]. The first three cases were travel-related [10]. "As emphasised in my statement, the Health of Namibians is the highest t priority. It is why on March 17, 2020, the Government declared the State of Emergency and responded with urgent and aggressive measures to contain the spread of the novel Corona Virus into our communities" [11].

In light of the rising travel-related six cases up to March 24, 2020, of COVID-19 disease in Namibia, Cabinet decided to strengthen the national response and some measures were adopted [11]. State of emergency—COVID-19 regulations: Namibian constitution was Proclamation by the President of the Republic of Namibia on Saturday 28 March 2020 [12]. The period of lockdown started on 28 March 2020 and ends on 17 April 2020, inclusive of the first and the last day. To date commutatively, 16 confirmed cases are reported in the country. No new confirmed case is reported from 2 April 2020. Three cases are related to local transmission, and 13 cases are imported [13].

3   Psychosocial Support

The coronavirus disease (COVID-19) has been spread in Namibia and all over the world. This COVID-19 pandemic has provoked attention countrywide. It is the need of the hour to look at the psychological effects of quarantines and their family members. People suffering from COVID-19 have psychological distress, and this leads to numerous problems like depression, anxiety, feeling of fear, aloneness, rejection and specially stigmatisation [14].

Besides physical distress, it is normal for COVID-19 patients to go through psychological distress and other mental and physical health-related complications. Psychologists and social workers are not the exceptions as they have to do counselling sessions with the infected patients, family members and relatives. The ministry of health and social services of Namibia has taken several steps to provide psychosocial support by arranging health education, psychosocial support and post counselling services to people under quarantine, COVID-19 confirmed cases and their families. The psychosocial support services are also available through radio talks [13].

As this pandemic is contagious, it is not possible to have one-on-one or face to face counselling sessions. So it is suggested to have online-based mental health intervention programs and counselling. This is feasible by incorporating technology, big data and AI for COVID-19 readiness and preparedness [15]. Mainly psychologists administer different types of psychological tests, assessments, and questionnaires to the patient suffering from COVID-19 to assess their mental state by having contact with each other, by doing this there are chances that the disease can spread vastly. Therefore, we can overcome this problem if all the assessments and their analysis are conducted and assisted with AI and ML algorithms. AI can also bring therapy to more people and at an affordable price [16]. Another difficulty the psychologists are facing in diagnosing the mental health status of the COVID-19 patients. To know about the mental state, regular interactions are needed as symptoms of these disorders change frequently. In this situation of a pandemic, it becomes difficult to have face to face counselling, and it is also not safe to be in contact with the patients frequently.

So there is a need to have additional approaches for counselling and analysing data using AI, such as audio and video analysis because these methods have better objectivity and also have good predictive value. These tools can also monitor the progress of patients. In this situation with limited resources, there is a need for various methods using AI for psychosocial counselling which are readily available and are more productive. By using AI, it becomes easy and fast to analyse extensive data and give a better prediction for the treatment [17].

If AI is successfully integrated into healthcare, it could improve the quality of care of the patients suffering from COVID-19 disease. By introducing AI in psychosocial interventions, this will lead to improving patient outcome like there mental state, and will also balance the workload of health care workers and also to analyse the big data in this situation. It will also be helpful to monitor the trend in which the disease is spreading [17].

Artificial intelligence can serve as an effective way for psychologists to make the best of the time they spend with their clients, and also to bridge any type of gap in access. Data analysis using artificial intelligence can assist psychologists in making their diagnosis faster and accurate and in giving the treatment as soon as possible. Besides this, other programs in which AI is incorporated will allow the psychologists to observe the patients remotely as the positive cases need frequent consultations and this regular touch with the psychologist the patients will feel safe. Programmes incorporating AI can also be helpful to collect data without getting in contact with the patients suffering COVID-19 and analysis can be done faster and accurate. At present, there is a need for such technology to be integrated into counselling sessions to provide psychosocial interventions so that both the patients and the clinicians can get all the benefits by maintaining social distance. For this study, the researcher could only analyse demographic data.

4 Statistical and Machine Learning Methods

The chapter analyses the patients infected by COVID-19 in Namibia. For this study, the author gathered the data for the *infected cases by COVID-19* and the *date of symptoms onset* within one month in Namibia. Patients data are collected from the Ministry of Health and Social Services, Republic of Namibia [13].

4.1 Statistical Models

Firstly the Statistical Package for the Social Sciences (SPSS), the software package is used to analyse the infected cases by COVID-19 and to find out the association between gender, age and citizen [18].

4.2 Machine Learning Models

Further, the researcher has developed the mathematical regression analysis model, which gives the relationship between infected cases by COVID-19, which is the dependent variable, and date of symptoms onset, which is the independent variable. This regression model is implemented with the help of Python 3.7, as it is an object-oriented and platform-independent programming language used for multi-disciplinary research and development in machine learning. In this study, Python3.7 and Jupyter Notebook are used to generate plots and establish regression model for COVID-19 data of Namibia [19]. This study has linear and quadratic regression and built a basic machine-learning model with COVID-19 dataset of Namibia.

The linear regression model is expressed as:

$$\hat{y} = b_0 + b_1 x \tag{1}$$

where x denotes the independent variable and the dependent variable is denoted by y. In regression, equation b_0 is the constant term, which intercepts the regression line on the vertical axis (y) and b_1 is called as the regression coefficient. The importing statements and codes of Python 3.7 for scatter plot and regression equation are:

Algorithm for scatter plot

```
#Import 'COVID-19 Patients' data from csv file to DataFrame
        import pandas as pd
#Import for creating plots.
                import matplotlib as mpl
# import formula api as alias sm
                import statsmodels.formula.api as sm
# Fitting linear regression model to training model
                from sklearn.linear_model import LinearRegression
#Perform statistical calculations
                from scipy import stats
#Import library for graphics
                import seaborn as sns
#Import library for scientific computing
                import numpy as np
#Import library for data visulation
                import matplotlib.pyplot as plt
#Read the csv file  contents into a DataFrame
                data=pd.read_csv("Namibia COVID-19.csv")
                data
                        data.plot('Date of Symptoms Onset','Patients',style='o')
                        plt.ylabel('COVID-19 Patients')
                        plt.title('COVID-19 Patients')
                        plt.show()
```

Algorithm for regression equation

```
#from pandas import DataFrame
        import statsmodels.api as sm
                date_sym=data['Date of Symptoms Onset']
                pat=data['Patients']
# Adding a constant
                date_sym=sm.add_constant(date_sym)
# Fit regression model
                model=sm.OLS(pat,date_sym)
                results=model.fit()
# Analysis result of the developed model
                print(results.summary())
```

5 Statistical Results and Discussion

Tables 1, 2 and 3 show that several COVID-19 infested males (75%) were significantly higher than females (25%) P = 0.043. Nevertheless, the difference between Namibian and non-Namibian citizens was non-significant P = 0.130. Though 68.8% infested persons were Namibians and 31.2% were non-Namibians. The trend was almost the same in both the genders. In males, 66.7% Namibians and 33.3% non-Namibians similarly in females, 75.0% were Namibians, and 25.0% were non-Namibians. This distribution was also independent as Fisher's exact probability was 1.00.

Table 4 shows that maximum infestation was in the age group 14–34 years (50%) it was followed by 35–59 (31.2%), 60–79 (12.5%) and was minimum in 1–14 (6.2%) age group.

Table 1 Males and females infested with COVID-19 in Namibia

	Female	Male	x^2	DF	P
Count	4	12	4.00	1	0.043
%	25.0	75.0			

Table 2 Namibian and non-Namibian citizens infested with COVID-19

	Non-Namibian	Namibian	x^2	DF	P
Count	5	11	2.250	1	0.130
%	31.2	68.8			

Table 3 Relationship between citizens and genders

Citizen		Gender	
		Male	Female
Non-Namibian	Count	4	1
	% within gender (%)	33.3	25.0
Namibian	Count	8	3
	% within gender (%)	66.7	75.0

Fisher's exact probability $= 1.00$

Table 4 Distribution of COVID-19 infestation in different age groups

Age (year)	1–14	15–34	35–59	60–79	x^2	DF	P
Count	1	8	5	2	7.500	3	0.056
%	6.2	50.0	31.2	12.5			

Table 5 indicates that in each age group, male were more infested than females. This distribution indicated that infestation was associated with the movement of persons.

The age group and gender are having more movement having more infestation and change according to the movement of other age groups. However, on account of a smaller sample, the x^2 test was not justified.

Table 6 presents the relationship between age and citizenship of the COVID-19 positive cases. The trend of infected patients was the same in both Namibians and non-Namibian citizens and was similar to the age group except a few exceptions. In Namibians, the maximum frequency was in the most active age group 15–34 (54.5%) followed by 35–59 (27.3%).

The age group 1–14 and 60–79 having an equal frequency, i.e. 9.1%. Similarly, in non-Namibians, more frequency was in the age group 15–34 and 34–59, i.e. 40%

Table 5 Relationship between age and gender

			Gender	
			Male	Female
Age in years	1–14	Count	1	0
		% within gender (%)	8.3	0.0
	15–34	Count	5	3
		% within gender (%)	41.7	75.0
	35–59	Count	4	1
		% within gender (%)	33.3	25.0
	60–79	Count	2	0
		% within gender (%)	16.7	0.0

Table 6 Relationship between age and citizen

			Citizenship	
			Namibian	Non-Namibian
Age in years	0–14	Count	1	0
		% within citizen (%)	9.1	0.0
	15–34	Count	6	2
		% within Citizen (%)	54.5	40.0
	35–59	Count	3	2
		% within citizen (%)	27.3	40.0
	60–79	Count	1	1
		% within citizen (%)	9.1	20.0

Table 7 The determinant of quadratic regression analysis

Sn	Type of patients	R square	Variability explained (%)
1.	All	0.980	98.00
2.	Male	0.992	99.20
3.	Female	0.977	97.70
4.	Namibian	0.956	95.60
5.	Non Namibian	0.825	82.50
6.	Age 14–34	0.972	97.20
7.	Age 35–59	0.902	90.20
8.	Age 60–79	1.000	100.00

in each. Rest of the 20% patients were in the age group 60–79 the youngest one age group 1–14 did not have any patient. Chi-square test again on account of a smaller sample size could not be justified.

From the Table 7 the determinant of quadratic regression analysis revealed that the date explains 98.00% of change in several patients. It was true in all the groups of patients but, varies from 90.2 (age 35–59) to 100% (age 60–79).

The analysis of variance for quadratic regression analysis (Table 8) revealed that regression explained the variability of patients significantly in all the groups except females, non-Namibian and age group 35–59.

6 Linear Regression for Machine Learning

Linear regression algorithm is one of the frequently used algorithm in statistics. It is a type of supervised machine learning and is used to create a linear regression model for the analysis of the tasks.

Table 8 ANOVA for quadratic regression analysis

Sn	Type of patients	DF Reg	DF Err	MS Reg	MS Err	P
1.	All	2	13	166.589	0.525	0.000
2.	Male	2	9	70.937	0.125	0.000
3.	Female	2	1	2.442	0.115	0.152
4.	Namibian	2	8	52.607	0.598	0.000
5.	Non Namibian	2	2	4.124	0.876	0.175
6.	Age 14–34	2	5	20.422	0.231	0.000
7.	Age 35–59	2	2	4.512	0.488	0.098
8.	Age 60–79	1	0	0.5	–	–

6.1 Regression Analysis

Linear regression model is used to express the association between the dependent and independent variables.

The use of a linear regression model is to describe the relationships between the dependent variable and a set of independent variables. The principle behind the simple linear regression model is that there is only one independent and one dependent variable.

The goodness-of-fit measure of the regression model measures with the help of the coefficient of determination called R-squared (R^2). So, the strength of the relationship between the independent variable and the dependent variable is measured by R-squared.

The estimated regression equation is used for estimation and prediction values. With the help of regression analysis, the model for significant can be tested. So it determines how well the model fits the data and can be used for the hypothesis testing. Thus, the regression analysis technique is beneficial where the cause and effect have to be measured between variables. This model can be used for process optimisation. If there are many independent variables, we can say which independent variable is a more important variable that affects the dependent variable.

The simple linear regression model shows the relationship between the dependent variable (y) and an independent variable (x) and also an error term.

The simple linear regression model is:

$$y = \beta_0 + \beta_1 x + \epsilon \tag{2}$$

where β_0 and β_1 are called parameters of the model, and ϵ is a random variable known as the error term.

Independent variable (x) itself is not enough to predict the dependent variable (y) as there may be some unknown variable other than x and the error due to that unknown variable is called error term.

The estimated linear regression equation is the expectation of $E(y) = \hat{y} = \beta_0 + \beta_1 x$, where β_0 is the y-intercept of the regression line, β_1 is the slope of the regression line, and $E(y)$ or $= \hat{y}$, is the expected value of y for a given x value.

When a comparison is made between the linear regression model and the estimated linear regression equation, an error term is also present in the equation because the error was minimised by using least squares method during the formation of the equation.

Least squares method

The principle behind the least square method is the sum of the square of the error has to be minimised so that line is the best.

$$\text{Least square criterion: min} \sum (y_i - \hat{y})^2 \tag{3}$$

where y_i is the observed value of the dependent variable for the ith observation and $\hat{y}$, is the estimated value of the dependent variable. Therefore, an error is the total of the square of the difference of actual value minus the predicted value of the dependent variable. This sum of the error square has to be minimised.

The beauty of this error squared the transformation is if there is a lesser deviation, there is a lesser penalty and if there is a larger deviation larger penalty. For example, for the low value the difference of $y_i - \hat{y}$, is 0.4 then the square is 0.16 but for high value, suppose the deviation is four then the square is 16.

6.2 Estimation Process

In Fig. 1, we assume a regression model $y = \beta_0 + \beta_1 x + \epsilon$ and this regression will be predicted with the help of regression equation, and that is expected value $E(y) = \hat{y} = \beta_0 + \beta_1 x$. In the population regression model $y = \beta_0 + \beta_1 x + \epsilon$ the unknown parameters are β_0, β_1, and ϵ. However, the unknown parameters are β_0 and β_1. Furthermore, there is no error term in the population regression equation.

We have to estimate the value of β_0 and β_1. If the estimated value of β_0 and β_1 that means there is no relation between the independent variable (x) and the dependent variable (y).

In this chapter, the gathered sample data for COVID-19 infested cases in Namibia are the date of symptoms onset (x) as an independent variable and patient (y) as the dependent variable. With the help of the data, a regression equation $\hat{y} = b_0 + b_1 x$ is developed and is applicable only for the sample data.

Hence, $\hat{y} = b_0 + b_1 x$, where x is an independent variable and $\hat{y}$ is the estimated dependent variable and b_1. is the slope of the sample regression equation line and b_0 is the intercept (the value of y when $x = 0$).

Now we have to estimate whether the value of the slope of the sample regression equation line b_1, and the intercept b_0 is valid even for the population (slope of the population regression model β_1, and the intercept β_0).

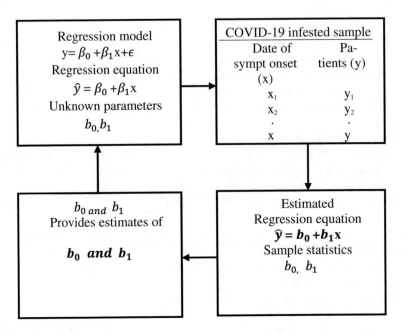

Fig. 1 Estimation process

So with the help of the sample regression equation, we can construct the population regression model. Expected regression equation at the population level is $\hat{y} = \beta_0 + \beta_1 x$ however, when we estimate the value of β_0, it may not be significant at population-level.

However, with the help of a sample mean $(\bar{x})$ we have predicted population parameter mean (μ), with the help of sample variance (s^2) we have predicted the population variance (σ^2) and with the help of sample proportion (p), we have predicted population proportion (P).

We have some x and y value from the sample and predicted regression equation $\hat{y} = \beta_0 + \beta_1 x$. Now we have to validate whether this relationship is valid even for the population.

Sometimes when a regression equation is constructed with the help of sample data, there is an association between an independent variable (x) and the dependent variable (y). However, when we test with the population, there is no relation between x and y.

Therefore, there is a difference between regression modelling and hypothesis testing. In hypothesis testing, only one parameter is tested at a time and can predict the mean or variance or population proportion.

6.3 Regression Model

Now a regression model is constructed with the help of sample data, and we will test this model in the population level. With the help of sample data, we have to find out the value of b_1 which is called the slope. The slope is the covariance divided by the variance of the independent variable. The slope (b_1) is calculated as:

$$\text{Slope } (b_1) = \frac{CoV(x, y)}{Var(x)} \tag{4}$$

$$\text{CoV } (x, y) = \sigma_{x,y} = \frac{\sum (x - \bar{x})(y - \bar{y})}{n - 1} \tag{5}$$

The variance formula includes only the independent variable (x).

$$\text{Correlation Coefficient} = \frac{CoV(x, y)}{\sigma_x \sigma_y} \tag{6}$$

$$\text{Variance}(x) = (s^2) = \frac{\sum (x - \bar{x})^2}{n - 1} \tag{7}$$

$$\text{Slope } (b_1) = \frac{CoV(x, y)}{Var(x)} = \frac{\frac{\sum (x - \bar{x})(y - \bar{y})}{n-1}}{\frac{\sum (x - \bar{x})^2}{n-1}}$$

$$= \frac{\sum (x - \bar{x})(y - \bar{y})}{\sum (x - \bar{x})^2} \tag{8}$$

Therefore, the slope (b_1) for the estimated regression equation is calculated by the following formula using least squares method:

$$\text{Slope } (b_1) = \frac{\sum (x - \bar{x})(y - \bar{y})}{\sum (x - \bar{x})^2} \tag{9}$$

Now we have to calculate y-intercept (b_0) for the estimated regression equation using the least squares equation:

$$\bar{y} = b_0 + b_1 \bar{x} \tag{10}$$

$$b_0 = \bar{y} - b_1 \bar{x} \tag{11}$$

where:

$\bar{x}$ mean value for independent variable
$\bar{y}$ mean value for dependent variable
n   total observations.

7 Results of Regression-Machine Learning

Linear regression or Ordinary Least Squares regression (OLS) results are shown in Table 9. The linear regression model is $\hat{y} = -4.5343 + 0.6320$ x, where x is the date of symptom and y is the patient (Table 9). Regression analysis will evaluate:

$$\hat{y} = -4.5343 + 0.6320x \tag{12}$$

7.1 Plot at Mean Value of Date of Symptoms Onset and Infected Cases

```
date_sym=data['Date of Symptoms Onset']
pat=data['Patients']

    plt.figure()
    sns.regplot(date_sym,pat,fit_reg=True)
    plt.scatter(np.mean(date_sym),np.mean(pat),color="green")
```

In Fig. 2, the X-axis is the date of symptoms onset (independent variable), and

Table 9 OLS regression results

Dep. variable:	Patients		R-squared:			0.954	
Model:	OLS		Adj. R-squared:			0.950	
Method:	Least Squares		F-statistic:			287.3	
Date:	Sat, 18 Apr 2020		Prob (F-statistic):			1.00e−10	
Time:	17:01:15		Log-likelihood: AIC:			−22.603	
No. observations:	16		BIC:			49.21	
Df residuals:	14					50.75	
Df model:	1						
Covariance type:	Nonrobust						
const	coef	std err	t	P>|t|	[0.025	0.975]	
Date of symptoms onset	−4.5343	0.814	−5.573	0.000	−6.279	−2.789	
	0.6320	0.037	16.949	0.000	0.552	0.712	
Omnibus:	1.160		Durbin-Watson:			0.457	
Prob(Omnibus):	0.560		Jarque-Bera (JB):			0.881	
Skew:	−0.291		Prob(JB):			0.644	
Kurtosis:	2.008		Cond. No.			67.0	

Note Standard Errors assume that the covariance matrix of the errors is correctly specified. Kurtosis test only valid for n ≥ 20

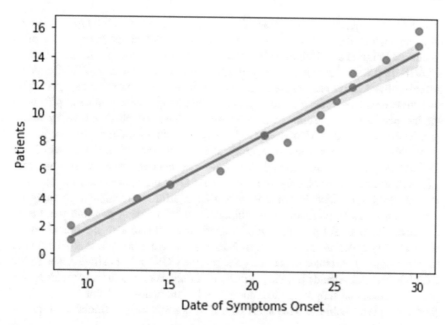

Fig. 2 Date of symptoms onset (March 2020) versus patients Linear regression

the Y-axis is the number of patients (dependent variable). The confidence interval is very narrow when $x = \bar{x}$. The estimated regression equation $-4.5343 + 0.6320\,x$ provides an estimate of the relationship between the dates of symptoms onset x and patients y. If the date is increased by one unit, patients will be increased by 0.6320 unit.

The F test value is 287.3 for the entire model, which shows the P-value $= 0.000$. The results show a statistically significant linear correlation between the two variables. Coefficient of determination (R squared) value tells how well the regression predictions estimate the actual data points.

The value for R squared is between 0 and 1 that states that how well the line fits the data set. An R^2 of 1 represents that the regression predictions fit the data perfectly. The value closer to 1, the better the line fits the data set and to draw correlation conclusions from the graph, so we want to be reasonably close to 1. So with an R^2 of 0.954 (Table 9), we can conclude that the variance of y (number of patients on the date) explains 95.4% by the x (date of symptoms onset).

8   Conclusions

In Namibia, the first COVID-19 infested patient was found on 9th March 2020. After that, the increase in the number of patients was reported with the increasing date following quadratic regression. This trend was true for all the type of patients viz., males, females, Namibian, non-Namibian and different age groups. Except for gender, no significant difference between the groups was there. The frequency of COVID-19 positive was significantly higher in males than in females. The frequency revealed that positive cases were more in the more exposer/ movable group. Further, this study develops a linear regression model, which gives the relationship between the independent variable and dependent variable. The available data is being used to predict the future value of infected COVID-19 cases in a similar environment.

In this study, the researcher mainly attempts to see the trend in which the COVID-19 pandemic will spread in future using machine learning and the analysis is conducted based on only one-month data. Overall, AI can benefit and support mental health specialists in doing their work. Algorithms are capable of analysing data much faster in comparison to humans, can recommend possible treatments, can easily keep an eye on a patient's recovery and can also alert the practitioner if there are any concerns. At present, in Namibia, there are no data available related to psychological variables to see the effect on the COVID-19 positive cases. In this COVID-19 crisis, AI and a human practitioner should work together to provide appropriate psychosocial support to the community. In future, this work can be extended if related data is available, and the analysis will be done by using artificial intelligence.

References

1. World Health Organization: Mental Health and Psychosocial Considerations During the COVID-19 Outbreak. World Health Organization, pp. 1–6 (2020)
2. Dhata, P. et al.: Mental Health Services in Namibia: Challenges and Prospects, vol. 4, no. 1, pp. 10–15 (2017)
3. Shangula, Kalumbi: Press briefing on confirmation of Covid-19 in Namibia. Minister of Health and Social Services, Republic of, Windhoek (2020)
4. The Presidency, Republic of Namibia: Confirmation of Two Cases of COVID-19 on Namibian SSoil, 14 March 2020
5. Rajinikanth, V., Dey, N., Raj, A.N.J., Hassanien, A.E., Santosh, K.C., Raja, N.S.M.: Harmony-Search and Otsu based System for Coronavirus Disease (COVID-19) Detection using Lung CT Scan Images. April 2020
6. Fong, S.J., Li, G., Dey, N., Gonzalez-Crespo, R., Herrera-Viedma, E.: Finding an accurate early forecasting model from small dataset: a case of 2019-nCoV novel coronavirus outbreak. Int. J. Interact. Multimed. Artif. Intell. 6(1), 132 (2020)
7. Mukherjee, H., Ghosh, S., Dhar, A., Obaidullah, S.: Shallow Convolutional Neural Network for COVID-19 Outbreak Screening Using Chest. pp. 1–10 December 2019
8. Fong, S.J., Li, G., Dey, N., Crespo, R.G., Herrera-Viedma, E.: Composite Monte Carlo decision making under high uncertainty of novel coronavirus epidemic using hybridised deep learning and fuzzy rule induction. Appl. Soft Comput. 106282 (2020)
9. Elghamrawy, S.: Diagnosis and prediction model for COVID-19 patient's response to treatment based on convolutional neural networks and whale optimization algorithm using CT images. medRxiv 2019, 23 (2020)
10. The Republic of Namibia: Update on COVID-19 in Namibia, Windhoek, 23 March 2020. Minister of Health and Social Services (2020)
11. The Presidency, Republic of Namibia: Briefing Statement on COVID-19 National Response Measures, 24 March 2020

12. The Presidency, Republic of Namibia: State of Emergency—COVID-19 Regulations: Namibian Constitution, Government Gazette of the Republic of Namibia, No. 7159, Windhoek, 28 March 2020. Republic of Namibia (2020)
13. Surveillance Team: Situation Report no. 24 for COVID-19 Namibia, 11 April 2020. Minister of Health and Social Service, Republic of Namibia
14. Li, W. et al.: Progression of Mental Health Services during the COVID-19 Outbreak in China, vol. 16 (2020)
15. Report of the WHO-China Joint Mission on Coronavirus Disease 2019 (COVID-19), vol. 2019, pp. 16–24 (2020)
16. What Is Artificial Intelligence For Psychology? [Online]. Available: https://becominghuman.ai/what-is-artificial-intelligence-for-psychology-6c5f3ee6f008
17. Lovejoy, C.A., Buch, V., Maruthappu, M.: Technology and mental health: the role of artificial intelligence. Eur. Psychiatry **55**, 1–3 (2019)
18. Jat, D.S., et al.: Applications of statistical techniques and artificial neural networks: a review. J. Stat. Manag. Syst. **21**(4), 639–645 (2018)
19. Solutions for Data Science Practitioners And Enterprise Machine Learning [Online]. Available: https://www.anaconda.com/

Role of the Accurate Detection of Core Body Temperature in the Early Detection of Coronavirus

Enas Selem and Sherine M. Abd El-kader

Abstract Recently, the COVID-19 virus appeared and threatened people's lives over the entire world. The danger of this virus is its rapid spread and there are no specific vaccines or treatments for COVID-19 at this time. One of the most important symptoms of the COVID-19 virus is the high temperature. Therefore, we must quickly discover people whose temperature has risen. So, the local manufacturing of medical non-contact thermometer is challenging requirement in this time. In this paper we outlined several core body temperature estimation techniques which is used in the manufacturing of the non-contact medical thermometers.

Keywords Corona virus · Non-contact thermometer · Core body temperature · Forehead · Internet of things (IoT) · Fifth generation (5G) · Local manufacturing

1 Introduction

The sudden appearance of the Coronavirus caused global panic and occupied the minds of all researchers around the world. Egypt is at the forefront of the world's countries that took all precautions and measures to face the Coronavirus crisis, and the Egyptian health system provided a model in dealing with the Coronavirus crisis professionally in accordance with the instructions of the World Health Organization (WHO). It also encourages researchers in all fields to confront the Coronavirus, many teams trying to produce respirators and others in the production of smart masks, or in the production of a non-contact thermometer.

E. Selem (✉)
Faculty of Science, Suez Canal University, Giza, Egypt
e-mail: enas.selem@yahoo.com

S. M. Abd El-kader
Department of Computers and Systems, Electronics Research Institute, Giza, Egypt
e-mail: Sherine@eri.sci.eg

A.-E. Hassanien et al. (eds.), *Big Data Analytics and Artificial Intelligence Against COVID-19: Innovation Vision and Approach*, Studies in Big Data 78, https://doi.org/10.1007/978-3-030-55258-9_14

Actually, there is a great need for the non-contact thermometer [1, 2] to early detect coronavirus by rapidly discovering the person who suffers from high temperature. It is used to remotely measure the core body temperature, it can measure the core body temperature within few seconds, few centimeters away from the body [3], records approximately 30 readings, and gives an alarm at 38 °C. The prices of this kind of thermometers are ranging from 100 to 200 dollars. IR thermometers have two types namely medical and industrial thermometer. Industrial thermometers [4] can be used as a medical thermometer [5], but it gives inaccurate readings [6]. Many companies in Egypt imported large quantities of thermometers with large amounts of money, and still, there is a need for more and more. So, we designed and manufactured non-contact IoT thermometer to help in the early detection of the coronavirus with reasonable cost.

Generally, the health care services are suffering from enormous challenges such as, high cost of the devices, the increase number of patients, a wide spread of chronic diseases, and a lack of healthcare management resources. The utilization of IoT & 5G in medical services [7, 8] will solve a lot of these problems by introducing the coming benefits:

Easy access to health care service by both of patients and doctors, smooth incorporation with several technologies, ensure the analysis and processing of massive data.

Effective utilization of healthcare resources, provide real time and remote monitoring established by the joint healthcare services, ensure real-time interaction between doctors and patients, and authorize health care services.

All of these benefits of the IoT & 5G services will improve the performance of healthcare applications by presenting different services to hospital, clinics and non-clinical patient environments.

1.1 Types of Thermometers

The non-contact thermometers are categorized into two types based on their purpose medical thermometers and industrial thermometers. Recently, medical thermometers manufacturing gained an enormous attention due to current events of appearance covid-19 virus.

Local manufacturing of Non-contact medical thermometer save money for the government and has a great role in tracking infected person with coronavirus as it gives an alarm when the person temperature is 38 °C or more. There are two kinds of medical IR thermometer: skin and ear. IR thermometry such as tympanic thermometry as shown in Fig. 1 can be used to measure the temperature rectally by placing the thermometer in the child's bottom, orally by placing the thermometer in the mouth under the tongue, axillary by placing the thermometer in the armpit. IR skin thermometry as shown in Fig. 2 is used to estimate the temperature of a certain place on the skin (e.g., axilla, forehead).

Fig. 1 tympanic
thermometry [9]

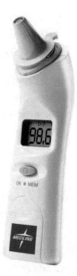

Fig. 2 Skin thermometer
[10]

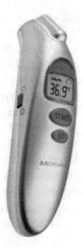

Any IR thermometer should satisfy these specifications [11].

- The Range of Displayed Temperature: In any display mode, an ear canal IR thermometer should show a volunteer's temperature over a minimum range of 34.4–42.2 °C (94.0–108.0 °F). On the other hand, a skin IR thermometer should show a volunteer's temperature over a minimum range of 22–40.0 °C (71.6–104.0 °F).
- Maximum Permissible Laboratory Error: for an Ear Canal IR Thermometer, for a blackbody temperature range from 36 to 39 °C (96.8 to 102.2 °F), the error should not be greater than 0.2 °C (0.4 °F), whereas for a Skin IR Thermometer, The laboratory error should be no greater than 0.3 °C (0.5 °F).

- Clinical Accuracy: The clinical accuracy is differentiated for different conditions such as device model, display mode, and for every age group of febrile and afebrile subjects on which the IR thermometer is intended to be used. Under no circumstances may the upper limit of the operating temperature range should be less than 35 °C (95 °F).
- Operating Humidity Range: The relative humidity range for the operating temperature range is up to 95%. The design of the IR thermometer to be used for medical purposes to detect a person who suffers from fever has great importance at this time.

1.2 Difference Between Industrial Thermometer and Medical Thermometer

Both of the industrial and medical infrared thermometers [12] are working by converting the analog signal to digital one. They consist of a thermopile sensor and microcontroller, power circuit, battery, memory, LCD monitor, alarm source and some buttons for measurement and operation. Generally, industrial thermometers are primary tools in observing experiments, assessing test materials, calibrating instruments, and other scientific procedures. Some researchers use them to ensure freezing and boiling points. Since they may be used for different kinds of solvents, the range is −10 °C to more than 300 °C as shown in Fig. 3. The material used in some thermometers is metal which is enriched via annealing or thermal tempering. While clinical thermometers (medical thermometers) as shown in Fig. 4 are used to measure the temperature of the human body. The range that they can assess is from 3510 to 4210 °C. Industrial thermometer can't be used as a clinical thermometer because the second one used for a fever to measure the internal core body temperature (hence the ear, mouth, or …). While the industrial IR thermometer is used in experiments, evaluating test materials, calibrating instruments, and other scientific procedure. If it used to measure core body temperature, it is only able to measure skin temperature which will vary more. As skin temperature is usually around 30–31 °C, but it mainly depends on the weared clothes and environment. While the core is generating energy, and because of thermal resistance, there will generally be a temperature decrease to your skin temperature. The core temperature is always kept at 37 °C (98.6 °F) as it is appropriate for normal body functions. It could be pointed to the ear but it would be pretty hard to get a reading from inside the ear, even if you centered it you wouldn't be sure of how accurate it would be. Table 1 summarizes the difference between clinical and industrial thermometers.

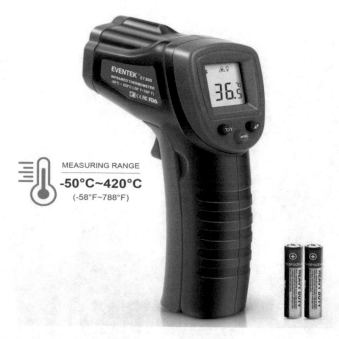

Fig. 3 Non-contact industrial thermometer [13]

2 Related Research

Measuring the core degree of core body temperature T_C without surgery (non-invasively) is one of the most important research topics. Conventional techniques of estimating T_C are usually not proper for the continual applications for the time of physical activity because it is invasive and it is not accurate enough. The rectal measurement of T_C or measuring at the bottom border of the esophagus (close to the heart) is annoying particularly in case of using sensors connected via wired connection. Axillary, orally, and ear (tympanic membrane) temperatures are not accurate especially through the practice of actions. The alternative method for measuring T_C is the use of ingestible telemetric thermometers but they are very expensive for daily use by a large number of persons. Although its great importance, the easy, cheap, and accurate measurement of T_C still a great challenge. Therefore, a lot of techniques have been investigated for the non-invasive T_C measurement. The invasively measurement of core body temperature is conducted using several experiments with varying assumption. The experiment is done in each method with a varying number of volunteers. The volunteers are varying in characteristics such as age, weight, height, and body fat. They wear different clothes with different thermal and vapor resistance. The volunteers were put under different test scenarios such as standing rest, walking on the treadmill for different times. The volunteers engaged in a different number of test sessions. The volunteers enter the test room with different room conditions

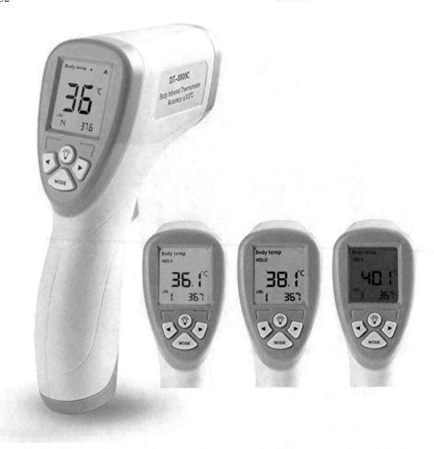

Fig. 4 Non-contact medical thermometer [14]

Table 1 Difference between clinical and industrial thermometers

Clinical thermometer	Industrial thermometer
Short range as it used for human body	Broad range as it used for different substance
Used for human body	Used for solid, liquid and gas substances
Used in hospitals, homes and airports	Used in laboratories and companies
The range from 35 degrees Celsius to 42 degrees Celsius	The range is −10 degrees Celsius to more than 300 °C
Give alarm at 38 °C.	No alarm
Measure core body temperature within 3 s, 10 cm away from the body	Measure the skin temperature which is differed approximately 3 °C from the core body temperature
Price is approximately 2000 L.E	300 L.E

such as snug [50% Relative Humidity (RH), 25 °C], hot-dry (20% RH, 40 °C), and hot-humid (70% RH, 35 °C)... etc. T_C was measured within different places such as pectoralis, sternum forehead, left scapula, left thigh, and left rib cage. The method that estimate T_C non-invasively are varying in the factors which T_C depends on such as skin temperature, ambient temperature, heat flux, heart rate...etc. The estimated T_C was compared to the observed T_C. The observed T_C is a rectal temperature or taken through a thermometer pill.

In [15] the protocol estimates the core body temperature T_C based on three factors which are skin temperature T_s, ambient temperature T_a and Heat Flux (HF) or Heat loss which is known as the heat transferred per unit time per unit area or from or to an object. Several linear regression techniques were presented to predict T_C which is dependent variables from two dependent variables HF and T_s. The system composed of T_C, T_s, and HF is regularly considered a dynamic system (the variables changes with time) as it affected by physical factors and physiological factors. The physical factors include the thickness of the tissue such as the thickness of the skin, fat, bone...etc. and the features of heat transfer of the tissue (e.g., thermal conductivity, heat capacity). The physiological factors including blood flow and sweat evaporation of the tissues. Metabolic heat is generated in the core of the body and is transported from the core to the skin by conduction over the tissue, after that it depletes from the skin to ambient (T_a) at a rate of heat flux (HF) by evaporation, convection, and radiation. The heat transfer resulted from the core to the skin through tissues is defined as follows:

$$\rho c \frac{\partial T}{\partial t} = \lambda \frac{\partial}{\partial x} \left(\frac{\partial T}{\partial x} \right) \tag{1}$$

where T is the temperature (°C), t is time in second (s), x is the distance from the core to the tissue in meter (m), q is the density in kg m^{-3}, c is the specific heat capacity in J kg^{-1} °C^{-1}, and k is the thermal conductivity in W m^{-1} °C^{-1}.

The heat exchange between the core surface and the skin surface is influenced by dynamic factors such as ambient temperature that change from time to time so the system is a varying system consists of steady state and dynamic state. The equation of heat transfer Eq. (1) is solved in the steady state as follows:

$$T_c = T_s + HF \frac{d}{\lambda} \tag{2}$$

where d is the shell thickness in m. This means that the derivation of T_c from T_s and HF in case of knowing d and k of the tissue is possible. The steady state is seldom in the human therefore, the process of heat transfer is usually varying. So, it is an important task to solve the steady state equation (Eq. 2) in varying conditions. Solving the steady state equation of the tissues (Eq. 1) means the varying temperature distributions over the tissue which indicates that the relation between T_C, T_s, and HF, is dynamic relation. The varying conditions were declared as follows:

The uniform temperature of the tissue is 33 °C, therefore, the initial condition at time t = 0 is T(x, 0) = 33 °C.

The dynamic process is begun when T_C (i.e., the core temperature at x = 0) is increased by 1–34 °C. So, the boundary condition at the core, (i.e., at x = 0 is T (0, t) = 34 °C at t > 0.

The boundary condition at the skin surface (i.e., at x = d) is heat loss via convection. The coefficient of heat transfer due to convective α is set at 10 Wm − 2 °C, and the initial ambient temperature T_a is 33 °C.

The mathematic description of these initial and boundary conditions are:

$$t = 0, T(x, 0) = 33 \,°\text{C};   \tag{3}$$

$$t > 0, x = 0, T(0, t) = 34 \,°\text{C};   \tag{4}$$

$$t > 0, x = d, -\lambda \frac{\partial T}{\partial t} = \alpha(T(x, t) - T_a)   \tag{5}$$

The temperature distribution T(x, t) changes little by little till it reaches another steady state [i.e., T(x, end)]. Within this transient time, the value of T_C in the steady state condition which is estimated by Eq. (2) will progressively converge to the perfect T_C. The results of the noticed T_C, T_s, and HF were taken from two places, the sternum and forehead and, at varying conditions (40 °C and 20% RH), the noticed T_C was taken by the telemetry pill or rectally and also it taken at different assumed condition and different assumed places (pectoralis, forehead, sternum,, left rib cage, left scapula, and left thigh) it was confirmed that the mechanisms for measuring T_C are based on the location of the sensor and their efficiency is varying based on the location of the sensor. For the placement studied, the best places are the sternum, or a collection of the sternum, scapula and rib sites.

Whereas in [16] estimate T_C exactly as [15] based on T_s, HF but the main difference that it take into consideration the Heart Rate (HR).

In [17] the core temperature is estimated using Kalman Filtering (KF) which consists of training and validation datasets. These data sets are consisting of the data from different persons. The parameters of KF model were predicted from the practice dataset using linear regression of T_C against T_s, HF, and HR. KF method used to estimate T_C consists of three states: state-transition state (A), noise correlated with each state and observation state (C).

First, the state-transition state shows the diversity in the state of the hidden variable T_c (x) from one time point to another as stated by:

$$xt = Axt - 1 + Wt   \tag{6}$$

where w is the transition state noise is assumed to be a zero means normal Gaussian distribution with covariance Q which depicted by:

$$Wt \sim N(0, Qt) \qquad (7)$$

Second, the observation state (C) compares full or a group of the observed variables T_s, HF, and HR (z) to the hidden variable of T_c from one time point to another as stated by:

$$Zt = Cxt + vt \qquad (8)$$

where v is the observation state noise and supposed to be a zero mean normal Gaussian distribution with covariance R which depicted by:

$$vt \sim N(0, Rt) \qquad (9)$$

T_c was the only hidden value, the matrix A composed of one value practiced using linear regression of time appeared in (minute to minute) to T_c values it means $(T_{c,t-1}, T_{c,t})$ from the practice dataset. Likewise, the matrix C composed of the weights practiced by linear regression of T_s, HF, and HR versus T_c. Variety of observation states were produced for each location of the HF sensor by using all sets of the T_s, HF, and HR as filter inputs for a total number of different states. The Q matrix consists of the variance of the differences of time showed in minutes in T_c whereas the values of the matrix R were practiced by utilizing the covariance of the minute differences of the various collection of T_s, HF, and HR. KF approach achieves perfect assessment of core body temperature in case of the availability of two of those three inputs (T_s, HF and HR).

In [18] a Kalman filter was used to suits the parameters of its model to each person and gives real-time T_c estimates. The model composed of, a mathematical model and a Kalman filter. This group was utilized wholly predict T_C through three steps as shown in Fig. 5.

This model uses the Activity (A_c) of the person, HR, and T_s, also uses two environmental variables, T_a and Relative Humidity (RH), to estimate the person's T_C in real time. The model consists of, a mathematical model and a Kalman filter. This combination was used altogether to give real-time individualized estimates of T_C via the following three procedures: First, in procedure 1, the calculated A_c and the environmental variables T_a and RH were utilized by the mathematical model for the estimation of the state variables, the actual estimated Heart Rate (HR) and the actual estimated core temperature $\left(\hat{T}_s\right)$. After that, in procedure 2, the difference (errors) between the measured values of T_s, HR and the actual estimated $\hat{T}_s$, $\hat{H}R$ were calculated. Lastly, in procedure 3, the Kalman filter utilizes these errors to justify the state variables and uses this repairing to update the mathematical model parameters. The mathematical model is formed of the following two sub models: a phenomenological element that connects A_c to HR and a first-principles macroscopic energy-balance element that relates HR to T_s and T_C. First, the framework of the phenomenological model was obtained by the observation of positive relationship between A_c and HR

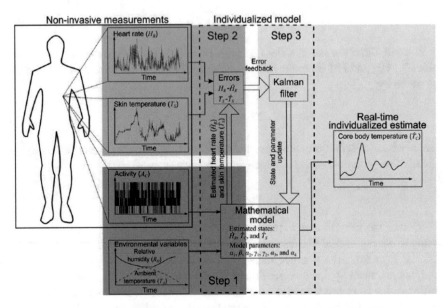

Fig. 5 The proposed model for individualized core body temperature estimation [18]

which means that the rise in A_c leads to a fast rise in HR, thereafter decreases exponentially when A_c decreases. This relationship was mathematically obtained by the next equation:

$$\frac{d\Delta HR}{dt} = -\alpha 1 \Delta HR + \beta A_c^4 \tag{10}$$

where ΔHR denotes the change in HR from a resting state HR0 (i.e., ΔHR = HR − HR0), $\alpha 1$ denotes the rate constant for HR, and β represents the gain in HR resulting from physical activity. Second, the first-principles component of the model consists of the core and skin-temperature compartments:

$$\frac{d\Delta T_c}{dt} = -\propto \Delta T_c + \gamma 1 S(\Delta HR)\Delta HR - \gamma 2(T_c - T_s) \tag{11}$$

where $\Delta T_c = T_c - T_{c0}$ and $\Delta T_s = T_s - T_{s0}$

T_{c0} is the initial core temperature, t_{c0} is the initial skin temperature, P_s denotes the vapor pressure of water for T_s, P_a represents the vapor pressure of water at a given T_a and RH, T_{c0} was set to 37 °C and T_{s0} is the mean of the measured T during the initial 10 min of data collection. The data is used from four studies to estimate the parameters $\alpha 1$ and β, which relate Ac to HR. Assessment of the performance of the model was evaluated by calculating the capability of the model to learn a person's heat-stress response under various experimental and environmental conditions by simulating the estimates of each T_C (i.e., $\hat{T}_C$) in continuous time and making a comparison between them. The accuracy of $\hat{T}_C$, was assessed by computing the square root of the mean squared differences between $\hat{T}_C$ and the T_C.

There are several methods of estimating core body temperature that has already experimentally applied as a patent [19, 20]. In [21], the patented introduce the procedure of estimating the core body temperature including: determining heat flux from an aimed surface area of the body that way giving the surface temperature; estimating the core temperature of the body based on two factors (ambient temperature and surface temperature), the function including the skin heat loss to the environment, for example the external ear canal or axilla, can be computed as follows:

$$q = hA(T_s - T_a) \tag{12}$$

where q is heat flow, A is surface area, T_s is the skin temperature and T_a is the ambient temperature, and h is an experientially calculated coefficient which comprises a radiation view factor between the ambient temperature and skin tissue. The heat flow process from the core arterial source to the skin is through the circulation of the blood, this model is very successful with comparison to the model of tissue conduction. Thermal transport through the circulation can be calculated as follows:

$$q = wc(T_c - T_s) \tag{13}$$

where q is heat flow, w is blood mass flow rate, c is blood specific heat, and T_c is the core body temperature and T_s, is the skin temperature. Therefore, the skin has a thermal view such as tissue being heated by its blood supply as shown in Eq. 13, keep balance by radiating heat to ambient as shown in Eq. 12. By solving Eq. 12. and Eq. 13. Generate the following equation:

$$hA(T_s - T_a) = wc(T_c - T_s) \tag{14}$$

Dividing by A (surface area):

$$h(T_s - T_a) = \rho c(T_c - T_s) \tag{15}$$

where ρ is blood flow per unit area, it can be named as termed perfusion rate as well.

Finally, our target is to estimate the core body temperature T_c is fulfilled by Eq. 15. in case of knowing the values of skin temperature T_s and ambient temperature T_a and also know their coefficients.

Determining T_c:

$$T_c = \frac{h}{\rho c}(T_s - T_a) + T_s \tag{16}$$

Where $h \backslash \rho c$, the weighting coefficient which weights the difference of ambient temperature and, the surface temperature is experimentally detected on a statistical basis over a set of patients and clinical states.

In [22], this invention is the thermometer that aimed to measure the body cavity temperature utilizing infrared sensing methods. Infrared radiation released by tissue surfaces gathered by an infrared lens and directed to an infrared sensor. This infrared sensor produces a signal voltage based on the difference of temperature between the body tissues being spotted and the infrared sensor. To detect the correct tissue temperature, a supplementary sensor is utilized to determine the ambient temperature of the infrared sensor and this ambient temperature is combined to the signal voltage. The relationship between the signals to produce exact tissue temperature is showed

$$T_s = G(E_s - E_a) + T_a \tag{17}$$

where E is the radiant energy from the body tissue, E_a is the radiant energy from the infrared sensor at ambient temperature.

In [23], this invention introduces a technique for the non-contact accurate and efficient measurement of the temperature of an object. By providing an infrared (IR) sensing assembly which determines the temperature of an object. This assembly consists of at least one IR sensing sensor which senses IR radiation and ambient temperature. Also, it consists of a processing circuit connected electrically to an IR sensing sensor. The processing circuit gains signals from the IR Sensing sensor and prophesies the temperature of the object.

In [24], this invention presents an IR thermometer which introduces a method for measuring core body temperature based on contact temperature, ambient temperature, and humidity degree.

In [25], this invention presents a forehead the non-contact thermometer that measures the core body temperature using the thermal radiation of the forehead. The core body temperature is calculated as a function of ambient temperature and skin temperature. The core body temperature is calculated as follows:

$$T_c = (1 + (h\backslash\rho c))(T_s - T_a) + T_a \tag{18}$$

T_s is the skin temperature, T_a is the ambient temperature, the function contains a weighted difference of the skin temperature and the ambient temperature with a weighting coefficient $h\backslash\rho c$.

3   Wireless Body Area Network

Wireless Body Area Network (WBAN) is used for medical systems. The main ides of WBAN is to monitor various biological functions by a variety of medical sensors that are placed inside or on the body as shown in Fig. 6. The medical sensors detect some signs that are important to follow up the status of the patient, such as temperature, heartbeats, blood pressure …etc. The medical sensors send the biological data using wireless connection to a gateway (e.g. IoT device) which in turn transmits it to a hospital server. The continual monitoring and diagnosing of patients can protect the

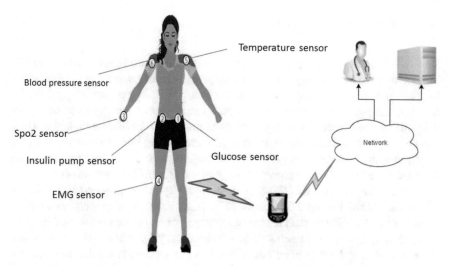

Fig. 6 WBAN system

lives of large number of patients particularly in the recent time because of the speed spread of coronavirus among people. Therefore, the fast detection of the peoples suffering from fever can help in preventing the fast spread of coronavirus. Thus, it demonstrates the significance of continuous communication between patients and medical servers. To ensure speedy delivery of the medical data to the medical servers, 5G technology can be used for this mission. Because of the features of 5G technology, it is considered the best technology used in WBAN systems to transfer the medical data to the medical server.

3.1 5G Technology

The fifth generation 5G wireless network is the upcoming fulfillment in the mobile communications. The main goal of this generation is to host variety devices with different types and large number, with the major increase of the number of different devices, 5G networks will connect whole world. This connectivity is accomplishment of thanks to the extreme data rate, minimum latency, and a large number of hosted devices that 5G can possess. Basically, 5G can be used for a variety of applications that get the lives of people better, for example, homes automation, remote medical care, wireless robots and driverless vehicles.

3.1.1   Role of 5G in the defense of coronavirus

Recently, because of the appearance of covid-19 the health care afford unbearable load as the existence of large number of hospitals is considered a terrible dangerous for both patients and health care workers. Using WBAN network along with 5G network can produce efficient and real time remote health care systems that gives the patients the possibility to get care from their homes [26]. Recommendations can be offered to patients by health care providers using brief video call, and give recipe demand. Doctors can give accurate diagnoses to the patient by requesting from the patients to send the report or image of tests result. The transmission process of medical images such as CT scans or X-rays requires high-speed transmission which can fulfilled using 5G network [27]. Also, the remote monitoring of large number of persons is the main reason of increased stress on the networks, this cause overcrowding and decrease network speeds, especially for healthcare providers that might be offering help to hundreds of patients per day. Additionally, the late and low level of the quality of patient care, could damage results in the long time. 5G Network can reduce whole medical costs and it permits the doctors to give nursing to anybody at any place without the need to the existence of patients at hospitals which can decrease the danger of the infection of covid-19 [28]. The features of 5G technologies as, low latency reliability…etc., fulfill high development in remote health monitoring because it awards different features in remote health care systems such as, imaging, diagnostics, treatment and data analytics. 5G will be used in several health applications that demand wide bandwidth and reliable connectivity. Utilizing the high -speed of 5G technology the transmission of tremendous files of medical images is done in a quick and reliable way, as well as, it facilitate to the doctors gaining the real time data that is required to improve the health care quality.

3.1.2   Features of 5G Network

- Very low latency
- Very fast response time
- It can host large number of devices
- It can host several types of devices
- It used for different application
- Wide capacity
- Permanent connectivity.

3.2   Using IR Thermometer in a WBAN Network

We can use the non-contact thermometer [33] as a wireless temperature sensor in a WBAN system [29] that gives an alarm when the person temperature is 38 °C or

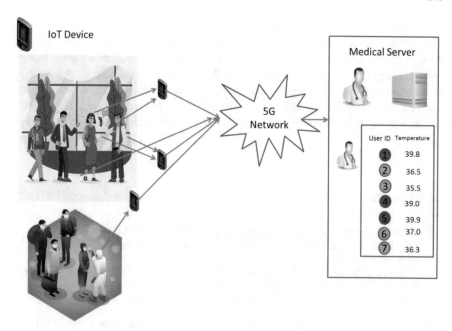

Fig. 7 Tracking of infected people with Coronavirus [33]

more. This IoT non-contact thermometer will be connected to the mobile gateway which is connected to a database in the medical server, the persons whose temperature is 37 °C will be colored with green mark while the assumed infected persons whose temperature exceed 38 °C will be colored with red as shown in Fig. 7. This medical server will be located in the ministry of health to continually follow up on the temperature of a large number of people. In order to meet the 5G and the IoT requirements [30, 31], The AESAS algorithm [32] will be used to increase the capacity and density of the network to serve a large number of devices effectively without any degradation in the quality of services, and to ensure that the priority is satisfied among all types of mobile gateways, increased the overall throughput of the network due to decreasing of the data drop rate, and decreased the delay or latency for sensitive-delay applications and services. The first part of the system will be achieved by designing the non-contact thermometer [33]; the second part will be the connection of all of these devices by a WBAN system [29] to ensure reliable and fast delivery of the medical data to the medical server [34–36].

4   Conclusions

In this paper we illustrate the role of non-contact thermometers in the early detection of coronavirus as well as the types of noncontact thermometers is explained. Several

method of estimating core body temperatures is surveyed. The role of 5G along with WBAN systems to face the danger of covid-19 was discussed. The IoT non-contact thermometer could be used as a part of WBAN system for early, real time detection and tracking of people suffers from a fever which might infected with corona virus. In the future work we will design a local manufactured IoT Non- contact thermometer and link it to our WBAN system that will be connected to a database in the medical server, and track the infected persons with corona virus whose have a fever with red color.

References

1. Sebban, E.: Infrared Noncontact Thermometer. U.S. Patent 549,114, issued Aug 21, 2007
2. Yelderman, M., et al.: Noncontact Infrared Tympanic Thermometer. U.S. Patent 5,159,936, issued Nov 3, 1992
3. Wenbin, C., Chiachung, C.: Evaluation of performance and uncertainty of infrared tympanic thermometers. Sens. (Basel, Switzerland) 10(4), 3073–3089 (2010)
4. Cascetta, F.: An evaluation of the performance of an infrared tympanic thermometer. Meas. 16(4), 239–246 (1995)
5. Jang, C., Chou, L.: Infrared Thermometers Measured on Forehead Artery Area. U.S. Patent US 2003/0067958A1, issued Apr 10, 2003
6. Teran, C.G., Torrez-Llanos, J., et al.: Clinical accuracy of a non-contact infrared skin thermometer in paediatric practice. Child: Care Health Dev. 38(4), 471–476 (2012)
7. Dhanvijay, M.M., Patil, S.C.: Internet of Things: A survey of enabling technologies in healthcare and its applications. Comput. Netw. 153(22), 113–131 (2019)
8. Alam, M.M., Malik, H., Khan, M.I., Pardy, T., Kuusik, A., Le Moullec, Y.: A survey on the roles of communication technologies in IoT-based personalized healthcare applications. IEEE Access 6, 36611–36631 (2018). https://doi.org/10.1109/ACCESS.2018.2853148
9. Edward, P., Alison, W., Billie, C.: Tympanic thermometry–normal temperature and reliability. Paediatric Nursing 21 (2009)
10. Thomas, F., Aaron, W., Rob, S., Graham, M.: Comparison of non-contact infrared skin thermometers. J. Med. Eng. Technol. 42, 1–7 (2018)
11. ASTM Standard E 1965. Standard Specification for Infrared Thermometers for Intermittent Determination of Patient Temperature (2003)
12. Fraden, J., Diego, S.: Medical Thermometer for Determining Body Core Temperature. U.S. Patent 7,785,266 B2, issued Aug 31, 2010
13. Xu, X., Karis, A.J., et al.: Relationship between core temperature, skin temperature and heat flux during exercise in heat. Springer 113, 2381–2389 (2013)
14. Welles, A.P., Xu, X., et al.: Estimation of core body temperature from skin temperature, heat flux, and heart rate using a Kalman filter. Comput. Biol. Med. 5(21) (2018)
15. TF-600 Thermometer Digital Body Temperature Fever Measurement Forehead Non-Contact Infrared LCD IR Thermometer Baby & Adult Review, Thermometers Beauty & Health, Health Care, Household Health Monitors, medek on January 23, 2019
16. Meco Irt550 Infrared Thermometer, Amazon
17. Eggenbereger, P., Macrae, B.A., et al.: Prediction of core body temperature based on skin temperature, heat flux, and heart rate under different exercise and clothing conditions in the heat in young adult males. Front. Physiol. 10(9) (2018)
18. Laxminarayan, S., Rakesh, V., et al.: Individualized estimation of human core body temperature using noninvasive measurements. J. Apll. Physoil. 124(6), 1387–1402 (2017)
19. Zou, S., Province, H.: Thermometer. U.S. Patent D837, 668 S, issued Jan 8, 2019

20. Roth, J., Raton, B.: Contact and Non-Contact Thermometer. U.S. Patent/000346, issued Jan 2, 2014

21. Pompei, F.: Ambient and Perfusion Normalized Temperature Detector, Boston, MA. EP 0 991 926 B1, issued Dec 12, 2005

22. Fraden, J., Jolla, L.: Infrared Thermometer, Calif. U.S. Patent 6,129,673, issued Oct 10, 2000

23. Fraden, J.: Infrared Thermometer, European Patent Application, EP 0 964 231 A2, issued Dec 1999

24. Jones, M.N., Park, L.F., et al.: Infrared Thermometer. U.S. Patent 0257469, issued Oct 15, 2009

25. Pompei, F.: Temporal Artery Temperature Detector, Boston, MA. U.S. Patent 6,292,685, issued Sep 18, 2001

26. Oleshchuk, V., Fensli, R.: Remote patient monitoring within a future 5G infrastructure. Wireless Personal Commun. **57**(3), 431–439 (2011)

27. West, D.M.: How 5G technology enables the health internet of things. Centre Technol. Innov. Brookings **3**, 1–20 (2016)

28. Magsi, H., Sodhro, A.H., Chachar, F.A., Abro, S.A.K., Sodhro, G.H., Pirbhulal, S.: Evolution of 5G in internet of medical things. In 2018 International Conference on Computing, Mathematics and Engineering Technologies (iCoMET), Sukkur, pp. 1–7 (2018)

29. Selem, E., Fatehy, M., Abd El-Kader, S.M., Nassar, H.: The (temperature heterogeneity energy) aware routing protocol for IoT health application. In IEEE Access, vol. 7, pp. 108957–108968 (2019)

30. Hussein, H.H., Abd El-Kader, S.M.: Enhancing signal to noise interference ratio for device to device technology in 5G applying mode selection technique. In 2017 Intl Conf on Advanced Control Circuits Systems (ACCS) Systems & 2017 Intl Conf on New Paradigms in Electronics & Information Technology (PEIT), Alexandria, pp. 187–192 (2017)

31. Salem, M.A., Tarrad, I.F., Youssef, M.I., Abd El-Kader, S.M.: An adaptive EDCA selfishness-aware scheme for dense WLANs in 5G networks. IEEE Access, vol. 8 (2020)

32. Salem, M.A., Tarrad, I.F., Youssef, M.I., Abd El-Kader, S.M.: QoS categories activeness-aware adaptive EDCA algorithm for dense IoT networks. Int. J. Comput. Netw. Commun. **11**(03), 67–83, May 2019

33. Selem, E., Gaber, A., AbdElkader, S.: Early detection of Covide19 using a non-contact fore-head thermometer. In: The 6th International Conference on Advanced Intelligent Systems and Informatics, AISI2020

34. Anar, F.H., Abd El-Kader, S., Eissa, H., Salem, A.: Multilevel minimised delay clustering protocol for wireless sensor networks. Int. J. Commun. Netw. Distrib. Syst. **13**(187) (2014). https://doi.org/10.1504/ijcnds.2014.064045

35. Selem, E., Fatehy, M., Abd El-Kader, S.M.: E-Health applications over 5G networks: challenges and state of the art. In: 2019 6th International Conference on Advanced Control Circuits and Systems (ACCS) & 2019 5th International Conference on New Paradigms in Electronics & information Technology (PEIT), Hurgada, Egypt, pp. 111–118 (2019). https://doi.org/10.1109/accs-peit48329.2019.9062841

36. Ullah, Z., et al.: DSCB: dual sink approach using clustering in body area network, vol. 12, pp. 357–370. Spinger, Peer-to-Peer Netw (2019)

The Effect CoronaVirus Pendamic on Education into Electronic Multi-modal Smart Education

Doaa Mohey El-Din, Aboul Ella Hassanein, and Ehab E. Hassanien

Abstract This paper presents how coronavirus drives education to smart education in interpreting multi-modals. It uses to improve the electronic learning in multiple data types. This paper is a survey paper about the importance of smart education and the effect of coronavirus on drives education into smart online education. It also presents many changes in the education vision around the world to utilize multi-modal for enhancing E-learning. The combination of artificial intelligence and data fusion plays a vital role in improving decision making and monitoring students remotely. It also presents benefits and open research challenges of a multi-modal smart education. This main objective of this paper is to highlight the deepening digital inequality in smart education in emergencies due to Coronavirus, the concept of digital equality has been defined as equal opportunities in accessing technology as hardware and software as well as equal opportunities in obtaining equal digital education through Ease of access to high-quality and interactive digital content based on the interaction

Keywords Coronavirus · Multi-modal · Fusion · Smart education ·
Internet-of-Things · Artificial intelligence · Fusion

D. M. El-Din (✉) · E. E. Hassanien
Information Systems Department, Faculty of Computers and Artificial Intelligence, Cairo
University, Cairo, Egypt
e-mail: d.mohey@alumni.fci-cu.edu.eg

E. E. Hassanien
e-mail: E.Ezat@fci-cu.edu.eg

A. E. Hassanein
Information Technology Department, Faculty of Computers and Artificial Intelligance, Cairo
University, Cairo, Egypt
e-mail: aboitcairo@gmail.com

© The Editor(s) (if applicable) and The Author(s), under exclusive license
to Springer Nature Switzerland AG 2020
A.-E. Hassanien et al. (eds.), *Big Data Analytics and Artificial Intelligence
Against COVID-19: Innovation Vision and Approach*, Studies in Big Data 78,
https://doi.org/10.1007/978-3-030-55258-9_15

1 Introduction

The Coronavirus pandemic forced the governments of the world to close educational institutions that caused 89% (more than 1.5 billion learners) from 188 countries to be forbidden access to educational institutions to receive face-to-face education as the UNESCO report in 2020 [1]. Many of these institutions are undertaking a large unplanned experience which is remote education in emergency situations, distance education in emergency situations [2] in order to limit the spread of the virus. The sudden transformation of smart education in emergency situations, to shock and tension among students and faculty members, whether on the personal or professional level, because of the process's need for redoubled efforts, or psychological instability due to the outbreak of the epidemic, as well as several unusual obstacles for school students And universities: such as lack of appropriate time, poor infrastructure, inadequate digital content, etc.

The disparity between countries in terms of technological development of technology operations in developing various fields in those areas to digital inequality and social justice, whether between countries with each other or within the countries themselves. The hypothesis that digital technology helps to achieve justice and social equality has been brought down, as in reality, digital inequality has deepened in distance teaching in emergency situations. Digital equality and the right to education is one of the United Nations' sustainable development goals. Previous researches reach the digital equality in education, especially higher education, which is a big obstacle that hinders the adoption of digital tools in higher education all over the world.

To achieve the goal of the paper, which is to highlight the deepening digital inequality in E-learning in emergencies due to Coronavirus, the concept of digital equality has been defined as equal opportunities in accessing technology as hardware and software as well as equal opportunities in obtaining equal digital education through Ease of access to high-quality and interactive digital content.

This paper presents a review paper of smart education in multi-modals of multiple data types. It shows the importance of smart education. It also presents many changes in the education vision around the world to utilize multi-modal for enhancing E-learning. The combination of artificial intelligence and data fusion plays a vital role in improving decision making and monitoring students remotely. It also presents benefits and open research challenges of a multi-modal smart education. It presents the advantages and challenges of implementation the smart education system in various countries. It also shows open research challenges of smart education.

The rest of the paper is organized as the following: Sect. 2, the effect Coronavirus on Education and discusses the importance of smart education, Sect. 3, Presents a discussion of Smart Education and previous works in this area, Sect. 4, benefits and challenges of smart education, Sect. 5, open research challenges and research directions in smart education, section Finally, Sect. 6, targets the conclusion outlines.

2   The Effect CoronaVirus on Education

Coronavirus becomes a global pandemic around the world. The World Health Organization (WHO) reports that the number of confirmed cases by a coronavirus (COVID-19) reaches 4,993,470. And the number of deaths reaches 327,738 deaths that achieves more than 15.3% [3]. It has a big spreading rapidly in all Continents. The United Nations Educational, Scientific and Cultural Organization estimates that 192 countries have closed schools across the country [4] and that many other countries have implemented regional or local closings. It causes of closed schools, educational institutions, faculties, Scientific organizations, and universities. Millions are forbidden from their education suddenly due to protect their lives and their families.

The educational institutions are under the closure's role of the United Nations Educational and World Health Organization for 80% of students worldwide. That causes several challenges for applying smart education applications due to the poverty and lack of automated applications of smart education and the available internet for all students concurrently. It also requires the effectiveness application based on various data types such as video, audio, and text. The development of applications not only for education but also used for training in many domains such as medical schools about how to deal with Coronavirus disease.

UNESCO recommends for all countries to turn to infer the technology in the automated education remotely. It depends on the reliability of Internet-of-things for smart education [5]. So, smart education becomes a new trend to benefit from the combination of internet-of-things and artificial intelligence in smart education. Millions of petabytes of data are used for smart applications based on the combination of artificial intelligence and internet-of-things. The artificial intelligence is utilized for interpreting big volume of extracted data, fusing heterogeneous data with multiple data formats, and understanding the velocity of the interpreting data. The fusion process between huge sensed data allows the capture of complementary information or trends [6]. The simulation of multimodal application is described by high exciting, fast, and high quality.

The properties of smart education, self-directed, motivated, adaptive, resource-enriched, and technology-embedded [6]. A smart education environment presents access to ubiquitous resources and interacts with learning systems anytime and anywhere. The vital learning orientation, suggestions, or helpful tools to them in the right form, at the right time and in the right place.

Smart education environments can provide accurate and rich learning services by using learning analytics. It depends on many important features for any education application, location, context-aware, social relationship, Interoperability, Adaptability, flexibility, Flexibility, Adaptability, Ubiquitous, Human computer interaction multimodal, and High Engagement. Sensed Locations, it can determine the location of each learner remotely from the location sensor in real-time. These sensors often are based on mobile sensors such as GPS in the mobile that use for detecting and tracking locations. Context-Aware, it examines various scenarios in various contexts and their information about each activity. There are several targets and properties for each educational scenario such as lectures, exams, student affairs, Graduate Studies, Make certificates, etc. Social Relationship Awareness, it discovers the social relationship from used sensors. Flexibility, it is high flexible to fuse multiple information from multiple sensors. Interoperability, it puts many standard roles that depends on various resources, activities, or services. It is considered an important step and obstacle till now to fuse multiple data source with one or variant data formats. Adaptability, it infers the education access, preference, and demand from education resources. Ubiquitous, it is based on the predication of education demand to construct system clear and visualized to access education resource to the learner. Human Computer Interaction (HCI) multimodal, it is based on the fusion between sensed multimodal interactions that consists of the position and facial expressions. High Engagement, it enters a multidirectional interaction for education experience with a technology-riches environment. The interconnected and interoperable education experience are considered high significant issues in a smart education system in the future.

3   Smart Education

Smart education or E-learning is the process of exploiting technology in communicating with the elements of the educational process among them as shown in the main architecture in Fig. 1. Electronic learning is a complex process that starts with planning to design decisions based on the needs of the target group. The evaluation process was designed and then the course was published. Although there are many benefits to simulating smart education as shown in Fig. 4 [7–9], for example, facing increasing student numbers, reducing the financial burden on educational institutions

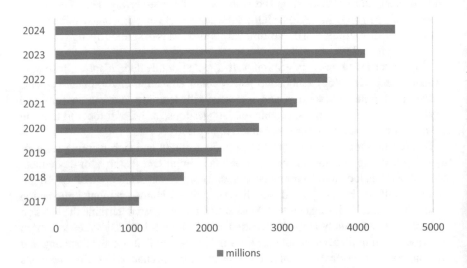

Fig. 1 The number of used smart devices in multimodal smart environments [31]

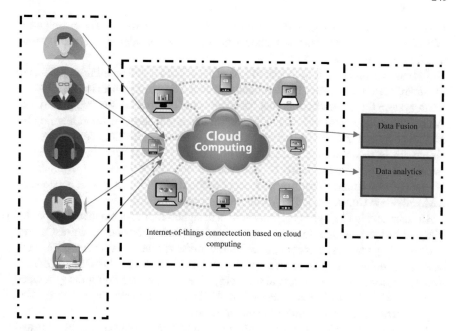

Fig. 2 The main architecture of smart education

resulting from this by reducing the numbers of students in its facilities, as well as the number of employees in them, and providing an opportunity for students who live Far areas of enrollment without having to change the place of residence, or refrain from sending children to school, and finally the inevitable solution to dealing with the problems that resulted from the closure of schools and universities in light of the spread and spread of the Corona virus.

The smart education is designed based on the combination of artificial intelligence and internet-of-things. The powerful role is shown in interpreting big data and data fusion as shown in Fig. 2 [9]. Smart education includes multi-data fusion in various data types from various sources that may be sensors or smart devices on education applications. It provides educational services such as digitalized context awareness, adaptive content, collaborative and interactive tool, rapid evaluation, and real-time feedback. Online smart education applications are effective and efficient in meaningful learning. It depends on the combination of increasing the effective of many interfaces, using smart IoT sensors or devices, and different education scenarios with various features and data [7, 8].

(A) *Related works of smart education*

Previous motivations in the implementation of smart education, Researchers in [9], presents a framework of a Smart Education Environment System (SEES), that support the integration database based on the incorporating three core sub-systems. These sub-systems include 'Electronic Bookshelves', use for the automation access and remotely for each book shelve that is entitled 'Virtual White Space'. The examination of library data includes Database for social network. It is considered integrated system that improves adaptive system.

Researchers in [10], present a stem education system based on multimodal fusion for smart classes to improve management and analytics. Researchers in [11], shows a smart system for generative learning based on cloud computing, fog computing, and swarm computing. Researchers in [12], present an application for smart learning for multiple contexts that can fuse several virtual education applications from a physical classroom. A recent idea of Education is considered it is as a Service, so it includes many challenges for the markets. Researchers in [13], create a new Application Framework for Smart Education System as entitled SES Framework. It depends on a Model-View-Controller (MVC) with multi-aspect model.

Researchers in [14], present the system is designed for the open-source technologies and services in order to make it capable of supporting the open IT-infrastructure and providing from various commercial hardware/sensor vendors furthermore open-source solutions. The application is developed for offer new app-that relies on educational solutions for various educational objectives or for controlling the efficiency remotely. The application is described by replicable and adaptable to settings that may be various than the scenarios envisioned here.

Researchers in [15], present a university model that reduces complexity and high adaption, which requires improving performance. Multimodal data contains the expressions of facial and review when the students monitor online videos and label them with two dimensions (interestingness, difficulty) in the subjective learning status. Then after pre-processing such as face recognition from video screenshots and normalization of review, they constructed a new model for fusion based on artificial neural network methods to compute the real-time learning status in the two dimensions. Smart education includes multi-data fusion in various data types from various sources that may be sensors or smart devices on education applications. It provides educational services such as digitalized context awareness, adaptive content, collaborative and interactive tool, rapid evaluation and real-time feedback. Online smart education applications are effective and efficient in meaningful learning. It depends on the integration of increasing interfaces, smart devices, and different learning data [7] (Table 1).

(B) *Related works of Multimodal fusion techniques*

Using Multimodal for smart education applications has a great effect on predication and making decisions [16]. The construction of multimodal is based on fusing data from multiple sensors. It improves predictions and detecting changes from various sources. the multimodal for Audiovisual properties that are fused for detecting the depression symptoms in [17] based on using a constructed dataset from dyadic interactions between an interviewer and paid participants.

Several fusion techniques are constructed based on the properties of video, audio, and transcripts [18]. The dataset is made through interviews conducted by an animated virtual interviewer managed by a human in another room.

Table 1 A comparative study between previous motivations of smart education

Reference No.	Year	Target	Pros	Cons
[9]	2014	Integrated system for education	High adoption system	Improve performance
[10]	2015	STEM education in Estonia	Provide analytics accuracy	Multimodal smart classes
[11]	2016	A smart system for generative learning	It is based on tri-tier computing, cloud computing, fog, swarm computing to improve management and analysis	Hardness of apply this system
[12]	2017	Education Context aware system	High flexible and effectiveness	Complex
[13]	2017	Creating a new Application Framework for Smart Education System: SES Framework is based Model-View-Controller (MVC) with multi-aspect model	High effectiveness	High complexity
[14]	2017	Faculty model and schools	Comprising 700 IoT points for fusing sensory data and improving remote decision making and monitoring students. High scalable and simplicity	Complex implementation
[15]	2018	University model	Reduce complexity and high adoption	Requires improving performance
[16]	2020	Creating smart deep multi-modal for education	Precision 92% Recall 69%	Complex

Researchers in [19], present a survey paper about a comprehensive study of recent motivations on multimodal deep learning from three dimensions: learning multimodal representations, fusing multimodal signals at various levels, and multimodal applications. The construction of multimodal is based on determining types of data formats and determining the fusion technique, signals, text, video, and image. Researchers in [20], multimodal learning analytics is presented by recent insights into student learning trajectories in more complex and open teaching applications. Many models based on deep learning are used for extracting powerful data from multiple modalities. The applications rely on Convolutional Neural Networks (CNNs) use for extracting the visual and audio properties and a word embedding model for textual analysis [21]. Researchers in [21], present a novel fusion technique for integrating different data representations in two levels, namely frame-level and video level. The results reach enhancing accuracy by more than 16% and 7% compared to the best results from single modality and fusion models.

The fusion process of modalities from various data formats is a very significant process in order to reach the highest performance and harvest relevant data. Classical data fusion techniques often contain the level of fusion, early, late, or middle fusion [22]. The existing studies of multimodal fusion studies contain the fusion level, but are not limited to, video (audio-visual) analysis [23], social networks [24], or human-computer interaction [25]. Researchers in [24] show a modal for analyzing sentiments that is based on tri- modalities textual, video, and audio. It uses a tri-modal Hidden Markov Model (HMM) for classifying models and determining the hidden interaction among them.

Deep learning techniques have been recently proposed and applied in many research, competitions, and real-world applications [26, 27]. The researchers in [23] presents a deep learning model as entitled Microsoft Residual Networks (ResNet) that solves the overfitting and vanishing gradients challenges. Researcher [28] presented a simple CNN based on word vectors for sentence-level classification. The proposed sentiment application targets analyzing sentiments and questions. Recurrent Neural Network (RNN) and its extended version Long Short-Term Memory (LSTM) has also been leveraged to classify speech [29] and text.

Although the fusion topic is an old topic, it has recent motivations especially in smart environments. Multimodal is the essential topic of research in fusion in Internet-of-things due to the massive extracted of sensory data. The used techniques of multi-modal fusion target fusing multiple data types from multiple resources.

4 Benefits and Challenges of Smart Education Applications

The implementation of smart education applications is very powerful and useful for electronic learning. This section discusses the benefits and challenges of smart education applications.

(A) Benefits of smart Education

The smart education has several advantages as shown in Fig. 3.

(1) Saving time

Electronic learning is described by quick communication, save time in asking lecturer, save time in mobility or transportation. The E-learning enables students to make online presentations and get the review about their work concurrently.

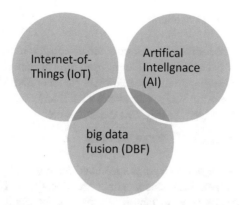

Fig. 3 The smart education application is constructed based on three levels (AI, IoT, and BDF)

(2) Increased productivity

Productivity is raised by sharing information based on multiple data formats from multiple data sources. The good smart education system aims to increase the productivity of lecturers and students [30].

(3) High flexibility

The interaction between student and lecturer becomes high flexible in requirements achievement [31].

(4) Improving Learning performance

Using smart education online technology is higher performance of understanding photos, maps, graphs, flowcharts and animated videos. This makes learning more attractive, interesting, and easy to understand. It encourages the ability of students to learn and memorize the topic for a prolonged period.

It is a universal truth, when we learn through visuals, we grab the subject easily rather than just looking into the blackboard & listening.

(5) Interactive Reliability

The interactive process between lecturers and students become reliable for smart technology by 55% [32]. The smart education system becomes easy and simple to construct a fast FAQ session between lecturers and students that makes a wonderful learning environment in the electronic classrooms.

(6) High interactive Access system

A smart interactive system is constructed based on some practical solutions. This system becomes adoptive to reach 70% of smartboards. This is an obvious indication that educational institutes are embracing this advanced technology.

(B) Challenges of Smart Education

The world countries are forced to construct smart education systems although the variant of availability of capabilities, training, and fund in each country. These smart educations become very important due to protect students' lives. So, the implementation of smart education in various countries face many obstacles and challenges are classified intro three types as Fig. 4 as the following:

(1) Technical challenges in Hardware, software and the availability of the internet

The internet services are not enough in speed and quality in all students and states whether that serves universities' students or schools' students. That requires to find suitable hardware as computer or laptop or mobile to be available online, present work and share assignments online.

(2) The digital content challenge

It includes three problems in the lack of the digital content in high-quality for various student's levels, Suitable, centralized digital content with many local languages, The

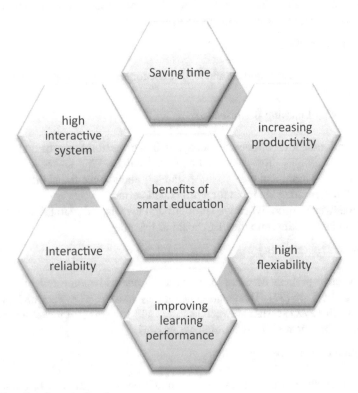

Fig. 4 Benefits of smart education

variety of importance of specific branches in explanations in high school or universities, and hardness of implementation the unification multi-modal of education system.

The lack of the digital content in high-quality for various student's levels, that challenge shows the problem in construction digital quality digital educational tutorials, assignments, and projects. It also the processes of the exchanging file between lecturer or teacher and students or other lecturers. That requires a huge database and complementary tutorials to cover changes in lecturers' tutorials and exploitations. A large percentage of teachers are unable to use digital tools in teaching, which reflects negatively on controlling the digital class through remote teaching in emergency situations.

Suitable, centralized digital content with many local languages as found in many countries that have multiple local languages, so there is a need to constructing digital content with many local languages to be suitable with people's expectations due to the lack of appropriate time for the lecturer/teacher to teach.

The variety of importance of specific branches in explanations in high school or universities. Each education level has one subject, or more is very important. So, most of teachers or lecturer's emphasis on these scientific explanations and ignoring emergency situations. Finally, the challenge of construction interpreting multi-modal for interpreting or summarize contents and evaluating students in multiple data types.

(3) Human-Computer Interaction (HCI) challenge

That is shown in two problems, the hardness or follow students in schools from parents and the difficulty of monitoring student progress in cumulative exams, assignments, and summaries.

The Hardness of follows school's students from Parent. The technical inability of parents follows their school student's children in their homework at home. The hardness of learning parents' new smart educational models in the digital equality process. The second problem is shown in the difficulty of monitoring student progress in cumulative exams, assignments, and summaries.

5 Open Research Directions of Smart Education

This paper presents an open research direction to implement and improve the construction of smart education systems. these systems can benefit from the artificial intelligence and internet-of-things in high-quality digital content for electronic education and monitoring the students' progress based on fusion multi-modals of their data. E-learning has become a refuge for any educational system in the world, and its officials must quickly make a decision to impose e-learning within our teaching methods. If the society was ready for e-learning, moving to it in the event of suspending the study for any reason would be easy for everyone, and when e-learning took all this debate from educators.

The open research directions divide into two essential dimensions:

(A) **The Multi-modal for constructing a summary of the Electronic Digital content**

A Flexibility of constructing a multi-modal [33] for digital content. The process of preparing curriculum components fuses multiple data sources from multiple teachers in various tools or from various sensors such as mobile sensors. The data fusion is a vital opportunity to build multi-modal smart education applications. The proposed multi-modal systems are based on flexibility to fusing and interpreting data from various sources in multiple data sources as shown in Fig. 5.

(B) **Multi-modal for monitoring and evaluating multiple students in smart Education**

The implementation of multi-modal smart education applications for monitoring the students' level and their progress in multiple exams, assignments, or delivery reports in the two dimensions parents/them or lecturers. These applications can reduce the effect of digital inequality in remote teaching in emergency situations, it is preferable to use an open-source that allows the creation of responsive interactive digital content. Another target of these applications achieve justice in evaluating the students from multiple deliveries in multiple data types such as video format, online broadcast, or text reports as shown in Fig. 6.

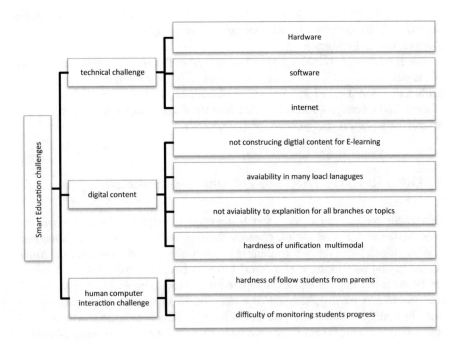

Fig. 5 The smart education challenges

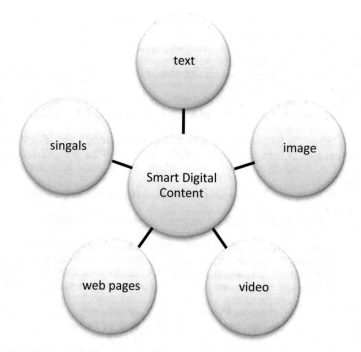

Fig. 6 Fusion between multiple data sources

6 Conclusion

CoronaVirus makes smart education becomes a hot trend in the implementation these applications whether for faculties or schools. This paper presents the effect of coronavirus on education and the importance of using Internet-of-things in automated remote education systems. It presents the discussion of smart education n and the importance of uses it. It also shows the obstacles and open research challenges in the multimodal fusion of smart education. The objective of smart education is to improve learner's quality of lifelong learning. It focuses on contextual, personalized and seamless learning to promote learners' intelligence emerging and facilitate their problem-solving ability in smart environments.

References

1. https://en.unesco.org/covid19/educationresponse
2. Martín, A. C., Alario-Hoyos, C., Kloos, C. D.: Smart education: a review and future research directions. Proceedings **31**(57), 1–10 (2019)
3. Ha, I., Kim, C.: The research trends and the effectiveness of smart learning. Int. J. Distrib. Sensor Netw. **4**, 1–9 (2014)

4. Gul, S., et al.: A survey on role of internet of things in education. IJCSNS Int. J. Comput. Sci. Netw. Security **17**(5), 159–165 (2017)
5. Yadegaridehkordi, E., et al.: Affective computing in education: a systematic review and future research. Comput. Educ. **142** (2019)
6. Hoel, T., Mason, J.: Standards for smart education—towards a development framework. Smart Learn. Environ. **5**(3), 1–25 (2018)
7. Uskov, V.L., Bakken, J.P., Pandey, A.: Smart education and smart e-learning. In: Uskov, V.L., Howlett, R.J., Jain, L.C. (eds.) The Ontology of Next Generation Smart Classrooms, p. 41. Springer, Heidelberg (2015)
8. Gunn, C., Raven, J.: Smart education: introducing active learning engineering classrooms in the Middle East. In: Conference: 2017 Fourth HCT Information Technology Trends (ITT 2017)
9. AlMajeed, S., Mirtshulava, L., Srim Naji, AlZubaidy, M.J.: Smart Education Environment System (2014)
10. Prieto, L.P., Rodr´ıguez-Triana, M.J., Kusmin, M., Laanpere, M.: Smart School Multimodal Dataset and Challenges (2018)
11. Zhu, Z.-T., Yu, M.-H., Riezebos, P.: A research framework of smart education. Smart Learn. Environ. **3**(4) (2016)
12. Soikova, E., Nikolov, R., Kovatcheva, E.: Conceptualising of Smart Education (2017)
13. Kobayashi, T., Sato, H., Tanimoto, S., Kanai, A.: An application framework for smart education system based on mobile and cloud systems. IEICE Trans. Inf. Syst. E100–D(10) (2017)
14. Amaxilatis, D., et al.: An IoT-based solution for monitoring a fleet of educational buildings focusing on energy efficiency. Sensors (2017)
15. Rico-Bautista, D.W.: Conceptual framework for smart university. In: Journal of Physics: Conference Series, vol. 1409, Sixth International Meeting of Technological Innovation (6th IMTI) (2019)
16. Mann, P., Paes, A., Matsushima, E.H.: Detecting Depression Symptoms in Higher Education Students Using Multimodal Social Media Data. arXiv:1912.01131v,2 (2020)
17. Blikstein, P., Worsley, M.: Multimodal learning analytics and education data mining: using computational technologies to measure complex learning tasks. J. Learn. Anal. **3**(2), 220–238 (2016)
18. Morales, M., Scherer, S., Levitan, R.: A linguistically-informed fusion approach for multimodal depression detection. In: Proceedings of the 5th Workshop on Computational Linguistics and Clinical Psychology: From Keyboard to Clinic, pp. 13–24 (2018)
19. Zhang, C., Yang, Z., He, X., Deng, L.: Multimodal Intelligence: Representation Learning, Information Fusion, and Applications. Arxiv (2019)
20. Blikstein, P., Worsley, M.: Multimodal learning analytics and education data mining: using computational technologies to measure complex learning tasks. J. Learn. Anal. **3**(2), 220–23 (2016)
21. Tian, H., Tao, Y., Pouyanfar, S., Chen, S.-C., Shyu, M.-L.: Multimodal deep representation learning for video classification. World Wide Web **22**, 1325–1341 (2019)
22. Atrey, P.K., Hossain, M.A., El Saddik, A., Kankanhalli, M.S.: Multimodal fusion for multimedia analysis: a survey. Multimed. Syst. **16**(6), 345–379 (2010)
23. He, K., Zhang, X., Ren, S., Sun, J.: Deep residual learning for image recognition. In: IEEE Conference on Computer Vision and Pattern Recognition, pp. 770–778 (2016)
24. Morency, L.P., Mihalcea, R., Doshi, P.: Towards multimodal sentiment analysis: harvesting opinions from the Web. Int. Conf. Multimodal Interfaces ACM **2011**, 169–176 (2011)
25. Panic, M., Sebe, N., Cohn, J.F., Huang, T.: Affective multimodal human-computer interaction. In: ACM International Conference on Multimedia, ACM 2005, pp. 669–676 (20050
26. Pouyanfar, S., Chen, S.C.: Automatic video event detection for imbalance data using enhanced ensemble deep learning. Int. J. Semant. Comput. **11**(01), 85–109 (2017)
27. Shahbazi, H., Jamshidi, K., Monadjemi, A.H., Manoochehri, H.E.: Training oscillatory neural networks using natural gradient particle swarm optimization. Robotica **33**(7), 1551–1567 (2015)

28. Kim, Y.: Convolutional neural networks for sentence classification. In: Conference on Empirical Methods in Natural Language Processing, pp. 1746–1751 (2014)
29. Aypdele, I., et al.: Artificial intelligence, smart classrooms and online education in the 21st century: implications for human development. J. Cases Inf. Technol. **21**(3), 66–79 (2019)
30. Peng, Q., Qie, N., Yuan, L., Chen, Y., Gao, Q.: Design of an online education evaluation system based on multimodal data of learners. In: International Conference on Human-Computer Interaction, HCII, Cross-Cultural Design, Culture and Society, pp. 458–468 (2019)
31. Perez, G., Amores, G., Manchon, P.: Two Strategies for Multimodal Fusion (2018)
32. https://www.abiresearch.com/blogs/2019/10/10/multimodal-learning-artificial-intelligence/
33. Vielzeuf, V., Lechervy, A., Pateux, S., Jurie, F.: CentralNet: a multilayer approach for multimodal fusion. In: European Conference on Computer Vision Workshops: Multimodal Learning and Applications (2018)

Deep Learning Against COVID-19

An H₂O's Deep Learning-Inspired Model Based on Big Data Analytics for Coronavirus Disease (COVID-19) Diagnosis

Sally Elghamrawy

Abstract The outbreak of coronavirus diseases (COVID-19) has rabidly spread all over the world. The World Health Organization (WHO) has announced that coronavirus COVID-19 is an international pandemic. Big Data analytics tools must handle and analyse the massive amount of big medical data, generated daily, quickly due to the fact that time is very significant issue in healthcare applications. In addition, several deep learning algorithms are used along with big data analysis processes to help in detecting COVID-19 outbreaks and predicting their worldwide spread. Many researchers developed their models to diagnosis COVID-19 using Computed Tomography (CT) or X-ray imaging. This chapter presents a detailed discussion of Deep Learning and Big Data Analytics effects in containment of the disease. In addition, an H2O's Deep-Learning-inspired model based on Big Data analytics (DLBD-COV) is proposed for early diagnosis of COVID-19 cases using CT or X-ray images. The proposed diagnosis model is build based on the machine learning framework (H2O) for scalable processing. The Generative Adversarial Networks (GAN) and the Convolutional Neural Networks (CNNs) are used and their classification results are compared. The experimental results emphasize the superiority of DLBD-COV when using H₂O framework for scalable COVID19 classification. The results obtained, using a dataset with thousands of real data and images, show encouraging performance using the automated feature extraction of deep learning techniques used in DLBD-COV.

Keywords Coronavirus disease (COVID-19) · CT imaging · X-Ray · Big data analytics · H₂O · Deep learning technique · Generative adversarial networks (GAN) · Convolutional neural networks (CNNs)

S. Elghamrawy (✉)
Computer Engineering Department, MISR Higher Institute for Engineering and Technology, Mansoura, Egypt
e-mail: sally_elghamrawy@ieee.org

Scientific Research Group in Egypt (SRGE), Cairo, Egypt

A.-E. Hassanien et al. (eds.), *Big Data Analytics and Artificial Intelligence Against COVID-19: Innovation Vision and Approach*, Studies in Big Data 78, https://doi.org/10.1007/978-3-030-55258-9_16

1 Introduction

The outbreak of an infectious pneumonia produced by the severe acute respiratory syndrome coronavirus 2 (SARS-COV-2) has initiated a universal panic. In Mar 28th 2020 [1], there have been 597,458 confirmed cases and 27,370 deaths. To the date (April 28th 2020), there have been 3,064,837 confirmed cases and 211,609 deaths all around the world [2]. It is obvious that in one month, the number of confirmed cases is increased by 5 times. These situation reports, announced by the World Health Organization (WHO), indicates that a rapid spread of the virus is forthcoming and COVID-19 is tremendously spreadable between people via respiratory droplets. As a result, it is critical to early detect infected cases for preventing the transmissible of the disease. The early diagnosis of COVID-19 helps the healthcare workers for applying appropriate treatment and quarantine procedures.

A number of researches [3–10] presented several COVID-19 diagnosis models using different Deep Learning techniques with Big Data analytics. These models are used for early discovery of COVID-19 to contribute in its containment. Several studies [5, 8–10] have proved that the chest Computed Tomography CT and X-ray images has high sensitivity over the Reverse Transcription Polymerase Chain Reaction RT-PCR test [7], which gives high false negative results. Accordingly, a CT and X-ray based diagnosis models are critically needed for precisely detecting COVID-19 cases.

In this chapter, an H_2O's Deep-Learning-inspired model based on Big Data analytics (DLBD-COV) is proposed for early diagnosis of COVID-19 using CT or X-ray images. H_2O [11] is implemented during the different phases of DLBD-COV for scalable and speedy processing. The Convolutional Neural Networks (CNNs) [12] and the Generative Adversarial Networks (GAN) [13] are used for segmentation and augmentation process of the model. The diagnosis results obtained from these networks are then classified and their classification results are compared.

The rest of the chapter is organized as follows: Sect. 2 shows the main big data analytics frameworks. Section 3 presents the Deep Learning techniques: Convolutional Neural Networks (CNNs) and Generative Adversarial Networks (GAN). Section 4 summarizes the main fields of Big Data Analytics in containment of COVID-19. In Sect. 5, a detailed discussion of recent Deep learning techniques used against COVID-19. The proposed DLBD-COV diagnosis model is presented in Sect. 6. Section 7 presented the experimental results of DLBD-COV. Section 8 summarizes the conclusions and presents future work.

Main Contributions of the Proposed DLBD-COV Model

DLBD-COV model is proposed to exploit different deep learning techniques along with big data analytic tools to improve the diagnosis utility. The main advantage of DLBD-COV model is presented as follows:

I. DLBD-COV supports either X-ray or CT images for diagnosing COVID-19 cases.
II. DLBD-COV applies pre-processing techniques to remove noise or missing data.

III. The Generative Adversarial Networks(GAN) is used for X-ray images and the Convolutional Neural Networks (CNNs) is implemented for the CT images.

IV. The results obtained from the GANs and CNNs are classified and validated using three different classifiers.

V. Using H$_2$O in the DLBD-COV reduces the computational time needed for diagnosis process.

VI. A comparison is made between the results obtained from DLBD-COV when using H$_2$O and Spark. The results obtained showed that H$_2$O proved an improved performance in terms of computational time over Spark. This is due to the availability of supported deep learning (Neural networks) algorithms in H$_2$O.ai [14].

2 Big Data Analytics

Big Data is collected from numerous sources e.g. sensors, social media and digital images and videos. Big data analytics is used to analyze Big Data in order to extract motivating patterns and hidden relationships. The companies can process more date for the same price, which will increase their offer in the market. There-fore, they potentially can increase the total amount of sales. Finally, a large panoply of competitive advantages can be reached by companies [15]. There are thousands of Big data analytics tools that is employed for different tasks [16], as shown in the Table 1.

There are two well-known frameworks for big data analysis, namely H$_2$O [11] and Apache Spark [17]. H$_2$O is considered as the new generation of Machine learning technology. It proved its effective performance over different open source machine learning. It gives users the ability to discover patterns in data using huge numbers of models. H$_2$O supports several types of Deep Learning algorithms [18–20] such as Convolutional Neural Networks (CNNs). In H$_2$O's Deep learning, the data is divided into partitions and then each partition is analyzed concurrently. Using this method provide H$_2$O the ability to process and analyze all the data instead of neglecting most of it.

Table 1 Big data analytics tools and their corresponding tasks

Task	Big data analytics tools
Data storage and management	Hadoop, MongoDB, Cassandra [51]
Data cleaning	OpenRefine, DataCleaner
Data mining	Rapid Miner, Waikato Environment for Knowledge Analysis (Weka), Oracle data mining, IBM Modeler
Data analysis	Qubole, BigML, Statwing.
Data visualization	Tableau, Silk, Charito, Plot.ly
Data integration	Blockspring, Pentaho
Data collection	Import.io

When the data is well stored and partitioned, an advanced analytics tools can be implemented to analyze this data using techniques of data mining and deep learning [21]. Data mining techniques are used to detect relationships and patterns in data. Deep learning develops a suite of algorithms for analyzing big data.

3 Deep Learning

Deep Learning (DL), hierarchical learning or Deep Neural Network is a branch of Machine Learning (ML) which is based on artificial neural networks. Its main goal is to model high-level abstractions in data [22–24]. DL uses several layers to gradually extract upper level features from the raw input data, as shown in Fig. 1. In this Chapter, different DL techniques are presented which are used for processing COVID19 images. In DL techniques, the lower layers possibly will detect edges, but upper layers will detect the features (signs) diagnosing COVID19.

There are different types of Deep learning architectures concerned with computer vision and Image processing such as Convolutional Neural Networks [12, 25], Generative Adversarial Networks (GAN) [13, 26] and Deconvolutional networks [27].

3.1 Convolutional Neural Networks (CNN)

It is a recent Deep Learning algorithm, first proposed by Badrinarayanan [12]. It's widely used in the fields of image processing, computer vision and classification. CNN primarily comprise of three kind of layers: convolutional, nonlinear and pooling layers. The convolutional layer is used for extracting the relevant features based on the weights assigned. The nonlinear layer is used to model any nonlinear function on feature maps. The pooling layers reduce the resolution of imaged by providing numerical information of a feature map. CNNs has advantage over other fully connected

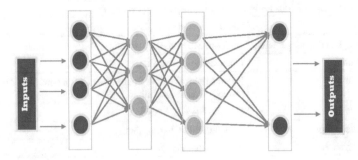

Fig. 1 The neural network

neural networks, is that the parameters' number in each field is reduced due to the ability of nodes in each layer to share weights. ResNet [28], VGGNet [29], GoogLeNet [30] and DenseNet [31] are most common CNN architectures.

3.2 Generative Adversarial Networks (GANs)

The Generative Adversarial Network (GAN) first introduced by Goodfellow [13] on 2014. GAN is a deep learning model, it is considered as a double framework that consists of generator and discriminator networks. The generative network created new objects while the discriminative network evaluates these newly generated objects. For this reason, GANs is widely used in real images generation.

The generator network trains a mapping, with a predefined distribution, to the target distribution of the real objects. The discriminator network tries to differentiate the generated objects from the real ones. GAN can be considered as game between generator and discriminator, in which the discriminator network attempts to reduce the classification error in differentiate between false samples from true ones. On the other hand, the generator network attempts to reduce the loss function [32, 33].

4 Big Data Analytics Against COVID-19

Recent studies used big data analysis tools to decrease the chance of spreading COVID-19 by monitoring COVID-19 disease and detecting the possible areas of infection. It is thus vital to utilize Big Data and intelligent analytics tools for monitoring COVID-19 disease to improve the community health. Many researchers exploit bid data and intelligent tools to monitor COVID-19 disease in different ways, as shown in Fig. 2.

- Data Tracking:

A recent study [34] has presented an approach for tracking passengers' data traffic from a big-data source. This tracking will show the probability of forecasting [35] COVID-19 and prevent the further spread of novel coronavirus (2019-nCoV). They collect tracking data from the official flight companies and digital big data sources extracted from data from citizens' mobile phones from the WeChat app, in order to provide information for risk management.

- Data Prediction

Leung et al. [36], at Wuhan city, uses big data storage tool to store and estimate number of travellers from Wuhan by using three different sources: the global flight bookings, the daily number of foreign and the domestic passenger volumes from

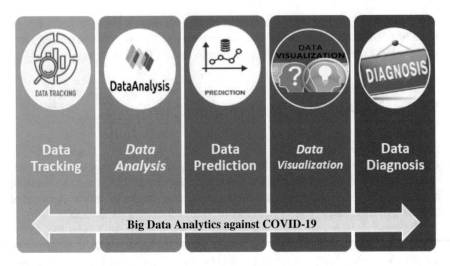

Fig. 2 Big data analytics against COVID-19

and to Wuhan. These data are then used to predict the forecasting of the epidemic in Wuhan based on the number of cases transferred from Wuhan to other cities.

- Data Analysis:

Coronavirus (Covid-19 outbreak has proved the need for proactive containment. All countries must rapidly utilize their resources to save their people lives and their economic stability. Taiwan [37] has been alerted from china epidemics and acted early to contain the crisis. The authors in [37] stated that Taiwan used big data analytic tools to present different approached to identify and contain COVID-19 cases early to protect the public health. They stated that they use big data storage advantage to apply integration between national health insurance database and immigration database. This huge database and its tools are used to dynamically generate alerts of COVID-19 confirmed cases and severe cases during the medical examination of the patient, thus identify and diagnosis Taiwan's cases and take rapid action.

- Data Visualization:

Zhou et al. [38] used the geographic information systems (GIS) and big data technologies to aggregate different big data sources and quickly create visualization for COVID-19 outbreak information. They stated that the tools used helped in predicting the risk allocation and regional transmissions.

- Data Diagnosis:

An integration between Big Data and artificial intelligence tools is a critical issue in detecting and preventing the spread of novel coronavirus. The authors in [39] investigated the importance of AI techniques with big data tools. They stated that using the 3 V's of Big data helped in creating different datasets that are used by many researchers and models. They reviewed a number of models that used AI and big data tools to contain the diseases like GoogleFlue [40] and BlueDot [41] that predicted the COVID-19 outbreak and sent alerts on December 31.

5 Deep Learning Against COVID-19

Due to the rapid development of deep learning technology that has been commonly implemented in the health arena, different studies [42–44] were conducted, based on deep learning technologies, for diagnosing and classifying different diseases like viral pneumonias and organs' tumours.

Currently, due to the COVID-19 outbreak disaster, many researchers have been motivated to develop models for early diagnosing and detecting COVID-19 as follows: Authors in [3] proposed a 3D deep convolutional neural Network to Detect COVID-19 from CT volume, namely DeCoVNet. But, the algorithm worked in a black-box manner when diagnosing COVID-19, since the algorithm was based on deep learning and its explain ability was still at an early stage. COVNET [4] developed a framework to detect COVID-19 using chest CT and evaluate its performances. The authors proposed a three-dimensional deep learning framework to detect COVID-19 using chest CT. Community acquired pneumonia (CAP) and other non-pneumonia exams were included to test the robustness of the model.

In addition, Yang et al. [5] investigated the diagnostic value and consistency of chest CT as compared with comparison to RT-PCR assay in COVID-19. Their analysis suggests that chest CT should be considered for the COVID-19 screening, comprehensive evaluation, and following-up, especially in epidemic areas with high pre-test probability for disease. Jiang et al. [6] proposed established an early screening model to distinguish COVID-19 pneumonia from Influenza-A viral pneumonia and healthy cases with pulmonary CT images using deep learning techniques. The authors used multiple CNN models to classify CT image datasets and calculate the infection probability of COVID-19. The findings might greatly assist in the early screening of patients with COVID-19 by deep learning technologies. The authors proposed a location-attention mechanism and uses it in the classical ResNet for feature extraction. The authors in [7] constructed a system based on deep learning for identification of viral pneumonia on CT. AIMDP model proposed in [9] utilized different AI techniques to enhance the diagnosis and prediction function of the model.

6 The Proposed H_2O's Deep-Learning-Inspired Model Based on Big Data Analytics (DLBD-COV) for COVID-19 Diagnosis

A novel Deep-Learning-inspired model (DLBD-COV) for COVID-19 diagnosis based on Big Data analytics tools is introduced in this section. The model consists of four main layers based on H_2O architecture to deal with large scale data collected, as shown in Fig. 3. DLBD-COV is used for early COVID-19 diagnosis using either X-ray or CT images based on Deep learning techniques.

At the beginning, the COVID-19 datasets are collected. As a starting point, in the pre-processing layer, the X ray and CT dataset are loaded from the HDFS, of the H_2O Architecture, and stored as RDD object. An RDD wrapper is created using RDD method by the H_2O architecture. The RDD is used to improve the distributed parallel computation and to provide H_2O the ability to implement the iterative algorithms with effective fault tolerance. In this layer the test and train datasets are splitted for both X-ray and CT images.

Then, the dataset analyzer phase handles the noise and corrupted files for each dataset, separately, by the stability manager module. The DLBD-COV model will detect the type of the image loaded either it's an X-ray or CT image using the Class detector. Finally, the number of images in each class is detected. The classes in the training dataset are stored in the images/classes repository. If the detected image belongs to the X-Ray class, then the GAN layer will handle these types of images. And if the detected image is in the CT class, then the CNN Layer will handle it, as shown in Fig. 3.

In general, H_2O's Deep Learning is implemented for feedforward and multi-Layer neural networks models. In Deep learning techniques, the networks may consist of huge number of hidden, ReLU and Tanh Layers. Each layer comprises of number of nodes and neurons and thousands of features and parameters. These parameters are trained by nodes with the parallel computing feature of H_2O to parallelize the DL algorithms processes, which leads to reducing the overhead and computational time.

The H_2O's Generative Adversarial Network layer is used for segmentation and for generating new X-ray images. Many researces [10, 13, 26] proved the superity of using GAN with X-ray images. The generated data by GAN provides the model with large scale data for training the neural networks. This will lead to a significant improvement in the deep learning performance for classifying the new COVID-19 cases. In this layer, the generative network provides additional X-ray images that will be stored in genertaed images respoitory, as shown in Fig. 3. The data collector mixes the generated images with the original training data. The dataset is then augmented based on the generated dataset. Finally, the discriminator network detect each image whether its a real image or generated one. The results obtained will be evaluated in the classification layer by testing the accuracy of the generated data.

On the other hand, the CT images are handled by the H_2O's Convolutional Neural Networks (CNNs). COVID-19 CT images contains specific features that uniquely identifies this pneumonia. CNNs applies number of filters to detect the COVID19

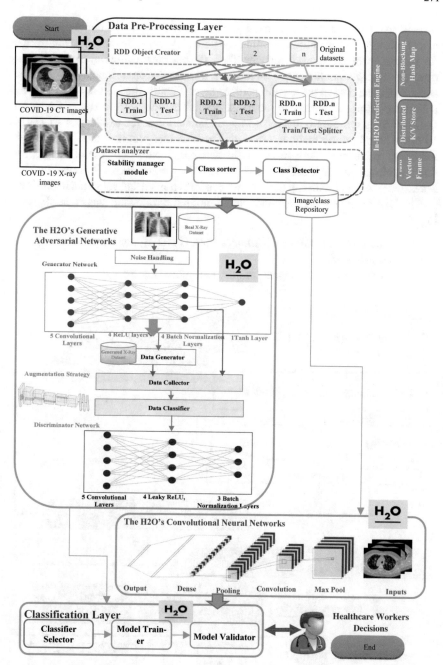

Fig. 3 The Proposed H₂O's deep-Learning-inspired model based on Big Data analytics (DLBD-COV)

associated features from image. In the proposed model, the CNNs contains four main layers: Max Pool, convolution, Pooling and dense layers [9]. In the first pooling layer, the features in the CT image is reduces. Then, the relevant features are extracted using predefined weights in the convolution layer. The resolution of images is minimized using statistical data in the second pooling layer. Finally, the features with identical patters are grouped together in the dense layer. The output from H_2O's CNNs and H_2O's GAN's are then delivered to the classification layer to diagnosis COVID-19 cases based on the features selected. The classifier picker is used to select the most appropriate classifiers, based on the delivered feature and type of image, from different classifiers: Support Vector Machine(SVM), Naive Bayes (NB) and Random Forest (RF). After classifying the data, the model is trained and validated in this layer.

The DLBD-COV model is conducted through the following stages, as shown in Fig. 4:

I. The dataset of X-ray or CT images for COVID-19 confirmed and suspected cases is loaded.
II. Applying pre-processing techniques to remove missing data.

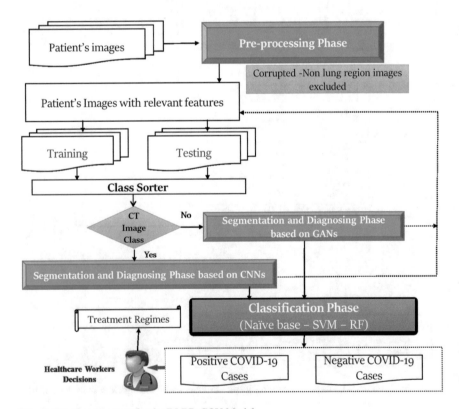

Fig. 4 The Flow diagram for the DLBD-COV Model

III. The type of images is detected to determine the most appropriate Deep learning technique that best handle this type of image.
IV. The GAN is used for diagnosing the X-ray images.
V. Implementing the CNNs for the CT images.
VI. The results obtained from the GANs and CNNs are classified and validated using different classifiers.
VII. Using H$_2$O in the DLBD-COV reduces the computational time needed for the diagnosis process.

7 The Experimental Results

A number of experiments were conducted to validate the proposed DLBD-COV's effectiveness. The model was implemented in MATLAB R2019a and are executed on a windows 10 PC with Intel(R) Core (TM) i7 CPU, with 16 GB RAM and 2.81 GHz clock speed. In the following experiments, a 10-fold cross validation is used. The stated results were taken as averages of the ten partitions. The CT scans chest dataset were collected from different resources [45–47]. The X-ray Images were collected from [48–50].

To validate the effectiveness of proposed model over other deep learning models, the accuracy, precision, recall(Sensitivity) and the computational time were used as the evaluations metrics, where:

$$Overall Accuracy = \frac{TP + TN}{TP + FP + TN + FN} \tag{1}$$

where TP, TN, FP and FN are true positive, true negative, false positive, and false negative respectively. The significant measures of the performance are: True Positive Rate (TPR), True Negative rate (TNR) and, Positive Predictive Value (PPV), defined as follows,

$$Recall(Sensitivity) = TPR = \frac{TP}{TP + FN} \tag{2}$$

$$Specificity = TNR = \frac{TN}{TN + FP} \tag{3}$$

$$Precision = PPV = \frac{TP}{TP + FP} \tag{4}$$

7.1   Experiment 1: Compare Between GAN and CNN Implemented in DLBD-COV

In order to validate the choice of choosing CNNs in diagnosis CT images and GAN for diagnosing X-ray images, the overall precision, recall and accuracy of DLBD-COV model is tested when diagnosing CT images only using GAN and CNN, as shown in Fig. 5. In addition, the overall precision, recall and accuracy of DLBD-COV model is tested when diagnosing X-ray images only using GAN and CNN, as shown in Fig. 6. The results obtained proved that the accuracy of diagnosing CT

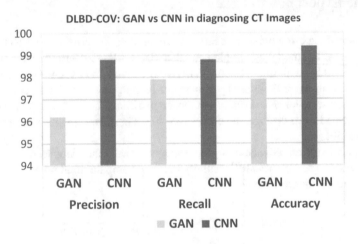

Fig. 5 Comparison between GAN and CNN in diagnosing CT Images in DLBD-COV

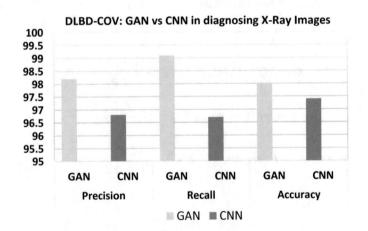

Fig. 6 Comparison between GAN and CNN in diagnosing X-Ray Images in DLBD-COV

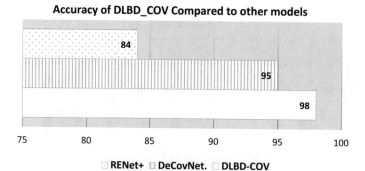

Fig. 7 The overall accuracy for DLBD-COV model compared to other models

images is better when using CNN while the accuracy of diagnosing X-ray images is better when using GAN.

7.2 Experiment Two: Evaluate the Overall Accuracy of DLBD-COV Model

In this experiment, the overall accuracy of DLBD-COV model is tested using three different classifiers as mention in the previous section. The results obtained are compared to the result obtained from recent deep learning models, namely, DeConNet [3] and ReNet + [6], as shown in Fig. 7.

It is obviously shown from Fig. 7 that the proposed DLBD-COV model achieved a superior accuracy over DeConNet and ReNet + . To perform this comparison, the same threshold values, classifiers and datasets are used for different models.

7.3 Experiment Three: Evaluate the Computational Time of DLBD-COV Model

This experiment main goal is to test the computational time needed for DLBD-COV model for diagnosing COVID-19 images and compare the time taken by DLBD-COV with the time needed for other deep learning models, DeConNet and ReNet + , for diagnosing, as shown in Fig. 8. In addition, three different classifiers are used in testing, namely SVM, NB and RF.

The results obtained proved that using H$_2$ O for parallel processing along with GAN and CNN fasten the diagnosing process compared to other models when using the three classifiers.

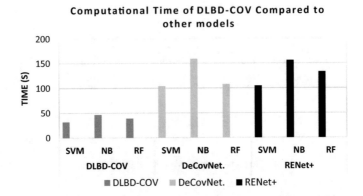

Fig. 8 The computational time of DLBD-COV compared to other models

7.4   Experiment Four: Test the Impact of Using H_2O on DLBD-COV Performance

In addition, in order to validate that H_2O is the optimum choice to be used in DLBD-COV model to deal with large scale data, this experiment has been conducted. A comparison is made, in this experiment, between the results obtained from DLBD-COV when using H_2O and Spark, as shown in Table 2. The results obtained showed that H_2O proved an improved performance in terms of computational speed over Spark. This is due to the availability of supported deep learning (Neural net-works) algorithms in H_2O.ai.

Table 2   The computational time of DLBD-COV Model when using H_2O and SPARK

Dataset type	No. of maps	DLBD-COV based spark time (s)	DLBD-COV based H_2O time (s)
X-Ray	512	31.8436	13.0986
	1024	35.5862	13.1081
	2048	46.6194	13.1275
CT images	512	31.7255	13.0876
	1024	36.1147	13.1024
	2048	42.0057	13.1371
Both X-Ray and CT images	512	34.264	13.2942
	1024	36.7934	13.3566
	2048	48.424	13.2739

8 Conclusion

WHO organization announced that COVID-19 disease as a pandemic. It leads to thousands of death in short time. Fast and accurate diagnosis of COVID-19 shows a crucial role in its containment. In this context, an H$_2$O's Deep-Learning-inspired model based on Big Data analytics (DLBD-COV) is proposed in this chapter for early diagnosis of COVID-19 cases. The DLBD-COV model supports two types of COVID-19's lung-region images: CT and X-ray images. H$_2$O is used for scalable processing that leads to speed the diagnosing process. The Generative Adversarial Network (GAN) had proved to perform better in diagnosing x-ray images, and the Convolutional Neural Network (CNN) are used for CT images. And their classification results are compared using three different classifiers: SVM, NB, RF. A classifier picker is implemented to select from these three classifiers, the most suitable classifier based on the lowest classification error obtained.

Number of experiments, using thousands of real and generated images, were performed to validate DLBD-COV performance. The obtained results proved that using H$_2$O framework speedup the diagnosing process which time is a critical issue in COVID-19 containment. In addition, the DLBD-COV achieves high accuracy, precision and recall compared to other diagnosing model. As a future work, a plan is made to use genetic algorithm (GA) for optimizing the parameters to improve the classifier performance

References

1. WHO: Coronavirus disease 2019 (COVID-19) Situation Report—66. 2020. https://www.who.int/docs/default-source/coronaviruse/situation-reports/20200326-sitrep-66-covid-19.pdf?sfvrsn=81b94e61_2. Accessed 27 Mar 2020
2. WHO: Coronavirus disease 2019 (COVID-19) Situation Report—66. 2020. https://www.who.int/docs/default-source/coronaviruse/situation-reports/20200427-sitrep-98-covid-19.pdf?sfvrsn=90323472_4. Accessed 27 Apr 2020
3. Zheng, C., Deng, X., Fu, Q., & Zhou, Q.: Deep Learning-based Detection for COVID-19 from Chest CT using Weak Label, pp. 1–13 (2020)
4. Hou, H., Lv, W., Tao, Q., Hospital, T., Company, J.T., Ai, T., Hospital, T., Wuhan, T., Hospital, T. (2019). Press In Pr. (2019)
5. Ai, T., Yang, Z., Hou, H., Zhan, C., Chen, C., Lv, W., Tao, Q., Sun, Z., Xia, L.: Correlation of chest CT and RT-PCR testing in Coronavirus Disease 2019 (COVID-19) in China: a report of 1014 cases. Radiology **2019**, 200642 (2020). https://doi.org/10.1148/radiol.2020200642
6. Xu, X., Jiang, X., Ma, C., Du, P., Li, X., Lv, S., Yu, L., Chen, Y., Su, J., Lang, G., Li, Y., Zhao, H., Xu, K., Ruan, L., Wu, W.: Deep Learning System to Screen Coronavirus Disease 2019 Pneumonia, pp. 1–29 (2020). http://arxiv.org/abs/2002.09334
7. Corman, V.M., Landt, O., Kaiser, M., et al.: Detection of 2019 novel coronavirus (2019-nCoV) by real-time RT-PCR. Euro. Surveill. **25**(3) (2020). https://doi.org/10.2807/1560-7917.es.2020.25.3.2000045
8. Lei, J., Li, J., Li, X., Qi, X.: CT Imaging of the 2019 Novel Coronavirus (2019-nCoV) Pneumonia. Radiology 200236 (2020)

9. ELGhamrawy, S.M.: Diagnosis and Prediction Model for COVID19 Patients Response to Treatment based on Convolutional Neural Networks and Whale Optimization Algorithm Using CT Images. medRxiv. 2020 Jan 1

10. Khalifa, N.E., Taha, M.H., Hassanien, A.E., Elghamrawy, S.: Detection of Coronavirus (COVID-19) Associated Pneumonia based on Generative Adversarial Networks and a Fine-Tuned Deep Transfer Learning Model using Chest X-ray Dataset. arXiv preprint arXiv:2004.01184. 2020 Apr 2

11. https://www.h2o.ai/blog/h2o-architecture/

12. Badrinarayanan, V., Kendall, A., Cipolla, R.: SegNet: A Deep Convolutional Encoder-Decoder Architecture for Image Segmentation. arXiv preprint arXiv:1511.00561 (2015)

13. Goodfellow, J., Pouget-Abadie, M., Mirza, B., Xu, D., Warde-Farley, S., Ozair, Courville, A., Bengio, Y.: Generative adversarial nets. In: Advances in Neural Information Processing Systems, pp. 2672–2680 (2014)

14. http://docs.h2o.ai/h2o/latest-stable/h2o-docs/data-science.html. Accessed 27 Apr 2020

15. Almeida, F.: Benefits, Challenges and Tools of Big Data Management, pp. 12–20 (2017)

16. Abdel-Hamid, N.B., ElGhamrawy, S., Desouky, A.E. et al.: A dynamic spark-based classification framework for Imbalanced big data. J Grid Computing **16**, 607–626 (2018). https://doi.org/10.1007/s10723-018-9465-z

17. Ed-daoudy, A., Maalmi, K.: Application of machine learning model on streaming health data event in real-time to predict health status using spark. In: 2018 International Symposium on Advanced Electrical and Communication Technologies (ISAECT) (2018)

18. Tripathi, R.; Kumari, V., Patel, S., Singh, Y., Varadwaj, P.: Prediction of lncRNA using deep learning approach. In: International Conference on Advances in Biotechnology (BioTech). Proceedings, pp. 138–142. Global Science and Technology Forum, Singapore (2015)

19. Candel, A., Parmar, V., LeDell, E., Arora, A.: Deep learning with h2o (2015)

20. Mehmood, R., Alam, F., Albogami, N.N., Katib, I., Albeshri, A., Altowaijri, S.M.: Utilearn: a personalised ubiquitous teaching and learning system for smart societies. IEEE Access **5**, 2615–2635 (2017)

21. Dey, N., Hassanien, A.E., Bhatt, C., Ashour, A., Satapathy, S.C. (eds.): (2018). Internet of Things and Big Data Analytics Toward Next-Generation Intelligence, pp. 3–549. Springer, Berlin, For COVID-19

22. Hinton, G.E., Osindero, S., Teh, Y.W.: A fast learning algorithm for deep belief nets. Neural Comput. **18**(7), 1527–1554 (2006)

23. Bengio, Y.: Learning deep architectures for AI. Foundations Trends® Mach. Learn. **2**(1), 1–127 (2009)

24. Lan, K., Wang, D.T., Fong, S., Liu, L.S., Wong, K.K., Dey, N.: A survey of data mining and deep learning in bioinformatics. J. Med. Syst. **42**(8), 139 (2018)

25. Krizhevsky, A,, Sutskever, I., Hinton, G.E.: Imagenet classification with deep convolutional neural networks. In: Advances in Neural Information Processing Systems, pp. 1097–1105 (2012)

26. Radford, A., Metz, L., Chintala, S.: Unsupervised Representation Learning with Deep Convolutional Generative Adversarial Networks. arXiv preprint arXiv:1511.06434. 19 Nov 2015

27. Zeiler, M.D., Krishnan, D., Taylor, G.W., Fergus, R.: Deconvolutional networks. In 2010 IEEE Computer Society Conference on Computer Vision and Pattern Recognition, 13 June 2010, pp. 2528–2535, IEEE

28. He, K., Zhang, X., Ren, S., Sun, J.: Deep residual learning for image recognition. In: Proceedings of the IEEE Conference on Computer Vision and Pattern Recognition, pp. 770–778 (2016)

29. Simonyan, K., Zisserman, A.: Very Deep Convolutional Networks for Large-Scale Image Recognition. arXiv preprint arXiv:1409.1556 (2014)

30. Szegedy, C., Liu, W., Jia, Y., Sermanet, P., Reed, S., Anguelov, D., Erhan, D., Vanhoucke, V., Rabinovich, A.: Going deeper with convolutions. In: Proceedings of the IEEE Conference on Computer Vision and Pattern Recognition, pp. 1–9 (2015)

31. Huang, G., Liu, Z., Van Der Maaten, L., Weinberger, K.Q.: Densely connected convolutional networks. In: Proceedings of the IEEE Conference on Computer Vision and Pattern Recognition, pp. 4700–4708 (2017)

32. Radford, A., Metz, L., Chintala, S.: Unsupervised Representation Learning with Deep Convolutional Generative Adversarial Networks. arXiv preprint arXiv:1511.06434 (2015)

33. Mirza, M., Osindero, S.: Conditional Generative Adversarial Nets. arXiv preprint arXiv:1411. 1784 (2014)

34. Wu, J.T., Leung, K., Leung, G.M.: Nowcasting and forecasting the potential domestic and international spread of the 2019-nCoV outbreak originating in Wuhan, China: a modelling study. The Lancet **395**(10225), 689–697 (2020)

35. Shinde, G.R., Kalamkar, A.B., Mahalle, P.N., Dey, N., Chaki, J., Hassanien, A.: Forecasting Models for Coronavirus (COVID-19): A Survey of the State-of-the-Art. TechRxiv (2020). Preprint. https://doi.org/10.36227/techrxiv, 12101547, v1

36. Zhao, X., Liu, X., Li, X.: Tracking the Spread of Novel Coronavirus (2019-nCoV) Based on Big Data. medRxiv (2020)

37. Wang, C.J., Ng, C.Y., Brook, R.H.: Response to COVID-19 in Taiwan: Big Data Analytics, New Technology, and Proactive Testing. JAMA (2020)

38. Zhou, C., Su, F., Pei, T., Zhang, A., Du, Y., Luo, B., Cao, Z., Wang, J., Yuan, W., Zhu, Y., Song, C.: COVID-19: challenges to GIS with big data. Geogr. Sustain. (2020)

39. Long, J.B., Ehrenfeld, J.M.: The Role of Augmented Intelligence (AI) in Detecting and Preventing the Spread of Novel Coronavirus (2020)

40. Lazer, D., Kennedy, R.: What We Can Learn from the Epic Failure of Google Flu Trends: WIRED (2020). https://www.wired.com/2015/10/canlearn-epic-failure-google-flu-tre nds/. Published 2015. Accessed 31 Jan

41. Niller, E.: An AI Epidemiologist Sent the First Warnings of the Wuhan Virus: WIRED (2020). https://www.wired.com/story/aiepidemiologist-wuhan-public-health-warnings/. Published 2020. Accessed 31 Jan

42. Salehinejad, H., Valaee, S., Dowdell, T., Colak, E., Barfett, J.: Generalization of deep neural networks for chest pathology classification in x-rays using generative adversarial networks. In: 2018 IEEE International Conference on Acoustics, Speech and Signal Processing (ICASSP), 15 Apr 2018, pp. 990–994, IEEE

43. Chen, C., Dou, Q., Chen, H., Heng, P.A.: Semantic-aware generative adversarial nets for unsupervised domain adaptation in chest x-ray segmentation. In: International Workshop on Machine Learning in Medical Imaging, 16 Sept 2018, pp. 143–151. Springer, Cham

44. Madani, A., Moradi, M., Karargyris, A., Syeda-Mahmood, T.: Semi-supervised learning with generative adversarial networks for chest x-ray classification with ability of data domain adaptation. In: 2018 IEEE 15th International Symposium on Biomedical Imaging (ISBI 2018), 4 Apr 2018, pp. 1038–1042, IEEE

45. https://github.com/ieee8023/covid-chestxray-dataset. Accessed 27 Apr 2020

46. https://github.com/UCSD-AI4H/COVID-CT. Accessed 27 Apr 2020

47. https://www.sirm.org/en. Accessed 27 Apr 2020

48. https://www.kaggle.com/paultimothymooney/chest-xray-pneumonia. Accessed 27 Apr 2020

49. Kermany, D., Zhang, K., Goldbaum, M. (2018). Large Dataset of Labeled Optical Coherence Tomography (OCT) and Chest X-Ray Images. Mendeley Data, v3. http://dx.doi.org/10.17632/rscbjbr9sj.3

50. https://www.kaggle.com/bachrr/covid-chest-xray. Accessed 27 Apr 2020

51. Elghamrawy, S.M., Hassanien, A.E.: A partitioning framework for Cassandra NoSQL database using Rendezvous hashing. J. Supercomput. **73**, 4444–4465 (2017). https://doi.org/10.1007/s11 227-017-2027-5

Coronavirus (COVID-19) Classification Using Deep Features Fusion and Ranking Technique

Umut Özkaya, Şaban Öztürk, and Mucahid Barstugan

Abstract COVID-19, which appeared towards the end of 2019, has become a huge threat to public health. The solution to this threat, which is defined as a global epidemic by the World Health Organization (WHO), is currently undergoing very intensive studies. There is a consensus that the use of Computed Tomography (CT) techniques for early diagnosis of pandemic disease gives both fast and accurate results. This study provides an automated and highly effective method for detecting COVID-19 at an early stage. CT image features are extracted using the convolutional neural network (CNN) architecture, which is the most successful image processing tool of today, for the detection of COVID-19, where early detection is vital for human life. Representation power is increased by combining features from the output of four CNN architectures with data fusion. Finally, the features combined with the feature ranking method are sorted, and their length is reduced. In this way, the dimensional curse is saved. From 150 CT images, 16×16 (Subset-1) and 32×32 (Subset-2) patches were obtained to create a subset. Within the scope of the proposed method, 3000 patch images are labeled as "COVID-19 (coronavirus)" or "No finding" for use in training and test stages. The Support Vector Machine (SVM) method then classified the processed data. The proposed method shows high performance in Subset-2 with 98.27% accuracy, 98.93% sensitivity, 97.60% specificity, 97.63% sensitivity, 98.28% F1 score and 96.54% Matthews Correlation Coefficient (MCC) metrics.

Keywords Coronavirus · COVID-19 · CT images · Deep learning · Feature fusion · Ranking

U. Özkaya (✉) · M. Barstugan
Electrical and Electronics Engineering, Konya Technical University, Konya 42250, Turkey
e-mail: uozkaya@ktun.edu.tr

M. Barstugan
e-mail: mbarstugan@ktun.edu.tr

Ş. Öztürk
Electrical and Electronics Engineering, Amasya University, Amasya 05001, Turkey
e-mail: saban.ozturk@amasya.edu.tr

© The Editor(s) (if applicable) and The Author(s), under exclusive license to Springer Nature Switzerland AG 2020
A.-E. Hassanien et al. (eds.), *Big Data Analytics and Artificial Intelligence Against COVID-19: Innovation Vision and Approach*, Studies in Big Data 78, https://doi.org/10.1007/978-3-030-55258-9_17

1 Introduction

COVID-19 has become an epidemic similar to some other pandemic diseases, causes patient deaths in China, according to the World Health Organization (WHO) [1–3]. Early application of treatment procedures for patients with COVID-19 infection increases the patient's chances of survival. The rapid diagnosis of the disease is one of the most critical facts to prevent the spread of the disease. Pathological tests performed in laboratories take time. A fast and accurate diagnosis is necessary for a productive struggle against COVID-19. For this reason, experts have been started to use radiological imaging methods. These procedures are performed with computed tomography (CT) or X-ray imaging techniques. COVID-19 cases have similar features in CT images in the early and late stages. It shows a circular and inward diffusion from within the image [4]. Therefore, radiological imaging provides early detection of suspicious cases with an accuracy of 90%.

Computer-aided diagnosis (CAD) methods have been used in the diagnosis of various diseases for many years. It is automatically interpreted by removing many human features such as the processing of images taken from the diseased areas by the computer and the interpretation of the audio signals. CAD systems have become the most prominent assistant of specialists by speeding up and facilitating many procedures. In the past, CAD systems were manually used for performing simple tasks. With the development of technology and the spread of computers, the direction of CAD systems has changed. Many processes, such as counting of cells, detection of organs, detection of diseased areas, have become automated. Although this development is due to the strength of the proposed algorithms each period, the CNN algorithm has affected the entire image processing area in recent times. It has mostly resolved the automatic image analysis problem in the medical field.

This study used 150 CT images to classify COVID-19 cases. Two different datasets were generated from 150 CT images. These datasets include 16×16 and 32×32 patch images. Each dataset contains 3000 number of images labeled with COVID-19 and No findings. Deep features were obtained with pre-trained Convolutional Neural Network (CNN) models. These deep features were fused and ranked to train Support Vector Machine (SVM). The proposed method achieved high performance for early diagnosis of COVID-19 cases. The most important of the main contributions of this study is the use of high-level deep features obtained from different pre-trained CNN networks. Another contribution is to increase the performance of the SVM classifier by giving inputs as the deep features obtained through fusion and ranking. The proposed method has a limitation for image classification. t-test feature ranking can be only used in binary classification. It is not appropriate for multi-class problems. When the proposed method results are examined, it is seen that it shows higher performance than other pre-trained CNN networks.

1.1 The Literature Review

Various COVID-19 dataset started to be shared on the internet, recently. Some studies [5–8] classified Chest X-ray images to detect the coronavirus disease. Some [9–12] studied on forecasting of the coronavirus spread. Some studies [13, 14] used blood test results to detect the coronavirus disease. The literature studies use deep learning methods, mostly. Shan et al. [15] proposed a neural network model called VB-Net to segment the COVID-19 regions in CT images. The proposed method has been tested on 300 new cases. A recommendation system has been used to make it easier for radiologists to mark infected areas within CT images. Xu et al. [16] analyzed CT images to determine healthily, COVID-19, and other viral cases. The dataset included 219 COVID-19, 224 viral diseases, and 175 healthy images. The study achieved an 87.6% general classification accuracy with the deep learning method. Li et al. [17] classified three different coronavirus situations such as mild, common, and severe-critical. The study used CT images of 78 patients, and the number of each class is 24, 46, and 8, respectively. The clinical classification method achieved 82.6% sensitivity, 100% specificity, and 0.918 AUC values. Tang et al. [18] used 176 chest CT images that consisted of two different classes as severe and non-severe. The study extracted 63 quantitative features on images, and the random forest algorithm classified the features. 3-fold cross-validation method was used during the classification process. The proposed method achieved 87.5% classification accuracy and 0.91 AUC value. Fong et al. [19] proposed a Composite Monte-Carlo (CMC) simulation to predict COVID-19 distribution. An increase in the number of cases in nearby cities was tried to be estimated by using the temporal-spatial data related to the city of Wuhan which is the source of the virus. Elghamrawy et al. [20] represented a method as Artificial Intelligence-inspired Model for COVID-19 Diagnosis and Prediction for Patient Response to Treatment (AIMDP). The proposed method was based on prediction on the spread of COVID-19 cases by using feature selection using the Whale Optimization Algorithm. Fong et al. [21] used data mining technique with polynomial neural network with corrective feedback (PNN + cf). This method had acceptable results to predict COVID-19 outbreak. Rajinikanth et al. [22] proposed a segmentation technique to analysis COVID-19 textures. It consisted of four parts as threshold filter, image enhancement, image segmentation and region-of-interest (ROI) extraction. The method has ability to extract infected regions from lung background. Our previous study used 126 chest X-ray images that have six different classes such as ARd, Covid-19, neumocystis-pneumonia, Sars, streptococcus, and no finding. The study extracted features on images with different methods and combined the features. Then, the feature set was shrunk by different methods and SVM classified the shrunken feature set. The best classification performance was obtained as 94.23%.

This study consists of six sections. The properties of obtained patch images are visualized in Sect. 2. In Sect. 3, the basics of deep learning methods, feature fusion, and ranking techniques are mentioned. Comparative classification performances are given in Sect. 4. Section 5 and Sect. 6 include discussion and conclusion.

Table 1 Properties of two different patch subsets

Subset	Patch dimension	Number of COVID-19 patches	Number of no finding patches
Subset 1	16×16	3000	3000
Subset 2	32×32	3000	3000

2 Material

2.1 Statistical Features of Dataset

Totally 53 infected CT images were accessed to the Societa Italiana di Radiologia Medica e Interventistica to generate datasets [23]. Patch images obtained from infected and non-infected regions from CT images. Table 1 presents the properties of two different subsets.

2.2 Visual Features of Dataset

The images in the dataset were acquired by different CT imaging tools. Thus, it caused a different infected grey level region in the CT images. This situation affects the classification process and performance quite negatively. CT images have different grey levels. Image patches of 16×16 and 32×32 dimensions with different characteristics were obtained from CT images. Figure 1 shows the process of patch creation.

3 Method

3.1 Deep Learning

Deep learning, which has become quite popular recently, has been used in many areas. Academic studies have been pioneers for their use in e-mail filtering, search engine matching, smartphones, social media, e-commerce areas, etc. [24]. Deep learning is also used for face recognition, object recognition, object detection, text classification, and speech recognition. In machine learning, Deep Belief Networks (DBN) is a productive graphical model or a class of deep neural networks consisting of multiple layers in hidden nodes. When trained on a series of unsupervised samples, the DBN can learn to reconfigure its entries as probabilistic. The layers then act as feature detectors. After this learning phase, a DBN can be trained with more control to make the classification. DBNs can be seen as a combination of simple, unsupervised

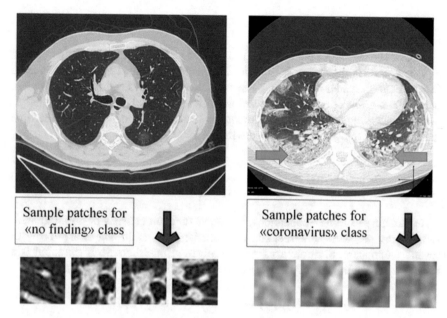

Fig. 1 Data generation for No finding and COVID-19 patches

networks, such as restricted Boltzmann machines (RBMs) or auto-encoders, which serve as the hidden layer of each subnet, the visible layer of the next layer.

3.2 Convolutional Neural Network

Convolutional neural networks (CNN) are a type of neural network with at least one layer of convolution. It has some layers such as convolution, ReLU, pooling, normalization, fully connected, and a softmax layer. Generally, convolution is a process that takes place on two actual functions. To describe the convolution operation, for example, the location of a space shuttle with a laser is monitored. The laser sensor produces a simple $x(t)$ output, which is the space of the space shuttle at time t. Where X and t are actual values, for example, any t is a different value received at a snapshot time. Also, this sensor has a bit noisy. To carry out a less noisy prediction, the designer can take the average of several measurements together. This can be done with the weighting function $w(a)$, which is a measurement period. If a weighted average operation is applied at all times, a new function is obtained, which allows estimating the position more accurately (see Eq. 1):

$$S(t) = \int X(a)W(t-a)da \tag{1}$$

The convolution process is represented by a star sign (see Eq. 2):

$$S(t) = (X * w)(t) \tag{2}$$

In CNN terminology, the first argument in X function at Eq. 2 is the input matrix, and the second argument for W function is called the kernel. The output is called a feature map. In the above example, the measurement is made without interruption, but this is not realistic. Time is parsed when working on the computer. To realize realistic measurement, one measurement per second is taken. Where t is the time index and is an integer, so X and W are integers (see Eq. 3).

$$S(t) = (X * W) = \sum_{a=-\infty}^{\infty} x(a)w(t-a) \tag{3}$$

In machine learning applications, the input function consists of a multidimensional array set, and the kernel function consists of a multidimensional array of several parameters. Multiple axes are convolved at one time. So if the input is a two-dimensional image, the kernel becomes a two-dimensional matrix (see Eq. 4).

$$S(i, j) = (I * K)(i, j) = \sum_{m} \sum_{n} I(i - m, j - n)K(m, n) \tag{4}$$

The above equation means shifting the kernel according to the input. This increases the invariance of convolution [25]. Many machine learning libraries process the kernel without inversion, which is called as cross-correlation that is related to convolution. Because it looks like a convolution, it is called a convulsive neural network (see Eq. 5):

$$S(i, j) = (I * K)(i, j) = \sum_{m} \sum_{n} I(i + m, j + n)K(m, n) \tag{5}$$

Convolution provides three essential thoughts to improve a machine learning system: infrequent interactions, parameter sharing, and covariant representations. Furthermore, the convolution process can be worked with variable-sized inputs. Convolution neural network layers use a matrix parameter that includes different kinds of the link between each input unit and each output unit. It means that each output unit connects with each input unit. However, CNN typically has infrequent interactions (also called sparse links or sparse weights).

A pooling function changes the output of the network at a specific location with summary statistics of nearby outputs. The pooling process consists of outputs from specific regions. When several parameters in the next layer depend on the input image or feature map size, any reduction in input size also increases the statistical efficiency and reduces the memory requirements for storing parameters.

The Rectified Linear Unit is an activation function type. The Rectified Linear Unit calculates the function $F(x) = \max(0, x)$. In other words, activation is thresholded equal to zero. There are several pros and cons to the use of ReLU. ReLU units can become sensitive during the training phase. For example, a large gradient scale flowing through neuron with a ReLU activation function can cause weights to be updated so that the neuron is not reactivated at any data point. That is, it can kill units irrevocably during training because data replication can be disabled. For example, if the learning rate is too high, 40% of the network may be dead. This is a less frequent occurrence with an appropriate adjustment of the learning rate.

In fully connected layers, a reduction of nodes below a certain threshold increased the performance. So it is observed that forgetting the weak information increases learning. Some properties of dropout value are as follows. The dropout value is generally selected as 0.5. Different uses are also common. It varies according to the problem and data set. The random elimination method can also be used for the dropout. The dropout value is defined as a value in the range [0, 1] when used as the threshold value. It is not necessary to use the same dropout value on all layers; different dilution values can also be used.

The softmax function is a sort of classifier. Logistic regression is a classifier of the classifier, and the softmax function is a multi-class of logistic regression. $1/\sum_j e^{f_j}$ term normalizes the distribution. That is, the sum of the values equals 1. Therefore, it calculates the probability of the class to which the class belongs. When a test input is given x, the activation function in $j = 1,...,k$ is asked to predict the probability of p $(y = j \mid x)$ for each value. For example, it is desirable to estimate the probability that the class tag will have each of the different possible values. Thus, as a result of the activation function, it produces a k-dimensional vector, which gives us our predictive possibilities. The error value must be calculated for the learning to occur, and the error value for the softmax function is calculated by the softmax loss function.

3.3 Feature Fusion and Ranking Technique

VGG-16, GoogleNet, and ResNet-50 models were used for feature extraction. The obtained feature vectors with these models were fused to obtain higher dimensional fusion features. In this way, the effect of insufficient features obtained from a single CNN network is minimized. Also, there is a certain level of correlation and excessive information among the features. This also increases consuming time and computational complexity. Therefore, it is necessary to rank the features. *t-test* technique was used in feature ranking. It calculates the difference between the two features and determines its differences statistically [26]. In this way, it performs the ranking process by taking into account the frequency of the same features in the feature vector and the frequency of finding the average feature.

3.4   Support Vector Machines (SVMs)

After the feature fusion and ranking functions were performed, the binary SVM classifier was trained for classification. SVM transfers feature into space where it can better classify features with kernel functions [27]. Linear kernel function was used in SVM. The SVM classifier was trained to minimize the squared hinge loss. The squared hinge loss is given in Eq. 6.

$$\min_w \frac{1}{2} w^T w + C \sum_{n=1}^{N} \max\left(1 - w^T x_n t_n, 0\right)^2 \tag{6}$$

Here, x_n represents the fusion and the ranking feature vector. The wrong classification penalty is determined by the C hyperparameter in the loss function.

3.5   Proposed Method

In the proposed method, pre-trained CNN networks were trained for Subset-1 and Subset-2, separately. VGG-16, GoogleNet, and ResNet-50 models were used as a pre-trained network. Patch images were given as input to pre-trained CNN structures. A discriminative method is used to obtain high-level features from pre-trained CNN feature vectors. This process is performed by Canonical Correlation Analysis (CCA) fusion method [28]. CCA is a widely used method that examines the degree of relationship between variables. If X and Y define vectors as matrices containing n features, S_{xx} and S_{yy} represent the in-class covariance matrix, $S_{xy} = S_{yx}$ inter-class covariance matrix. The vector S is expressed as in Eq. 7.

$$S = \begin{pmatrix} S_{xx} & S_{xy} \\ S_{yx} & S_{yy} \end{pmatrix} \tag{7}$$

It is challenging to understand the correlation between feature vectors from this matrix. Therefore, the correlation between the two properties is obtained by Eqs. 8 and 9 in the CCA fusion method.

$$X^* = W_x^T X, \ Y^* = W_y^T Y \tag{8}$$

$$\text{corr}(X^*, Y^*) = \frac{\text{cov}(X^*, Y^*)}{\text{var}(X^*). \text{var}(Y^*)} \tag{9}$$

Combining and vectorizing features in the fusion process is obtained as CCA feature vectors Z.

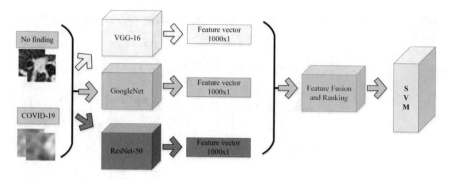

Fig. 2 Proposed method

$$Z = X^* + Y^* = W_x^T X + W_y^T Y \tag{10}$$

The *t-test* evaluates the statistical difference between the two classes. Mean feature frequency and variance are evaluated for each class by Lindeberg-Levy theorem [29]. *t-test* equation for feature rankings showed as in Eq. 11.

$$t - test(t_i, C_k) = \frac{|tZ_k - tZ_i|}{s.m} \tag{11}$$

where t is the frequency term, C_k is the number of k classes, tZ_k feature frequency of between classes, and tZ_i in-class frequency. s is the standard deviation and m is equal to $\sqrt{1/N_k - 1/N}$. N_k is the number of features in the kth class. N indicates the total number of features. t values for class can be performed as in Eq. 12 t-test

$$t - test_{avg}(t_i) = \sum_{k=1}^{K} t - test(t_i, C_k) \tag{12}$$

Correlation values between features were taken into consideration in the fusion process. The obtained features were ranked by the t-test method. In the t-test ranking process, features close to each other were eliminated according to feature frequency. In the last stage, fusion and ranking deep features were evaluated with the SVM classifier. The method proposed in Fig. 2 is visualized.

4 Experimental Results

This study presents the classification of COVID-19 texture for two different size data sets. First of all, the features obtained from CNN structures have been passed through fusion and ranking processes and classified. Six different metrics were used to evaluate the proposed method. These metrics are sensitivity (SEN), specificity (SPE), accuracy (ACC), precision (PRE), F-score, and Matthews Correlation Coefficient (MCC).

$$Sensitivity = TP/(TP + FN) \tag{13}$$

$$Specificity = TN/(TN + FP) \tag{14}$$

$$Accuracy = (TP + TN)/(TP + FN + TN + FP) \tag{15}$$

$$Precision = TP/(TP + FP) \tag{16}$$

$$F-score = (2xTP)/(2xTP + FN + FP) \tag{17}$$

$$MCC = \frac{TP \times TN - FP \times FN}{\sqrt{(TP + FP)(TP + FN)(TN + FP)(TN + FN)}} \tag{18}$$

TP, TN, FP, and *FN* values are the number of true positives, true negatives, false positives, and false negatives, respectively [30].

4.1 Classification Results of Subset 1

There are 6000 pieces of 16×16 CT patches in Subset-1. Data distribution between classes is equal. 75% of these images were used for training and 25% for testing. Table 2 shows comparatively classification performance pre-trained CNN networks and of the proposed method.

Table 2 The classification results for Subset-1

Methods	Evaluation metrics (%)									
	TP	TN	FP	FN	ACC	SEN	SPE	PRE	F1-score	MCC
VGG-16	716	653	97	34	91.27	95.47	87.07	88.07	91.62	82.83
Resnet-50	742	682	68	8	94.3	**98.93**	90.93	91.60	95.13	90.16
GoogleNet	631	742	8	119	91.53	84.13	**98.93**	**98.75**	90.86	83.99
Proposed method	700	734	16	50	**95.60**	93.33	97.87	97.77	**95.50**	**91.29**

Table 3 The classification results for Subset-2

Methods	Evaluation metrics (%)									
	TP	TN	FP	FN	ACC	SEN	SPE	PRE	F1-score	MCC
VGG-16	744	710	40	6	96.93	**99.20**	94.67	94.90	97.00	93.96
Resnet-50	744	716	34	6	97.33	**99.20**	95.47	95.63	97.38	94.73
GoogleNet	727	741	9	23	97.87	96.93	**98.80**	**98.78**	97.85	95.75
Proposed method	742	732	18	8	**98.27**	98.93	97.60	97.63	**98.28**	**96.54**

4.2 Classification Results of Subset 2

Subset-2 includes 3000 COVID-19 and 3000 No finding 32×32 CT patches. Comparative classification results of Subset-2 are given in Table 3.

4.3 Performance Evaluation

Table 2 shows that the best performance in Subset-1 was obtained as 95.60%. The highest performance belongs to ResNet-50 models with 98.93% in the sensitivity metric. In specificity and precision metrics, GoogleNet performed best with 98.93% and 98.75%, respectively. The proposed method in F1-score and MCC metrics is the most successful among pre-trained CNN structures with 95.50% and 91.29%, respectively.

Comparative performance metrics for Subset-2 are given in Table 3. The proposed method stands out with its 98.27% performance in accuracy metric. In the sensitivity metric, VGG-16 and ResNet-50 models show the highest performance with 99.20%. In the precision and F1-score metrics, the GoogleNet model achieved 98.80% and 98.78%, respectively. The proposed method achieved the highest metric performance in F1-score and MCC metrics with 98.28% and 96.54%, respectively. Figures 3, 4 presents the confusion matrices of the proposed method for Subset-1 and Subset-2.

The confusion matrix was obtained for the proposed method using Subset-1 in Fig. 3. When the confusion matrix was evaluated in class, the COVID-19 class was classified with an accuracy rate of 97.9%. Performance of No findings class was lower than COVID-19. 93.3% accuracy rate was obtained for this class. Classification accuracy of 93.6% was obtained in the analysis of positive class. In the negative class, this rate is higher and had a value of 97.8%.

Subset-2 was used in the training and testing process for the proposed method. In Fig. 4, a confusion matrix was obtained for test data. In-class analysis, a 97.6% accuracy rate of COVID-19 class was obtained. The performance was increased compared to Subset-1 in the No findings class. The accuracy rate was 98.9% for this class. In the positive and negative class evaluation, a classification accuracy of 98.9% and 97.6% were obtained, respectively. Also, the test time of the proposed method for each image is 0.34 s.

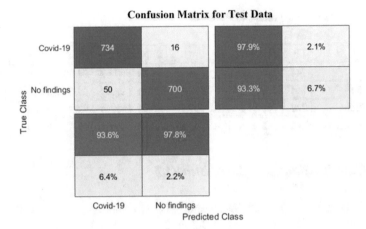

Fig. 3 Confusion matrix of the proposed method for Subset-1

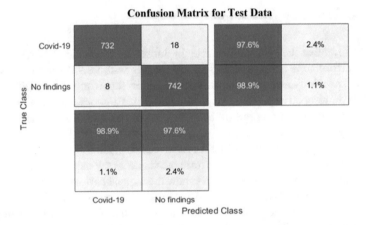

Fig. 4 Confusion Matrix of Proposed Method for Subset-2

5 Discussion

The first case of COVID-19 was found in the Wuhan region of China. COVID-19 is an epidemic disease and threatens the world's health system and economy. COVID-19 virus behaves similarly to other pandemic viruses. This makes it challenging to detect COVID-19 cases quickly. Therefore, COVID-19 is a candidate for a global epidemic. Radiological imaging techniques are used for a more accurate diagnosis in the detection of COVID-19. Therefore, it is possible to obtain more detailed information about COVID-19 using CT imaging techniques. When CT images are examined, shadows come to the fore in the regions where COVID-19 is located. At the same time, a spread is observed from the outside to the inner parts.

Table 4 The literature comparison

Study	Dataset	Method	ACC (%)	AUC
[5]	X-ray, 100 images	ResNet50	98	–
[6]	X-ray, 260 images	CNN	100	–
[7]	X-ray, 1427 images	Transfer learning	96.78	–
[8]	X-ray, 1431 images	CNN	–	0.934
[13]	Blood test, 404 samples	XG-boost	97	–
[14]	Blood Test, 49 samples	Random forest	95.12	–
[16]	CT, 618 images	3D-CNN	86.7	–
[17]	CT, 78 images	Statistical analysis	–	0.918
[18]	CT, 176 images	Random forest	87.5	0.91
Proposed method	CT, 6000 images	CNN feature fusion and ranking	98.27	–

The images in this study were acquired with different CT devices. Different characteristics of CT devices cause that the grey-levels of the similar part of the images are different. This complicates the analysis of the images. In the study, deep features were obtained by using pre-trained CNN networks. Then, deep features were fused and ranked. The data set was generated by taking random patches on CT images. Pre-trained CNN networks were trained using the transfer learning method in the Subset-1 and Subset-2 datasets. With the proposed method, 95.60% accuracy and 91.29% MCC metric performance were obtained for Subset-1. In Subset-2, the proposed method showed 98.27% accuracy, and 96.54% MCC metric performance. Table 4 presents the literature comparison.

Table 4 shows that all results are over 85%. The literature studies show that artificial intelligence can help experts to diagnose the coronavirus disease. The accuracy metric reached 100% in the literature [6]. The proposed method is in the second-best place in state-of-the-art methods. The worst performance belongs to 86.7% accuracy [16]. In the literature, most of the studies on COVID-19 are medical studies. The studies on classification and segmentation of COVID-19 on images will be increased. The need for coronavirus dataset is evident, especially for segmentation studies, because the target segmentation area is needed to be labeled by expert radiologists.

6 Conclusion

In this study, a method, which applies deep features fusion and ranking procedures features from pre-trained CNNs, was proposed for the early diagnosis of COVID-19 cases. In the proposed method, deep features were fused by CCA method, and ranking was performed with a t-test technique. SVM algorithm, a powerful classifier, was used to classify high-level features as a binary type. Also, the proposed method was evaluated on two different data sets as Subset-1 and Subset-2. It showed the highest performance on the Subset-2 dataset with 98.27% accuracy, 98.93% sensitivity, 97.60% specificity, 97.63% sensitivity, 98.28% F1 score and 96.54% MMC metric values. It is seen that the classification process was performed better and more effectively than other pre-trained CNNs. When comparing performance with other studies in the literature, it showed the second-highest performance. Thanks to this high performance, it has been proven to provide an accurate diagnosis of texture classification within CT images. It is foreseen that the early diagnosis of COVID-19 cases is carried out in time with the proposed method. Thus, it can be provided that the number of cases is under control.

References

1. Huang, C., Wang, Y., Li, X., Ren, L., Zhao, J., Hu, Y., et al.: Clinical features of patients infected with 2019 novel coronavirus in Wuhan. China. The Lancet. **395**(10223), 497–506 (2020)
2. Huang, P., Park, S., Yan, R., Lee, J., Chu, L.C., Lin, C.T., et al.: Added value of computer-aided CT image features for early lung cancer diagnosis with small pulmonary nodules: a matched case-control study. Radiology **286**(1), 286–295 (2018)
3. Esteva, A., Kuprel, B., Novoa, R.A., Ko, J., Swetter, S.M., Blau, H.M., et al.: Dermatologist-level classification of skin cancer with deep neural networks. Nature **542**(7639), 115–118 (2017)
4. Xie, X., Li, X., Wan, S., Gong, Y. (eds.) Mining X-ray Images of SARS Patients. Data Mining. Springer (2006)
5. Narin, A., Kaya, C., ZJapa, P.: Automatic detection of coronavirus disease (COVID-19) using X-ray images and deep convolutional neural networks. arXiv preprint arXiv:2003.10849 (2020)
6. Salman, F.M., Abu-Naser, S.S., Alajrami, E., Abu-Nasser, B.S., Ashqar, B.A.: COVID-19 detection using artificial intelligence. Int. J. Acad. Eng. Res. (IJAER) **4**(3), 18–25 (2020)
7. Apostolopoulos, I.D., Mpesiana, T.A.J.P.: Covid-19: automatic detection from x-ray images utilizing transfer learning with convolutional neural networks. Phys. Eng. Sci. Med. **1** (2020)
8. Zhang, J., Xie, Y., Li, Y., Shen, C., Xia, Y.: COVID-19 screening on chest X-ray images using deep learning based anomaly detection. arXiv preprint arXiv:2003.12338 (2020)
9. Grasselli, G., Pesenti, A., Cecconi, M.J.J.: Critical care utilization for the COVID-19 outbreak in Lombardy, Italy: early experience and forecast during an emergency response. JAMA **323**(16), 1545–1546 (2020)
10. Buizza, R.: Probabilistic prediction of COVID-19 infections for China and Italy, using an ensemble of stochastically-perturbed logistic curves. arXiv preprint arXiv:2003.06418 (2020)
11. Fanelli, D., Piazza, F.: Analysis and forecast of COVID-19 spreading in China, Italy and France. Chaos, Solitons & Fractals, **134**, 109761
12. Botha, A.E., Dednam, Japa, W: A simple iterative map forecast of the COVID-19 pandemic. arXiv preprint arXiv:2003.10532 (2020)
13. Yan, L., Zhang, H.-T., Goncalves, J., Xiao, Y., Wang, M., Guo, Y., et al.: A machine learning-based model for survival prediction in patients with severe COVID-19 infection. MedRxiv (2020)
14. Wu, J., Zhang, P., Zhang, L., Meng, W., Li, J., Tong, C., et al.: Rapid and accurate identification of COVID-19 infection through machine learning based on clinical available blood test results. MedRxiv (2020)
15. Shan, F., Gao, Y., Wang, J., Shi, W., Shi, N., Han, M., et al.: Lung infection quantification of COVID-19 in CT images with deep learning. arXiv preprint arXiv:200304655 (2020)

16. Xu, X., Jiang, X., Ma, C., Du, P., Li, X., Lv, S., et al.: Deep learning system to screen coronavirus disease pneumonia. Appl. Intell. **2020**, 1 (2019)
17. Li, K., Fang, Y., Li, W., Pan, C., Qin, P., Zhong, Y., et al.: CT image visual quantitative evaluation and clinical classification of coronavirus disease (COVID-19). Eur. Radiol. 1–10 (2020)
18. Tang, Z., Zhao, W., Xie, X., Zhong, Z., Shi, F., Liu, J., et al.: Severity assessment of coronavirus disease 2019 (COVID-19) using quantitative features from chest CT Images. arXiv preprint arXiv:2003.11988 (2020)
19. Fong, S.J., Li G., Dey N., Crespo, R.G., Viedma, E.H.: Composite monte carlo decision making under high uncertainty of novel coronavirus epidemic using hybridized deep learning and fuzzy rule induction. arXiv preprint arXiv:200309868 (2020)
20. Elghamrawy, S.M., Hassanien, A.E.: Diagnosis and prediction model for COVID19 patients response to treatment based on convolutional neural networks and whale optimization algorithm using CT. medRxiv. (2020)
21. Fong, S.J., Li, G., Dey, N., Crespo, R.G., Viedma, E.H.: Finding an accurate early forecasting model from small dataset: a case of 2019-nCoV novel coronavirus outbreak. Int. J. Interact. Multimedia Artif. Intell. **6**, 132 (2020)
22. Rajinikanth, V., Dey, N., Raj, A.N.J., Hassanien, A.E., Santosh, K.C., Raja, N.S.M.: Harmony-search and otsu based system for coronavirus disease (COVID-19) detection using lung CT scan images. arXiv preprint arXiv:200403431 (2020)
23. Societa Italiana di Radiologia Medica e Interventistica; 2020 [Available from: https://www.sirm.org/
24. Hinton, G.E., Srivastava, N., Krizhevsky, A., Sutskever, I., Salakhutdinov, R.R.: Improving neural networks by preventing co-adaptation of feature detectors. arXiv preprint arXiv:120 70580 (2012)
25. Matassoni, M., Gretter, R., Falavigna, D., Giuliani, D. (eds.) Non-native children speech recognition through transfer learning. In: 2018 IEEE International Conference on Acoustics, Speech and Signal Processing (ICASSP). IEEE (2018)
26. Zhou, N., Wang, L.: A modified T-test feature selection method and its application on the HapMap genotype data. Genomics, Proteomics Bioinform. **5**(3–4), 242–249 (2007)
27. Kulkarni, S.R., Harman, G.: Statistical learning theory: a tutorial. Wiley Interdisc Rev: Comput Stat. **3**(6), 543–556 (2011)
28. Sun, Q.-S., Zeng, S.-G., Liu, Y., Heng, P.-A., Xia, D.S.: A new method of feature fusion and its application in image recognition. Pattern Recogn. **38**(12), 2437–2448 (2005)
29. Zhou, N.N., Wang, L.P.: A modified t-test feature selection method and its application on the hapmap genotype data. Geno. Prot. Bioinfo. **5**(3–4), 242–249 (2007)
30. Ruuska, S., Hämäläinen, W., Kajava, S., Mughal, M., Matilainen, P., Mononen, J.: Evaluation of the confusion matrix method in the validation of an automated system for measuring feeding behaviour of cattle. Behav. Proc. **148**, 56–62 (2018)

Stacking Deep Learning for Early COVID-19 Vision Diagnosis

Ahmed A. Hammam, Haytham H. Elmousalami, and Aboul Ella Hassanien

Abstract early and accurate COVID-19 diagnosis prediction plays a crucial role for helping radiologists and health care workers to take reliable corrective actions for classify patients and detecting the COVID 19 confirmed cases. Prediction and classification accuracy are critical for COVID-19 diagnosis application. Current practices for COVID-19 images classification are mostly built upon convolutional neural network (CNNs) where CNN is a single algorithm. On the other hand, ensemble machine learning models produce higher accuracy than a single machine leaning. Therefore, this study conducts stacking deep learning methodology to produce the highest results of COVID-19 classification. The stacked ensemble deep learning model accuracy has **produced 98.6%** test accuracy. Accordingly, the stacked ensemble deep learning model produced superior performance than any single model. Accordingly, ensemble machine learning evolves as a future trend due to its high scalability, stability, and prediction accuracy.

Keywords Deep learning · Ensemble learning · Stacking · Classification · COVID-19 · Biomedical image processing

1 Introduction

The world health organization (WHO) declared that the COVID-19 outbreak is an international pandemic on 11th March 2020. On 24th April 2020, the number of confirmed cases has increased up to 3,042,444 cases and 211,216 deaths around more than 209 countries. The number of confirmed cases and deaths grow exponentially in our world. Therefore, all efforts should be integrated to fight COVID 19 pandemic. In the age of digital transformation, and machine learning (ML) play a key role in

A. A. Hammam (✉) · H. H. Elmousalami · A. E. Hassanien
Faculty of Computers and Artificial Intelligence, Cairo University, Cairo, Egypt
e-mail: ahmed.a.hammam@grad.fci-cu.edu.eg
URL: http://www.egyptscience.net

Scientific Research Group, Cairo, Egypt

© The Editor(s) (if applicable) and The Author(s), under exclusive license
to Springer Nature Switzerland AG 2020
A.-E. Hassanien et al. (eds.), *Big Data Analytics and Artificial Intelligence
Against COVID-19: Innovation Vision and Approach*, Studies in Big Data 78,
https://doi.org/10.1007/978-3-030-55258-9_18

processing the data to be converted into knowledge and decisions [1]. In the age of digital transformation, big data and machine learning (ML) play a key significant in processing the data to be converted into knowledge and decisions [2]. Several means of COVID-19 diagnosis can be applied to identify the confirmed cases of COVID-19. Radiologist's diagnosis includes computed tomography (CT) scans; chest X-ray (CXR) radiographs [3]. In any case, CT scans and X-ray pictures are time expending and exhausted indeed for master radiologists. Computer vision and deep learning computing such as convolutional neural networks (CNN) can viably offer assistance radiologists for identifying COVID-19 affirmed cases.

Based on the chest CT scans, radiologists can detect the (COVID-19) pneumonia and the arrange of persistent recuperation or weakening. Computerized insights models can precisely produce early location for the conclusion of the patients of COVID-19 by detecting the early lung thermal signs within the X-ray images. A beginning inception neural model has been connected for two-fold classification for tainted with COVID-19 or wellbeing people utilizing 1119 CT pictures [4]. Using 6000 CT, U-Net++ system can distinguish the COVID-19 patients with 93.55 and 100% for specificity and sensitivity [5]. Feature Pyramid Network have been used for to distinguish the COVID-19 cases with an acceptable total accuracy of 86.7%. Accordingly, the fully-connected layers produced better results with sensitivity of 0.93 and AUC of 0.99 [6, 7].

2 Deep Learning Models

A convolutional neural network (CNN) is a deep neural network that is conducted for computer vision applications [8]. CNN architecture is commonly applied for biomedical processing, analysis and classifications. CNNs are consisted of regularized multi-layer perceptron and filters. The hidden layers of CNNs typically are represented of a series of convolutional layers where these convolutional layers convolve based on dot product to extract the features of each sample of images pixels. Each convolutional layer has the following parameters: Convolutional kernels, the number of input channels and output channels, the depth of the convolution filter. CNNs includes pooling layers to reduce the dimensions of the data by converting the neuron outputs to one layer based on mathematical voting such as average. Multi-layer perception neural network (MLP) can be used as a Fully connected to classify the images as displayed in Fig. 1.

MobileNets proved its efficiency in several applications for embedded vision applications and mobile applications. MobileNets applies streamlined architecture based on depthwise convolutions for developing light weight model. MobileNets optimizes the global parameters by trading off accuracy and latency [9]. The key advantage of MobileNets is using limited hardware resources for computing by reducing the network parameters and maintains the model accuracy.

MobileNets needs 1/33 of parameters needed for VGG-16 to achieve the same classification accuracy [10]. Inception is a deep convolutional neural network (CNN)

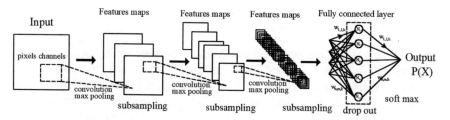

Fig. 1 CNN architecture

Fig. 2 A building block of
residual learning

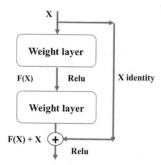

architecture used for detection and classification applications. Inception architecture expands width and depth of the network with saving the computational cost. The Inception architecture optimizes quality of the architecture design using multi-scale processing and Hebbian principle [11]. Training deeper neural networks is a high computational process. Therefore, residual learning model has been developed to substantially train deeper models using residual functions related to the input layer as showed in Fig. 2. The key advantage of Residual nets is improving accuracy with depth of neural model and easier for optimization. Residual nets model has achieved a first place on the ILSVRC 2015 classification task [12].

3 Research Methodology

Model ensemble is a technique in which the predictions of a collection of models are given as inputs to a second-stage learning model. Ensemble learning helps improve machine learning results by combining several models. This approach allows the production of better predictive performance compared to a single model.

3.1 Stacking Ensemble Deep Learning

The ensemble ML algorithms are depending on ensemble voting such as majority, plurality voting, "hard", or "soft" voting. In hard voting, the final class label is predicted as the class label that has been predicted most frequently by the classification models. In soft voting, the class labels are predicted by averaging the class-probabilities. The soft voting is only recommended if the classifiers are well-calibrated [13, 14]. In majority voting (Hard Voting) can be formulated as the following formula:

$$\hat{y}_i = mode \ \{C_1(X), C_1(X), \ldots, C_m(X)\} \tag{1}$$

The weighted majority vote can be computed by associating a weight wj with classifier C_j as the following formula:

$$\hat{y}_i = \arg\max \sum_{j=1}^{m} W_j(C_j(X) \tag{2}$$

where (i) is the outcome of the classifier or class labels. In soft voting, the class labels are predicted based on the predicted probabilities pj for classifier. This approach is only recommended if the classifiers are well-calibrated.

$$\hat{y}_i = \arg\max \sum_{j=1}^{m} W_j P_j(X) \tag{3}$$

Stacking is to ensemble several classifications algorithms such as Bagging or Boosting techniques. Stacking (Stacked Generalization) is applying different algorithms to learn part of the problem space and combining these different algorithms. Stacking paradigm improves the overall accuracy than any other individual based learner [15]. As shown in Fig. 3, implementation of stacking models consists of two main levels; Level-0 is training base learners (model A, model B and model C) where each model produces different classifications. Level-1(generalizer) is collecting the classification of each based learner to make final classification.

3.2 Model

The scope of the current research will focus on development stacking ensemble deep learning model for early COVID-19 diagnosis prediction using deep stacking model to boost the accuracy of single computer vision algorithms. As illustrated in the Fig. 5. The research methodology can be conducted through the Algorithm 1 and the following steps:

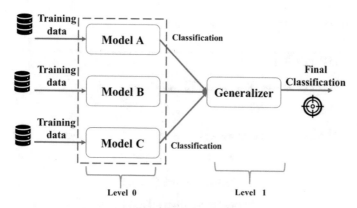

Fig. 3 A stacking ensemble learning

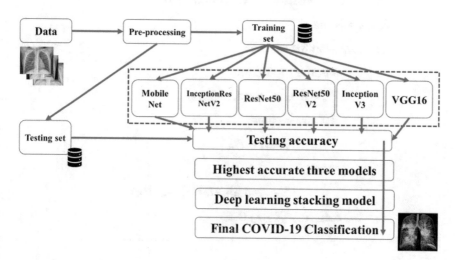

Fig. 5 Application methodology for deep stacking model

- Collecting data set of X-ray or CT scans for COVID-19 confirmed cases.
- Applying pre-processing techniques to remove missing data.
- Applying different classification computer vision models.
- Compare the results and performance of the applied model algorithms to rank using classification evaluation techniques.
- Apply the stacking ensemble deep learning using the best performance models.
- Compare the results of the stacking ensemble deep learning against the best single model using classification evaluation techniques.

Algorithm 1: Deep stacking Algorithm

OUTPUT P$_f$

INPUT D$_{train}$, D$_{test}$, D$_{Valid}$, X$_{Model\_Number}$

I=0

While (I< X$_{Model\_Number}$):

      I=I+1

      Train Model$_I$ (D$_{train}$)

      Valid Model$_I$ (D$_{valid}$)

MODELS = SELECT TOP 3 MODEL

X$_{stack}$ = None

For Model in MODELS:

      # make prediction

      P$_M$ = Model. predict (D$_{test}$)

      if X$_{stack}$ is None:

            X$_{stack}$ = P$_M$

      else:

            X$_{stack}$=data_stack(X$_{stack}$,P$_M$)

P$_f$ = Model$_{Stack}$.fit(X$_{stack}$, D$_{test}$)

---

4 Result

The data set consist of 500 X-ray images where the data set has been divided d into three subsets: training set (80%), validation set (10%) and testing set (10%). The whole X-ray images have two labels: 0 for positive COVID-19 case and 1 for negative COVID-19 case as shown in Fig. 4.

To compare machine learning algorithms, the identical blind validating cases used to test the performance of the algorithm. The data set has been dividing into a training set (80%), validation set (10%) and testing (10%) where the validation cases are excluded from the training data to ensure the generalization capability. Classification accuracy (Acc), specificity and sensitivity are scaler measures for the classification performance. Moreover, receiver operating characteristics (ROC) is a

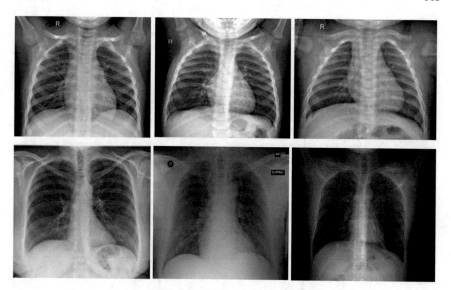

Fig. 4 A sample of X-ray images dataset for normal cases (first row) and COVID-19 patients (second row)

graphical measure for classification algorithm [16]. The receiver operating characteristics (ROC) curve is a two- dimensional graph in which the true positive rate (TPR) represents the y-axis and a false positive rate (FPR) is the x-axis. Classification accuracy (Acc) computes the ratio between the correctly classified instances to the total number of samples as the following equations:

$$TPR = \frac{TP}{TP + FN} \tag{4}$$

$$FPR = \frac{FP}{TN + FP} \tag{5}$$

$$Acc = \frac{TP + TN}{TP + TN + FP + FN} \tag{6}$$

where: true positive (TP); false positive (FP); true negative (TN); false negative (FN). Based on ROC, the perfect classification happens when the classifier curve possesses through the upper left corner of the graph.

The study applies six different deep learning models for COVID-19 classification. These models are MobileNet, InceptionResNetV2, ResNet50, ResNet50V2, InceptionV3, and VGG16. Table 1 shows the setting for each model used for training process; the number of epochs was 100, learning rate was 0.001, and the optimization algorithm was Adam.

Figures 6 and 7 illustrates the training accuracy and validation accuracy during for the applied models. Moreover, the corresponding confusion matrix to each frame

Table 1 Setting of algorithms training

Parameter	Setting
Epoch number	100
Learning rate	0.001
Optimization algorithm	Adam
Training sample size (%)	80
Testing sample size (%)	10
Validation sample size (%)	10

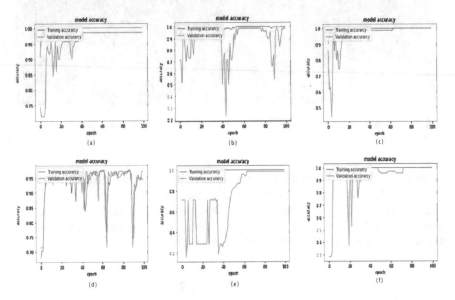

Fig. 6 Accuracy Comparison For each model **a** Mobile Net, **b** ResNet50V2, **c** Inception ResNetV2, **d** ResNet50V2, **e** VGG16 and **f** InceptionV3

woke have been displayed. All models presented acceptable accuracies ranging from 0.971 to 0.943 based on Testing accuracy. As shown in Table 2 and Fig. 8, the training, validation and testing accuracy for each model have been displayed. The results show that the MobileNet, InceptionResNetV2 and ResNet50 have 0.971 for testing accuracy. ResNet50V2, and InceptionV3 have 0.957 for testing accuracy. VGG16 have 0.943 for testing accuracy. As a result, the first three accurate models were MobileNet, InceptionResNetV2 and ResNet50. The next stage is applying stacking ensemble deep learning model to collect the results of MobileNet, InceptionResNetV2 and ResNet50. The stacked ensemble deep learning model accuracy has produced 0.986 test accuracy. Accordingly, the stacked ensemble deep learning model produced

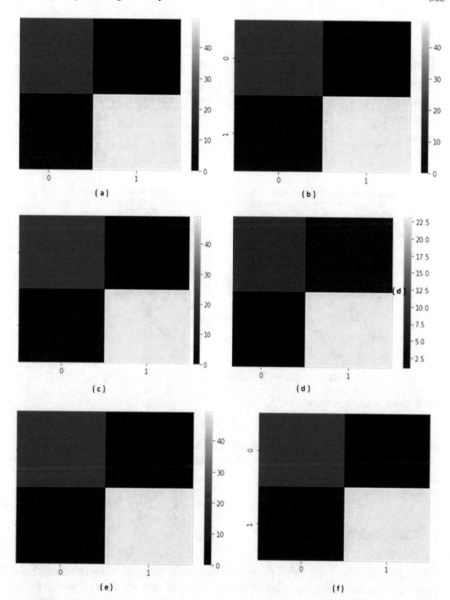

Fig. 7 Heat-map comparison for each model **a** MobileNet, **b** ResNet50V2, **c** InceptionResNetV2, **d** ResNet50V2, **e** VGG16 and **f** InceptionV3 where 0 = Positive and 1 = Negative

Table 2 Deep leaning models results

	Training accuracy	Validation accuracy	Testing accuracy
MobileNet	1	0.985	0.971
InceptionResNetV2	1	1	0.971
ResNet50	1	0.985	0.971
ResNet50V2	1	0.9857	0.957
InceptionV3	1	1	0.957
VGG16	0.977	0.971	0.943

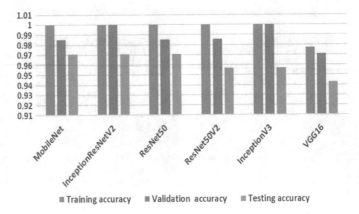

Fig. 8 Deep leaning models results

superior performance than any single model. The stacked model improves the accuracy of COVID-19 classification by 1.54% than other the highest accurate applied models.

5 Conclusion

We proposed stacked ensemble deep learning model by combining the predictions from multiple deep learning models on the same dataset, the models are typically different in architecture that are skilled on the dataset, but in different ways. Stacked is an ensemble method where model figures out how to best join the predictions from numerous current models. The stacked ensemble deep learning model accuracy has produced 0.986 test accuracy. The stacked ensemble deep learning model produced superior performance compared to any single model (top single model one is 0.971). The ensemble learning algorithms could be a future trend for prediction and classification applications where dataset have limited size. Moreover, we plan to further explore more ensemble deep learning approaches to produce higher predictive accuracy than single computer vision algorithm for classification.

References

1. Elmousalami, H.H., Hassanien, A.E.: Day level forecasting for coronavirus disease (COVID-19) spread: analysis, modeling and recommendations, arXiv preprint arXiv:2003.07778 (2020)
2. Elmousalami, H.H.: Comparison of artificial intelligence techniques for project conceptual cost prediction: a case study and comparative analysis. IEEE Trans. Eng. Manage. 1–14 (2020)
3. Hassanien, A.E., Mahdy, L.N., Ezzat, K.A., Elmousalami, H.H., Ella, H.A.: Automatic X-ray COVID-19 lung image classification model based on multi-level thresholding and support vector machine. medRxiv (2020)
4. Wang, S., Kang, B., Ma, J., Zeng, X., Xiao, M., Guo, J., Cai, M., Yang, J., Li, Y., Meng, X., et al.: A deep learning algorithm using CT images to screen for corona virus disease (COVID-19). medRxiv preprint medRxiv:2020.02.14.20023028 (2020a)
5. Chen, J., Wu, L., Zhang, J., Zhang, L., Gong, D., Zhao, Y., Hu, S., Wang, Y., Hu, X., Zheng, B., et al.: Deep learning-based model for detecting 2019 novel coronavirus pneumonia on high-resolution computed tomography: a prospective study. medRxiv preprint medRxiv:2020.02.25.20021568 (2020b)
6. Xu, X., Jiang, X., Ma, C., Du, P., Li, X., Lv, S., Yu, L., Chen, Y., Su, J., Lang, G., et al.: Deep learning model to screen coronavirus disease 2019 pneumonia. arXiv preprint arXiv: 2002.09334 (2020)
7. Song, Y., Zheng, S., Li, L., Zhang, X., Zhang, X., Huang, Z., Chen, J., Zhao, H., Jie, Y., Wang, R., et al.: Deep learning enables accurate diagnosis of novel coronavirus (COVID-19) with CT images. medRxiv preprint medRxiv:2020.02.23.20026930 (2020)
8. Krizhevsky, A., Sutskever, I., Hinton, G.E.: Imagenet classification with deep convolutional neural networks. In: Advances in Neural Information Processing Models, pp. 1097–1105 (2012)
9. Howard, A.G., Zhu, M., Chen, B., Kalenichenko, D., Wang, W., Weyand, T., Andreetto, M., Adam, H.: Mobilenets: efficient convolutional neural networks for mobile vision applications. arXiv preprint arXiv:1704.04861 (2017)
10. Li, Y., Huang, H., Xie, Q., Yao, L., Chen, Q.: Research on a surface defect detection algorithm based on MobileNet-SSD. Appl. Sci. **8**(9), 1678 (2018)
11. Szegedy, C., Liu, W., Jia, Y., Sermanet, P., Reed, S., Anguelov, D., ... & Rabinovich, A.: Going deeper with convolutions. In: Proceedings of the IEEE Conference on Computer Vision and Pattern Recognition, pp. 1–9 (2015)
12. He, K., Zhang, X., Ren, S., Sun, J.: Deep residual learning for image recognition. In: Proceedings of the IEEE Conference on Computer Vision and Pattern Recognition, pp. 770–778 (2016)
13. Dietterich, T.G.: Ensemble methods in machine learning. In: International Workshop on Multiple Classifier Models, pp. 1–15 (2000)
14. Goyal, A., Sardana, N.: Empirical analysis of ensemble machine learning techniques for bug Triaging. In: 2019 Twelfth International Conference on Contemporary Computing (IC3), pp. 1–6 (2019)
15. Deng, L., Yu, D., Platt, J.: Scalable stacking and learning for building deep architectures. In: 2012 IEEE International Conference on Acoustics, Speech and Signal Processing (ICASSP), pp. 2133–2136. IEEE (2012)
16. Tharwat, A.: Classification assessment methods. Appl. Comput. Inf. (2018)

Printed in the United States
by Baker & Taylor Publisher Services